SELF-HELP APPROACHES
FOR OBESITY AND EATING DISORDERS

SELF-HELP APPROACHES FOR OBESITY AND EATING DISORDERS

Research and Practice

Edited by
JANET D. LATNER
G. TERENCE WILSON

THE GUILFORD PRESS
New York   London

© 2007 The Guilford Press
A Division of Guilford Publications, Inc.
72 Spring Street, New York, NY 10012
www.guilford.com

Printed in the United States of America

This book is printed on acid-free paper.

Last digit is print number: 9   8   7   6   5   4   3   2   1

Library of Congress Cataloging-in-Publication Data

Self-help approaches for obesity and eating disorders : research and practice / edited by
Janet D. Latner and G. Terence Wilson.
    p. cm.
Includes bibliographical references and index.
ISBN-13: 978-1-59385-442-3 (hardcover : alk. paper)
ISBN-10: 1-59385-442-0 (hardcover : alk. paper)
1. Obesity.   2. Eating disorders.   3. Obesity—Popular works.   4. Eating disorders—
Popular works.   I. Latner, Janet D.   II. Wilson, G. Terence, 1944–
RC628.S445 2007
616.3'98—dc22

                                                            2006037398

About the Editors

Janet D. Latner, PhD, is Assistant Professor of Psychology at the University of Hawaii at Manoa. Her research is focused on the diagnosis, maintenance, treatment, and self-help treatment of obesity and eating disturbances, and on improving the long-term maintenance of weight loss through self-help. Dr. Latner has authored and presented over 40 articles and book chapters on eating disorders and obesity and has served as an investigator on several nationally funded research projects.

G. Terence Wilson, PhD, is the Oscar K. Buros Professor of Psychology at Rutgers, The State University of New Jersey. He has published numerous scientific articles and has written or edited a number of books, including *Binge Eating: Nature, Assessment, and Treatment* (with Christopher G. Fairburn). Dr. Wilson's research is focused on the development and evaluation of cognitive-behavioral treatments for eating disorders and obesity, and on the analysis of mechanisms of therapeutic change. He served as a member of the American Psychiatric Association's Eating Disorders Work Group, which developed the diagnostic criteria for eating disorders in the fourth edition of the *Diagnostic and Statistical Manual of Mental Disorders* (DSM-IV), and of the National Institutes of Health Task Force on the Prevention and Treatment of Obesity (1995–2002).

Contributors

Kelly C. Allison, PhD, Center for Weight and Eating Disorders, Department of Psychiatry, University of Pennsylvania School of Medicine, Philadelphia, Pennsylvania

Kelly D. Brownell, PhD, Yale Center for Eating and Weight Disorders, Yale University, New Haven, Connecticut

Meghan L. Butryn, PhD, Department of Psychology, Drexel University, Philadelphia, Pennsylvania

Janet D. Carter, PhD, Department of Psychology, University of Canterbury, Christchurch, New Zealand

Thomas F. Cash, PhD, Department of Psychology, Old Dominion University, Norfolk, Virginia

Emily Dionne, MS, RD, LDN, MGH Weight Center, Massachusetts General Hospital, Boston, Massachusetts

Meredith S. Dolan, MS, RD, LDN, Healthy Weight Program, The Children's Hospital of Philadelphia, Pennsylvania

Johanna Dwyer, DSc, RD, Frances Stern Nutrition Center, Tufts–New England Medical Center, Boston, Massachusetts

Myles S. Faith, PhD, Center for Weight and Eating Disorders, University of Pennsylvania School of Medicine, and The Children's Hospital of Philadelphia, Philadelphia, Pennsylvania

Stacy A. Gore, PhD, School of Medicine, University of Alabama at Birmingham, Birmingham, Alabama

Carlos M. Grilo, PhD, Department of Psychiatry, Yale University School of Medicine, New Haven, Connecticut

Miriam Grover, MSc, Section of Eating Disorders, Division of Psychological Medicine and Psychiatry, Institute of Psychiatry, King's College London; and Eating Disorders Services, South London and Maudsley NHS Foundation Trust, London, United Kingdom

Kathryn E. Henderson, PhD, Department of Psychology, Yale University, New Haven Connecticut

Joshua I. Hrabosky, PsyD, Department of Psychiatry, Yale University School of Medicine, New Haven, Connecticut

Megan Jones, BA, Department of Psychiatry, Stanford University School of Medicine, Stanford, California

Jennifer Jordan, PhD, Department of Psychological Medicine, Christchurch School of Medicine and Health Sciences, Christchurch, New Zealand

Janet D. Latner, PhD, Department of Psychology, University of Hawaii at Manoa, Honolulu, Hawaii

Natalie K. Lueders, BBA, Center for the Study of Obesity, University of Arkansas for Medical Sciences, Little Rock, Arkansas

Bess H. Marcus, PhD, Department of Psychiatry and Human Behavior, Brown Medical School and The Miriam Hospital, Providence, Rhode Island

Virginia V. W. McIntosh, PhD, Department of Psychological Medicine, Christchurch School of Medicine and Health Sciences, Christchurch, New Zealand

Vanessa A. Milsom, MS, Department of Clinical and Health Psychology, University of Florida, Gainesville, Florida

Michael G. Perri, PhD, Department of Clinical and Health Psychology, University of Florida, Gainesville, Florida

Suzanne Phelan, PhD, Brown Medical School and The Miriam Hospital, Providence, Rhode Island

Rebecca M. Puhl, PhD, Rudd Center for Food Policy and Obesity, Yale University, New Haven, Connecticut

W. Jack Rejeski, PhD, Department of Health and Exercise Science, Wake Forest University, Winston-Salem, North Carolina

Ulrike Schmidt, PhD, Section of Eating Disorders, Division of Psychological Medicine and Psychiatry, Institute of Psychiatry, King's College London; and Eating Disorders Services, South London and Maudsley NHS Foundation Trust, London, United Kingdom

Marlene B. Schwartz, PhD, Yale Center for Eating and Weight Disorders, Yale University, New Haven, Connecticut

Allison Stevens, MS, RD, LDN, Culinary Nutrition Consultant and Freelance Writer, Sublette, Kansas

Albert J. Stunkard, MD, Center for Weight and Eating Disorders, Department of Psychiatry, University of Pennsylvania School of Medicine, Philadelphia, Pennsylvania

Robyn Sysko, MS, Department of Psychology, Rutgers, The State University of New Jersey, Piscataway, New Jersey

C. Barr Taylor, MD, Department of Psychiatry and Behavioral Sciences, Stanford University School of Medicine, Stanford, California

Adam Gilden Tsai, MD, Center for Weight and Eating Disorders, University of Pennsylvania, Philadelphia, Pennsylvania

Thomas A. Wadden, PhD, Center for Weight and Eating Disorders, University of Pennsylvania, Philadelphia, Pennsylvania

Alison Wallace, PhD, New Zealand Institute for Crop and Food Research Limited, Canterbury Agriculture and Science Centre, Lincoln, New Zealand

B. Timothy Walsh, MD, Department of Psychiatry, Columbia University, and the New York State Psychiatric Institute, New York, New York

Delia Smith West, PhD, Center for the Study of Obesity, University of Arkansas for Medical Sciences, Little Rock, Arkansas

Jessica A. Whiteley, PhD, Department of Psychiatry and Human Behavior, Brown Medical School and The Miriam Hospital, Providence, Rhode Island

David M. Williams, PhD, Centers for Behavioral and Preventive Medicine, Brown Medical School and The Miriam Hospital, Providence, Rhode Island

G. Terence Wilson, PhD, Graduate School of Applied and Professional Psychology, Rutgers, The State University of New Jersey, Piscataway, New Jersey

Rena R. Wing, PhD, Brown Medical School and The Miriam Hospital, Providence, Rhode Island

Preface

Researchers and clinicians are increasingly recognizing that the high demand for professional health services cannot always be met; alternative options are needed. This is especially true for obesity and eating disorders; prevalence rates for the former are rising steeply, and increased awareness of the latter is bringing more and more patients into treatment. The result has been an upsurge in the practice of self-help for these problems and research into its efficacy. Consumers and patients are mobilized to help themselves and each other and to seek help from commercial products, programs, and technology.

What is self-help? Traditionally, self-help has been viewed as a modality of treatment that involves helping or improving oneself without relying on the assistance of anyone else. However, we define self-help more broadly to include any treatment or approach that views the person receiving help as the main instigator, driver, and agent of change. This does not preclude the use of manuals, commercial products, technology, supportive peers, or even a caring professional to assist the person's efforts. In each of these cases, the recipient of help can still be the major contributor to the change produced by treatment. However, the amount of assistance provided by these outside sources determines how much independent effort is required on the part of a self-help recipient. Self-help that is completely unassisted, for example, requires independent effort. Self-help assisted by an Internet-based treatment program may be aided by graded computer feedback, e-mails from a professional, or a chat room with peers. However, a great deal of independent work and effort is still required from the participant in such a program.

The purpose of this volume is to bring together the research on different forms of self-help for obesity and eating-related disturbances. We hope this book will provide a comprehensive resource that will allow practitioners to make knowledgeable recommendations to their clients and decisions about their care. Practitioners in settings that range from primary care to specialty clinics may often find it helpful to suggest to their patients self-care strategies and programs of known efficacy. We also hope this volume will serve as a guide for researchers seeking up-to-date reviews of the literature on self-help for weight control and eating disorders.

With these purposes in mind, we chose the topics covered in the book based on the research evidence behind them. A series of topic areas have been sufficiently researched to suggest a critical mass of empirical support for several particular approaches. The disorders covered in this book include obesity and overweight in adults and children, binge-eating disorder, bulimia nervosa, body-image disturbance, and night eating syndrome. In addition to being researched widely, these problems can often be treated through self-help or with minimal professional guidance. Popular programs and written manuals exist for all of these disorders, with varying degrees of empirical support (reviewed in this volume). In contrast, anorexia nervosa was deliberately left out of this volume. Because most experts agree that it necessitates professional care, anorexia nervosa is not suitable for self-help treatment.

The contents of the first four parts of this book cover the spectrum from purely self-directed strategies to interventions involving varying degrees of professionally assisted self-help. This continuum, from more to less independent, with progressively more professional or technological support, may be likened to a stepped-care model of treatment. As in a stepped-care treatment program, individuals may wish initially to use those strategies that are most independent, that involve the least cost or inconvenience, and that require the least specialist time. While monitoring their outcomes, they may discover that they are not benefiting from their current level of self-help. They may then move to another level of care, such as guided or computer-assisted self-help. Alternatively, other individuals may benefit most from starting immediately with higher levels of professional involvement if, for example, they have failed previous self-help attempts or their problems are severe. The first four parts of the book progress from the most independent forms of self-help to forms that utilize more assistance from external sources.

Independent effort at weight control, or unguided self-help, is discussed in Part I. Chapter 1 discusses self-guided dieters—the behaviors they engage in and the effectiveness of self-directed approaches for long-term weight control. Chapter 2 systematically analyzes the nutritional adequacy, safety, and efficacy of the major popular weight-loss diets available to the public.

Contents

PART I. INDEPENDENT (UNGUIDED) SELF-HELP   1

1   Self-Guided Approaches to Weight Loss   3
Meghan L. Butryn, Suzanne Phelan, and Rena R. Wing

2   Popular and Fad Diet Programs: Nutritional Adequacy,   21
Safety, and Efficacy
Allison Stevens, Emily Dionne, and Johanna Dwyer

PART II. PARTIALLY ASSISTED (GUIDED) SELF-HELP   53

3   Self-Help Strategies for Promoting and Maintaining   55
Physical Activity
Bess H. Marcus, David M. Williams, and Jessica A. Whiteley

4   Guided Self-Help for Binge-Eating Disorder   73
Carlos M. Grilo

5   Guided Self-Help for Bulimia Nervosa   92
Robyn Sysko and B. Timothy Walsh

6   Self-Help Treatment for Body-Image Disturbances   118
Joshua I. Hrabosky and Thomas F. Cash

PART III. COMPUTER-ASSISTED SELF-HELP   139

7   Internet-Based Prevention and Treatment of Obesity   141
and Body Dissatisfaction
C. Barr Taylor and Megan Jones

8   Computer-Based Intervention for Bulimia Nervosa and Binge Eating   166
Ulrike Schmidt and Miriam Grover

PART IV. GROUP SELF-HELP   177

9 Commercial and Organized Self-Help Programs   179
for Weight Management
Adam Gilden Tsai and Thomas A. Wadden

10 Guided Group Support and the Long-Term Management   205
of Obesity
Vanessa A. Milsom, Michael G. Perri, and W. Jack Rejeski

11 Continuing Care and Self-Help in the Treatment of Obesity   223
Janet D. Latner and G. Terence Wilson

PART V. PRACTICAL STRATEGIES   241
AND CONSIDERATIONS

12 Behavioral Obesity Treatment Translated   243
Delia Smith West, Stacy A. Gore, and Natalie K. Lueders

13 Prevention of Overweight with Young Children and Families   265
Meredith S. Dolan and Myles S. Faith

14 Treatment of Overweight Children: Practical Strategies for Parents   289
Kathryn E. Henderson and Marlene B. Schwartz

15 Self-Help for Night Eating Syndrome   310
Kelly C. Allison and Albert J. Stunkard

16 Appetite-Focused Cognitive-Behavioral Therapy for Binge Eating   325
*Virginia V. W. McIntosh, Jennifer Jordan, Janet D. Carter,
Janet D. Latner, and Alison Wallace*

17 Strategies for Coping with the Stigma of Obesity   347
Rebecca M. Puhl and Kelly D. Brownell

Index   363

In contrast to purely independent self-help, Part II reviews research on partially assisted self-help, also known as guided self-help. This form of self-help also involves a high degree of effort on the part of the consumer or client, but it is guided by periodic contacts with a professional or lay coach. Guided self-help strategies for increasing and maintaining physical activity and addressing binge-eating disorder, bulimia nervosa, and body-image disturbances are critically reviewed in Chapters 3–6.

Computer-directed self-help treatment is a new development that has the potential to reach countless numbers of individuals in need, including those in rural areas who may not have access to professional care. Part III considers research on treating and preventing obesity and body dissatisfaction through Internet-based programs (Chapter 7) and on addressing bulimia nervosa and binge eating through computer-based treatment (Chapter 8).

Group self-help is one of the most common forms of obesity treatment. Part IV reviews the literature on group programs and treatments for weight control. Chapter 9 reviews literature on the efficacy of commercial and organized self-help programs. Enhancing the long-term impact of treatment through guided group support is discussed in Chapter 10. Chapter 11 discusses the role of continuing care, or ongoing treatment, in self-help groups for weight control.

Whereas the first sections of the book are primarily descriptive, the fifth section is more prescriptive in its purpose and content. The chapters in Part V contain a collection of practical strategies and considerations for dealing with specific clinical issues. Their purpose is to assist practitioners, individuals, and families in making critical decisions about how to use self-help strategies. Chapter 12 is a step-by-step guide or "translation" of the effective strategies used in behavioral weight-loss treatment. The next two chapters address the prevention (Chapter 13) and treatment (Chapter 14) of overweight in children, presenting practical and helpful strategies for parents and families and the research supporting these techniques. Chapter 15 outlines strategies that can be used to address night eating syndrome, an eating disturbance that has recently received increased research and clinical attention. Chapter 16 presents an innovative set of procedures to correct the disturbances in appetite among individuals with binge-eating disorder and bulimia nervosa. Finally, being overweight often involves having to cope with repeated and distressing experiences of weight-based stigmatization; Chapter 17 presents the evidence for different strategies to deal with obesity stigma and discrimination.

We are extremely grateful to the distinguished leaders in the field who have generously contributed their time and expertise to writing this volume. The continual support and hard work of the staff of The Guilford Press have made this project possible. We also thank Ann W. Latner, JD, for her valuable assistance in the development of this project.

We hope that this book will be a valuable tool for researchers, clinicians, and students in the fields of obesity and eating disorders. By examining the research literature on self-help, as well as by describing practical strategies that may help individuals seeking care, we hope that this book will serve as a practical guide for clinicians seeking cost-effective or alternative means of delivering services and pointing patients in the direction of effective self-care. We also hope this volume will be helpful to lay practitioners and consumers of self-help treatments for weight and eating disorders.

SELF-HELP APPROACHES
FOR OBESITY AND EATING DISORDERS

PART I

INDEPENDENT (UNGUIDED) SELF-HELP

Many men and women attempt to lose weight on their own. Only a certain proportion of these succeed. Who are these "successful losers"? What behaviors and characteristics set them apart? What can others learn from them?

Chapter 1 reviews the literature on self-guided dieting: who succeeds at this approach, what characterizes the approach and those who benefit from it, and what clinicians can suggest to their overweight patients to increase the likelihood of their success with self-guided dieting. Chapter 2 analyzes the safety and efficacy of the fad diet programs that are currently popular and widely used by self-guided dieters. Accurate information about these programs' adequacy and likely effectiveness is essential to clinicians recommending them and to consumers considering them.

I

Self-Guided Approaches
to Weight Loss

MEGHAN L. BUTRYN, SUZANNE PHELAN,
and RENA R. WING

At any given time, a large number of U.S. adults are dieting. Although prevalence rates vary (likely according to how questions are phrased), high rates of dieting have been documented in several studies that have collected data from large, nationally representative samples of U.S. adults. The Behavioral Risk Factor Surveillance System, a telephone survey conducted by state health departments, found that 46% of women and 33% of men were dieting (Bish et al., 2005). The National Health Interview Survey, which conducted face-to-face interviews, found that 38% of women and 24% of men were dieting (Kruger, Galuska, Serdula, & Jones, 2004). Both the Continuing Survey of Food Intakes by Individuals, which conducted face-to-face interviews, and the National Health and Nutrition Examination Survey, which administered questionnaires during home visits, found lower rates of dieting—17% and 24%, respectively (Kant, 2002; Paeratakul, York-Crowe, Williamson, Ryan, & Bray, 2002). However, looking across these studies, it appears that at any time between 20 and 40% of adults are dieting.

Self-guided dieting may be one of the most common approaches that dieters in the general population are using for their weight-loss attempts. One national study found that 27% of dieters developed their diets themselves and that 15% followed a diet that they had read or heard about (Paeratakul et al., 2002). Research consistently indicates that a small proportion of dieters (5–13% of women and 1–5% of men) joined an organized weight-loss program for their most recent dieting attempt (Jeffery, Adlis, & Forster, 1991; Kruger et al., 2004; Levy & Heaton, 1993; Paeratakul et al., 2002). Thus many of these individuals may be losing weight on their own.

Given the prevalence of self-guided dieting, it is important to determine how successfully this approach promotes long-term weight control. However, little is known about these individuals, as they are losing weight on their own and thus are not part of the data collected by commercial programs or hospital-based clinics. This chapter summarizes the information that is available about the behaviors engaged in by self-guided dieters and the effectiveness of this approach for long-term weight control. It begins with a review of the data on self-guided dieting available from the National Weight Control Registry (NWCR), the largest study to date on successful weight-loss maintenance. Because many NWCR members report losing weight on their own, these data should be a valuable resource for information on self-help dieting. The behaviors of self-guided dieters who are successful at weight-loss maintenance are compared with those of dieters using more structured approaches and with the behaviors of self-guided dieters in the general population. Finally, the findings of experimental studies that approximate self-guided dieting are reviewed.

SELF-GUIDED DIETERS IN THE NWCR

In an effort to learn more about successful weight-loss maintenance, Wing and Hill (2001) established the NWCR in 1994. The NWCR enrolls individuals who are over 18 years of age and who report having lost at least 30 pounds and kept it off at least 1 year. The NWCR has received extensive media coverage, and individuals who read about the registry are invited to enroll. Thus the NWCR is a self-selected sample of successful weight losers; findings from this group cannot be assumed to generalize to the broader population of successful weight losers. However, the self-reported weights of NWCR members have been shown to be very accurate, and a population-based study of successful weight losers confirmed that the behaviors reported by registry members are also observed in the general population of successful weight losers (McGuire, Wing, Klem, & Hill, 1999). Participants in the NWCR complete a variety of questionnaires when they enroll and are then followed annually. At present, approximately 5,000 individuals are enrolled in the NWCR. The NWCR members are 77% women, 95% European American, 82% college educated, and 64% married; average age is 46.8 years. On average, NWCR members lost 70 pounds each and have kept at least 30 pounds off for an average of 5.7 years. They clearly have succeeded at long-term weight loss and maintenance. Because many dieters struggle with weight-loss maintenance, much can be learned from these unique individuals who have been so successful.

Prevalence of Self-Guided Dieting in the NWCR

On entry to the NWCR, participants are given a list of several common weight control strategies and are asked to check off all strategies that they used to attain their successful weight loss. Self-guided dieting is a common approach used by NWCR members to attain their weight loss. Approximately one-third of participants in the NWCR reported that their weight loss was achieved either (1) on their own (i.e., without the help of a specific program or contact with a health care professional) or (2) by following a diet program obtained from a book, magazine, or another person. These participants, hereafter referred to as "self-guided" dieters, used *only* these strategies for weight loss. The remaining two-thirds of participants used other approaches to achieve their weight loss, such as joining a commercial program (e.g., Weight Watchers, Jenny Craig), participating in a self-help group (e.g., Overeaters Anonymous, Take Off Pounds Sensibly), taking medication, or having individual contact with a psychologist or physician. The fact that one-third of all NWCR members report having used self-guided dieting for weight loss indicates that this approach has the potential to produce large weight losses that can be successfully maintained over time.

Characteristics of Self-Guided Dieters

The members of the NWCR who used only a self-guided strategy for weight loss have been compared with individuals who reported having used a more structured approach to determine whether there are differences between these groups (Wing, Phelan, Butryn, & Hill, 2006). Self-guided dieters (n = 1,286) were compared with participants who reported having used a commercial program for weight loss, without the additional use of medication or weight-loss surgery (n = 511). Self-guided and commercial program participants did not differ significantly in ethnicity, education level, or age. However, male participants made up approximately one-third of the self-guided group, whereas they made up only one-tenth of the commercial program group. These data are consistent with the finding from other samples of dieters showing that rates of joining an organized weight-loss program are significantly higher for women than men (Jeffery et al., 1991; Paeratakul et al., 2002). It is possible that men who try to lose weight are less likely than women to seek out the interaction, support, and monitoring that a commercial program offers. An alternative explanation is that dieters often seek out more structured approaches only after failing to lose weight or to maintain a weight loss on their own and that men may simply be more successful than women at self-guided weight loss and thus less likely to need a commercial program.

When they enrolled in the NWCR (i.e., after attaining their weight loss), self-guided participants had an average body mass index (BMI) of 24.4 kg/m^2, which was significantly lower than that of commercial program participants. The maximum BMI that the participants had previously reached also was significantly lower in the self-guided group than in the commercial program group. Participants in both groups lost approximately 30% of their maximum body weight in achieving their most recent successful weight loss. At entry to the NWCR, those in the self-guided group were maintaining their weight loss for an average of 6.5 years, significantly longer than those in the commercial program group (4.9 years). In sum, although the percentage of weight loss that these participants achieved is similar, self-guided participants had previously been less obese than their commercial program counterparts, and they entered the NWCR at lower BMIs. This is consistent with the finding from another sample of dieters that the likelihood of joining an organized weight-loss program was higher for individuals who were more overweight than for those who were less so (Jeffery et al., 1991).

The difference in maximum BMI that self-guided and commercial program participants previously reached suggests that individuals who seek out commercial programs have had more weight-control difficulty than those who use self-guided approaches. In fact, a greater proportion of self-guided participants (18%) than commercial program participants (7%) reported that they had never tried to lose weight prior to their recent successful weight loss. Self-guided participants also had a less extensive weight-cycling history than commercial program participants, as measured by the total kilograms that they intentionally lost in their lifetime (irrespective of regain). Thus commercial program participants were more likely to have previously tried to lose weight and failed. Additionally, scores on a measure of disinhibited eating were significantly lower for self-guided than for commercial program participants. The latter finding provides some support for the hypothesis that self-guided dieters may have more control over their eating than those individuals who seek out more structured programs for weight loss.

Behaviors during Weight Loss

At entry to the NWCR, participants provided retrospective information about the behaviors that they engaged in to attain their successful weight loss. Because the groups differed in some demographic characteristics, these analyses were adjusted for gender and maximum lifetime weight. To achieve their weight loss, self-guided participants in the NWCR were likely to have used strategies such as decreasing intake of unhealthy foods, controlling portion size, and engaging in high levels of physical activity. Approximately 90% of self-guided participants reported that they limited their intake of certain types of food (e.g., fats or sugars) or classes of food (e.g., desserts), a rate higher than that reported by commercial program participants. Two other common strategies, each reported by about half of self-guided dieters, were decreasing the quantity of all types of food eaten and using fat- or calorie-modified foods, but each of these strategies was reported by a higher proportion of commercial program dieters. Fewer than half of participants in both groups reported limiting the percentage of their daily calories from fat, counting fat grams, or counting calories. Self-guided participants reported that during their weight loss they engaged in approximately 6.5 hours per week of physical activity. Commercial program participants reported engaging in physical activity for approximately 1 hour less per week than self-guided participants.

Behaviors during Maintenance

Participants in the self-guided and commercial program groups also provided information on the strategies they used to maintain their weight loss. All of these analyses, as well as those examining weight change after enrollment in the NWCR, were adjusted for gender, duration of weight loss, percentage of initial weight lost, and weight at entry to the NWCR. The most common weight-maintenance strategies reported by self-guided participants were keeping many healthy foods in the house, regularly monitoring their weight, and buying books or magazines that relate to nutrition or exercise. Self-guided participants reported using fewer strategies for weight maintenance than commercial program participants, suggesting that they may have used a simpler approach. Self-guided participants also were less likely than commercial program participants to report using some of the behavioral strategies that commonly are taught in commercial programs, such as stimulus control.

During weight maintenance, self-guided participants continued to engage in high levels of physical activity; they reported expending significantly more calories than commercial program participants (approximately 2,630 kcal/week and 2,300 kcal/week, respectively). The caloric intake and macronutrient composition of self-guided and commercial program participants' diets also differed during weight maintenance. Self-guided participants reported that they ate a diet consisting of approximately 1,500 kilocalories per day, whereas commercial program participants ate approximately 1,300 kcal per day. Self-guided participants consumed 32% of calories from fat, whereas commercial program participants consumed 25% of calories from fat. Carbohydrate intake was lower for self-guided participants than for commercial program participants (48 vs. 54%), but protein intake did not differ between groups. NWCR participants, regardless of previous dieting strategy, seemed to succeed at long-term weight control by engaging in a high level of physical activity and restricting their intake to a moderate amount of calories and fat.

Weight-Maintenance Success

Self-guided participants were generally very successful at continuing to maintain their weight loss after entry to the NWCR. At 2-year follow-up, approximately 96% of self-guided participants maintained a weight loss that was at least 10% of their maximum body weight. During this follow-up period, they gained an average of 3.4 kg. There was no significant difference between self-guided and commercial program participants' trajectories of weight change after entry to the NWCR, and participants in both groups maintained the vast majority of their weight loss. These data indicate that NWCR participants who lost weight through self-guided approaches were no less successful at long-term maintenance than participants who lost weight with the more structured approach of a commercial program.

SELF-GUIDED DIETING IN THE GENERAL POPULATION

It is important to compare the experiences of NWCR participants with those of other dieters, because NWCR participants are, by definition, a unique group. Differences in the approaches that typical dieters and NWCR participants use may be indicative of the differential weight-control success that these groups have.

Weight-Loss Behaviors

A few studies have collected data on the type of behaviors that dieters in the general population are engaged in. Given that most dieters do not report joining formal programs, it seems reasonable to infer that many of the dieters in these samples are self-guided. Among individuals attempting to lose weight, about half reported eating a reduced-calorie or reduced-fat diet (Bish et al., 2005; Paeratakul et al., 2002). In the Continuing Survey of Food Intakes by Individuals, current dieters, across sex, reported a total energy intake of approximately 1,700 kcal per day, with 30% of energy from fat (Paeratakul et al., 2002). Male dieters who participated in the third National Health and Nutrition Examination Survey (NHANES III) reported an intake of approximately 2,400 kcal per day, with 34% of calories from fat, whereas female dieters reported an intake of 1,650 kcal per day, with 33% of calories from fat (Kant, 2002). Data from the NWCR indicate that the successful dieters, regardless of method of weight loss, reported a caloric intake during weight maintenance that was lower than this. Without sufficient caloric restriction, self-guided dieters in the general population may struggle to achieve or maintain a successful weight loss. In fact, although many individuals report that they are "dieting," many of them are not using an approach that would be expected to successfully produce weight loss.

Between one-half and two-thirds of adults in the general population who are trying to lose weight reported that they were engaging in some physical activity to assist in their weight-loss attempts (Bish et al., 2005; Kruger et al., 2004). However, only one-third of individuals trying to lose weight were combining physical activity with dietary change, and many dieters were not engaging in the high levels of physical activity necessary for weight loss (Kruger et al., 2004). One survey found that only one-quarter of dieters exercised at least 5 times per week (Paeratakul et al., 2002). Another found that women reported exercising approximately 160 minutes per week and that men reported exercising 260 minutes per week, with walking as the most common form of activity (Levy & Heaton, 1993). Whereas only one-fifth of dieters in the general population reported engaging in more than 150 minutes per week of physical activity and restricting their caloric intake, the majority of self-guided dieters in the NWCR reported doing so (Bish et al., 2005). Discrepancies such as this may explain why many individuals' efforts do not result in weight loss. (See also Chapter 3, this volume)

Although reducing caloric and fat intake and increasing physical activity are the most common approaches for weight loss among U.S. adults, other behaviors also are used. Data from the Weight Loss Practices Survey (Levy & Heaton, 1993), which administered questionnaires to a national sample of U.S. adults, found that among respondents attempting weight loss, 71% of women and 70% of men were regularly weighing themselves. Fewer reported taking vitamins and minerals (33% of women and 26% of men), skipping meals (21% of women and 20% of men), using commercial meal replacements (15% of women and 13% of men), recording food amounts (15% of women and 8% of men) and taking diet pills (14% of women and 7% of men). Another nationally representative study (Serdula et al., 1994) found that among adults attempting weight loss, few reported taking special diet supplements (10% of women and 7% of men), fasting (5% of women and 5% of men), or using diet pills (4% of women and 2% of men). The National Health Interview Survey (Kruger et al., 2004) found that few adults who were attempting weight loss were skipping meals (9% of women and 11% of men), using food supplements (6% of women and 5% of men), or taking diet pills (3% of women and 2% of men). Although it is encouraging that relatively few adults are using weight-control practices that have questionable effectiveness (e.g., food supplements, skipping meals), more individuals might benefit from engaging in behaviors such as recording food amounts or using commercial meal replacements, which appear to improve weight-loss outcomes.

Duration and Success of Self-Guided Diets

Little information is available on the duration and success of typical self-guided weight-loss attempts. One national sample of U.S. adults in the midst of weight-loss attempts found that participants had been dieting for approximately 6 months and that their self-reported weight loss to date was 6 kg (Levy & Heaton, 1993). In a sample of college students (Smith, Burke, & Wing, 2000), most participants who previously had dieted reported that their attempts had lasted between 1 and 3 months. The most common reasons for discontinuing the diets were losing interest in them or missing certain foods. Only one-third of participants reported that they discontinued their diets because they achieved their desired weight loss. Additional research is needed on the length of time that self-guided dieters attempt weight loss, their weight-loss success, and the reasons why they abandon their efforts.

Weight Maintenance Behaviors

A small sample of successful dieters ($n = 30$) recruited from health maintenance organization (HMO) clinics yielded additional information about weight-loss maintenance behaviors in successful dieters (Kayman, Bruvold, & Stern, 1990). The successful dieters were of average weight (as determined by the 1959 Metropolitan Life Insurance Tables), had previously been 20% overweight, and had maintained reduced weight for at least 2 years. To attain their weight loss, 73% of these participants devised a personal eating plan, an additional 10% followed a book or magazine diet, and 20% attended formal groups or weight-loss programs. Three-quarters reported that they had exercised as part of their weight-loss programs. They reported using several strategies to maintain their weight loss, including monitoring their weight (reported by 87% of participants), staying active (83%), eating less (83%), and monitoring intake (60%). These weight-maintenance behaviors are remarkably similar to strategies reported by NWCR participants.

EFFECTIVENESS OF WEIGHT-LOSS PROGRAMS THAT PROVIDE MINIMAL GUIDANCE

The research that has been conducted on self-guided dieting in the general population suggests that the weight-control strategies that individuals typically use may not be sufficient to promote substantial weight loss. However, no studies have prospectively measured weight change over time in self-guided dieters, making conclusions about success difficult to draw. In the absence of such research, it is useful to review the results of studies that provided participants with minimal support and structure, although the participants who joined such clinical research programs may differ from typical self-guided dieters. In this section, we review three categories of interventions, each of which is considerably less intensive than standard behavioral weight loss treatment: (1) minimal contact, (2) minimal contact plus bibliotherapy, and (3) minimal contact plus meal replacements.

Minimal Contact

To measure the weight-loss success of self-guided dieters, control groups from large clinical trials provide some useful data. Although these data capture a special group of dieters (i.e., those who volunteered for a clinical trial from which they may have hoped to receive an intensive intervention), these studies, unlike many others, typically have large samples and long follow-up periods.

For instance, individuals who enrolled in the Diabetes Prevention Program (Diabetes Prevention Program Research Group, 2002) were randomly assigned to receive either (1) a lifestyle modification program delivered through frequent individual and group sessions ($n = 1,079$); (2) the drug metformin plus lifestyle recommendations ($n = 1,073$); or (3) placebo plus lifestyle recommendations ($n = 1,082$). The lifestyle recommendations in the second and third groups consisted of written information and an annual 20- to 30-minute individual session during which they were encouraged to reduce their weight, increase their physical activity, and follow the Food Guide Pyramid and a low-fat, low-cholesterol diet. Participants were followed for an average of approximately 3 years; attrition was 9%, and only treatment completers were included in analyses. (*Note:* For all studies reviewed in the following sections, results are from intent-to-treat analyses unless otherwise noted.) Average weight loss at the conclusion of the study was 0.1 kg in the placebo-plus-lifestyle-recommendations group, significantly less than that achieved in the metformin-plus-lifestyle-recommendations group (2.1 kg) and the lifestyle-modification group (5.6 kg). The results of this study indicate that participants who were instructed to lose weight on their own were generally unable to achieve the substantial long-term weight losses demonstrated by those who received intensive guidance.

In another clinical trial, participants were randomly assigned to either a self-help control group ($n = 211$) or a commercial program ($n = 212$; Heshka et al., 2003). Self-help participants attended two 20-minute sessions with a dietitian (one at week 0 and one at week 12), were provided with publicly available printed materials on diet and exercise, and were directed to use additional educational resources (e.g., Internet websites) as needed. Participants in the commercial program group were given vouchers to attend as many Weight Watchers sessions as they wished during the 2-year study. The self-help participants maintained smaller weight losses than commercial program participants at both 1-year (1.3 kg and 4.3 kg, respectively) and 2-year assessments (0.2 kg and 2.9 kg, respectively). Of the self-help participants who completed the 2-year assessment ($n = 159$), 15% sustained a weight loss of between 5 and 10% of initial body weight, and 6% sustained a weight loss of more than 10%. In sum, the results of this study and the Diabetes Prevention Program indicate that when participants enrolled in clinical trials are encouraged to lose weight but given little guidance for doing so, most do not achieve meaningful weight losses, particularly over long periods of time.

Minimal Contact plus Bibliotherapy

More structured assistance may be offered to self-guided dieters by using bibliotherapy. Many interventions provide participants with guidance in the form of a weight-loss manual or book, and some also offer an orientation to the diet plan or brief visits or phone calls to review progress. Results of these bibliotherapy interventions may provide information relevant to the experiences of the large number of dieters who follow a diet program from a book or magazine.

In some studies, bibliotherapy participants simply are given a weight-loss manual. For instance, in one study (Wing, Venditti, Jakicic, Polley, & Lang, 1998), participants were randomly assigned to one of four groups: a diet intervention ($n = 37$), exercise intervention ($n = 37$), diet-plus-exercise intervention ($n = 40$), or bibliotherapy control group ($n = 40$). Participants in the bibliotherapy group were provided with a behavioral weight loss manual and encouraged to lose weight and exercise on their own, but they had no other contact with staff during the treatment period. Attrition was 15% at 6 months, 22% at 1 year, and 16% at 2 years; completer analyses were conducted for weight-loss data. Bibliotherapy participants lost 1.5 kg at 6 months and 0.3 kg at 1 year, significantly less at each time point than participants in the diet group (9.1 kg at 6 months and 5.5 kg at 1 year) and the diet-plus-exercise group (10.3 kg at 6 months and 7.4 kg at 1 year). However, at 2 years the weight loss in the bibliotherapy group (0.3 kg) did not significantly differ from that of other groups, although the diet-plus-exercise participants did maintain a significant decrease from baseline in body weight (2.5 kg). At 24 months, 19% of bibliotherapy participants achieved a weight loss of at least 4.5 kg. Characteristics of those who succeeded at weight loss and possible use of other weight-loss approaches in the year of follow-up were not evaluated.

Other studies have provided bibliotherapy participants with additional staff contact, often with better weight-loss results. In a study conducted with individuals who had previously been unsuccessful at self-administered weight loss, participants were randomly assigned to either a bibliotherapy condition ($n = 53$) or a wait-list control group ($n = 9$; Miller, Eggert,

Wallace, Lindeman, & Jastremski, 1993). Bibliotherapy participants were given a weight-loss workbook that emphasized self-monitoring of diet and exercise without severe restriction of energy intake. Participants were taught to use a behavioral score sheet, on which they could total 100 points, to evaluate their fat, carbohydrate, and sugar intake, water consumption, exercise, and eating behaviors (e.g., snacking, overeating). They participated in a 1-hour orientation to the workbook's approach and were instructed to mail in completed self-monitoring forms on a monthly basis (no feedback was provided about these forms). Control group participants had no contact with staff between baseline and 6-month assessments. Attrition in the intervention group was 34%; completer analyses were conducted. Bibliotherapy participants lost an average of 8.1 kg at 6 months, whereas the control participants did not show a significant weight change. Although this intervention offered minimal face-to-face contact with staff, this weight loss is among the largest observed for bibliotherapy, even if the weight losses are adjusted for high attrition. Follow-up data are not available to determine how well weight loss was maintained.

Face-to-face contact was more frequent in a study that randomly assigned participants to a bibliotherapy program ($n = 24$) or to a commercial Internet weight-loss program ($n = 23$; Womble et al., 2004). Participants in the bibliotherapy condition were given a behavioral weight-loss manual, as well as a manual providing guidance for weight maintenance. During the 1-year intervention, participants in both programs visited the clinic 10 times to be weighed and also participated in five 20-minute individual sessions with a psychologist in which the goals of the program were reviewed and progress was assessed. Attrition at 1 year was 34%, and analyses were done using the last-observation-carried-forward method. Bibliotherapy participants lost an average of 3.3 kg at 1 year, significantly more than the weight loss achieved by participants in the commercial Internet program (0.8 kg).

A similar amount of clinical contact was provided in a study that randomly assigned participants to receive dietary instruction in either a low-fat ($n = 30$) or low-carbohydrate ($n = 30$) diet and provided a corresponding diet book to guide their dietary change (Foster et al., 2003). Participants attended 15- to 30-minute sessions with a registered dietitian at baseline and at 3, 6, and 12 months and visited the clinic 11 times during the 1-year treatment period to have weight measured and other assessments completed. Attrition was 41% at 12 months; for participants who did not complete the study, data obtained at the time of the last follow-up visit were used. Percentage of initial weight lost was greater in the low-carbohydrate than in the low-fat group at 3 months (8.1 vs. 3.8%) and at 6 months (9.7 vs. 5.3%), but not at 12 months (7.3 vs. 4.5%). (Because participants averaged almost 100 kg at baseline, weight losses in kilograms would be similar to percentages of initial weight lost.) These results indicate that use of a low-carbohydrate or low-fat diet book, along with minimal contact with a clinician, can promote moderate weight losses that are maintained for up to 12 months.

Another study that provided participants with popular diet books and offered some additional support found that although modest weight losses could be achieved, attrition rates were similarly high. Participants (n = 160), all of whom had hypertension, dyslipidemia, or fasting hyperglycemia, attended four 1-hour group classes in the first 2 months of the study (Dansinger, Gleason, Griffith, Selker, & Schaefer, 2005). At these sessions they were provided with guidance about the popular diets that they were randomly assigned to follow (Atkins, Zone, Ornish, or Weight Watchers). Participants were advised to follow the diet as closely as possible for 2 months and to determine their own level of adherence thereafter. At 1 year, attrition was 42%, and missing data were replaced with baseline data. Weight loss at 1 year averaged 2.4 kg for women and 3.3 kg for men (there were no significant differences between diets). Of all participants originally enrolled in the study, 25% sustained a weight loss of more than 5% of initial body weight, and 10% of participants sustained a weight loss of more than 10%.

Some research has examined the addition of telephone contact to bibliotherapy. One study, conducted for 12 weeks with heart transplant candidates who were overweight or obese, randomly assigned participants to receive bibliotherapy alone (n = 22) or bibliotherapy in conjunction with telephone contact (n = 21; Park, Perri, & Rodrigue, 2003). All participants participated in one session of instruction in meeting calorie goals and self-monitoring and were given a manual with 20 lessons on cognitive-behavioral weight-loss strategies. They were instructed to return calorie- and fat-intake monitoring information on a weekly basis during treatment. Participants in the bibliotherapy-plus-telephone condition additionally received weekly 15- to 20-minute telephone calls from a therapist, during which manual lessons, strategies, and goals were reviewed. Weight loss was 1.0 kg in the bibliotherapy group and 2.8 kg in the bibliotherapy-plus-telephone group; weight change from baseline was significant only in the latter.

Another study examining the use of bibliotherapy and telephone contact randomly assigned participants to one of three groups: minimal contact (n = 22), weight-focused telephone contact (n = 21), or behavior-focused telephone contact (n = 21; Hellerstedt & Jeffery, 1997). All participants received two 1-hour behavioral weight-loss group sessions during which they were provided with instruction in reduction of calorie and fat intake, in regular exercise, in stimulus control, in relapse prevention, and in self-monitoring. All participants were given a weight-loss manual, self-monitoring records, and menu plans and were encouraged to contact the study nutritionist by telephone if they wanted to receive additional counseling (few calls were placed). Participants in the minimal-contact group received only those intervention components. Participants in the weight-focused-telephone-contact group also received weekly telephone calls from a research assistant asking them to report their current weight; those in the behavior-focused-telephone-contact group received weekly telephone calls asking them to report their current weight and the past week's caloric and fat intake and caloric expenditure. At the end of the 24-week intervention, attrition was 14%; completer analyses were conducted. Weight loss, which did not significantly differ between groups, was 5.7 kg in the minimal-contact group, 3.7 kg in the weight-focused-telephone-contact group, and 3.4 kg in the behavior-focused-telephone-contact group. These results indicate that the addition of scheduled monitoring telephone contact did not improve weight loss over that attained with the combination of bibliotherapy and brief instruction in behavioral weight-loss strategies.

In contrast to these results, another intervention produced much larger weight losses through the use of bibliotherapy and telephone contacts. In that study (Goulis et al., 2004), all participants were advised to create a caloric deficit of 500–600 kcal per day and to exercise 20 to 30 minutes at least 5 days per week in order to accomplish a 2- to 3-kg weight loss per month. Patients attended monthly clinic visits with a dietician and physician at which an examination was performed, weight was measured, and adherence to the diet was reviewed. Participants were randomly assigned either to receive only this usual care ($n = 77$) or to participate additionally in telephone-based monitoring ($n = 45$). During the 6 months of treatment, the latter group of participants was given an electronic blood pressure monitor and scale and instructed to submit information by telephone every 3 days on their self-monitored blood pressure, weight, and adherence to diet and exercise plan. The information was submitted to an automated call center according to a schedule given to participants. On average, at 6 months, participants who received usual care lost 2.0 kg, and those who received the increased contact lost 12.4 kg, a significant difference.

In general, the studies reviewed here indicate that when bibliotherapy is combined with some clinical contact, such as a few sessions of instruction on weight management or encouragement to report self-monitoring information to staff, the combination can promote modest weight losses. Maintenance of such weight loss, however, remains difficult and underassessed, and attrition rates for these programs are high. Contradictory findings across studies may reflect difference in sample characteristics, small sample sizes, or differences in intervention components. There is some indication that more frequent contact and greater structure may promote weight loss (Goulis et al., 2004; Miller et al., 1993) but this finding is not consistent across studies (e.g., Hellerstedt & Jeffery, 1997).

Minimal Contact plus Meal Replacements

Just as bibliotherapy is used by some self-guided dieters to add structure to their weight-loss programs, other individuals use meal replacements as part of their programs. Studies that have attempted to assess typical use of meal replacements (i.e., without additional intensive behavioral or nutritional intervention) have indicated that they may be an effective approach for achieving weight loss and weight-loss maintenance.

In one study, all participants ($n = 301$) were given free meal replacements and encouraged to follow the instructions on the package insert (Heber, Ashley, Wang, & Elashoff, 1994). Participants had weight measured on a weekly basis for the first 12 weeks of the study. Attrition at 12 weeks was 9%; completer analyses were conducted. Male and female participants lost an average of 8.3 kg and 6.3 kg, respectively, at 12 weeks. Participants who lost at least 4 kg in the 12-week program ($n = 238$) were encouraged to continue using one meal replacement per day and were weighed biweekly; only these participants were included in follow-up assessments. At 2 years, when attrition from this follow-up sample was 55%, males who completed the program lost an average of 6.3 kg and females 6.1 kg. However, if a conservative approach were used wherein missing data were replaced with baseline values, average weight loss would be approximately 3 kg.

In a second study, which also yielded promising weight-maintenance results, intervention participants ($n = 158$) were given free meal replacements and had their weight measured at a local community center weekly for 3 months and twice per year thereafter. During weight loss, they were encouraged to use two meal replacements per day. During weight maintenance, they were encouraged to use one meal replacement per day or to monitor their weight daily and resume regular use of meal replacements if they gained more than 1–2 kg. Attrition was 11% at 5 years, and an additional 4% of participants were excluded from follow-up analyses because they could not be matched with control participants; completer analyses were conducted. At 5 years, male participants lost an average of 5.8 kg and female participants lost an average of 4.2 kg, whereas male and female controls matched for age, BMI, and race gained an average of 6.7 kg and 6.5 kg, respectively, during this time period (Rothacker, 2000). These studies indicate that meal replacements may be an effective method that self-guided dieters can use to promote long-term weight control.

CONCLUSIONS AND FUTURE DIRECTIONS

Self-guided dieting is a common method of attempting weight lost in the general population. Between 20 and 40% of adults in the United States are dieting at any given time, and few of them are joining organized weight-loss programs. People may choose to diet on their own for any number of reasons: perhaps because it may seem more convenient, less expensive, or less time-consuming than organized programs; because they are skeptical about the effectiveness of organized programs; or because they are not comfortable seeking help from others for their weight-control difficulties. The high prevalence of overweight and obesity in the United States suggests that most of these self-guided dieting attempts are not producing substantial weight losses that are maintained over time. Indeed, many dieters in the general population are not engaging in the levels of caloric restriction and physical activity necessary to produce meaningful weight loss. Few are engaging in other behaviors that may improve their weight control, such as self-monitoring their food intake or using meal replacements. Nonetheless, these individuals should be encouraged by data from the NWCR that indicates that self-guided dieting has the potential to produce substantial weight loss than can be successfully maintained.

The individuals in the NWCR who lost weight on their own provide some suggestions about the characteristics of successful self-guided dieters. Given that men in the NWCR were much more likely to report using self-guided dieting than a commercial program to attain their weight loss, it is possible that men fare better than women with this approach. It also is possible that self-guided dieting is more likely to be effective for individuals who have had fewer weight-control difficulties in the past. Similarly, it is possible that individuals who have a greater predisposition toward obesity or who engage more frequently in disinhibited eating will have more success in a structured, guided program.

Clinicians should recommend that their patients who wish to lose weight on their own follow several recommendations. During weight loss, successful self-guided dieters tend to limit their intake of certain types of food, as well as to decrease the quantity of all types of food eaten. To lose weight, they also engage in high levels of physical activity, exercising approximately 1 hour per day. To maintain their weight loss, these dieters keep many healthy foods in their homes and regularly monitor their weight. They also maintain high levels of physical activity and consume a diet that is low in calories and fat. Individuals attempting to lose weight should be encouraged to emulate these successful self-guided weight losers. It is unclear whether or not individuals who are at high risk for failure with self-guided dieting should be encouraged by their physicians or other health care providers to seek out other approaches for weight loss before attempting a self-guided diet or whether a stepped-care model is most effective.

Clinicians may be able to provide their weight-loss patients with suggestions about how to maximize the likelihood of success with a self-guided diet. Although the experimental studies that have been conducted on minimally intensive weight-loss interventions have not generated a consistent pattern of results, the findings indicate that two elements of these interventions might be particularly effective: providing participants with regular contact with staff members and increasing structure in the diet plan.

When participants have regularly scheduled contact with clinical or research staff members, they may achieve greater weight losses, even if the contact does not provide them with additional skills or education. What such contact provides may be a sense of "accountability"; participants may find that knowing that their weight will be recorded by the staff increases their adherence to diet and exercise. Support for this hypothesis is found in the differential results of the studies conducted by Foster and colleagues (2003) and Dansinger and colleagues (2005), in both of which a group of participants was instructed to follow a low-carbohydrate diet and provided them with the same popular diet book detailing this approach. In Foster and colleagues' (2003) study, weight loss in the low-carbohydrate group was about 9.6 kg at 6 months and about 7.2 kg at 12 months, whereas in Dansinger and colleagues' (2005) study, weight loss was 3.2 kg at 6 months and 2.1 kg at 12 months. The amount of instruction that participants received in following the diet was similar in each study. However, in Foster et al.'s study, participants visited the clinic 11 times during the year for weight to be measured, whereas participants in Dansinger et al.'s study had four clinic visits for weight measurement. This differential contact may explain the superior results found by Foster and colleagues. Frequent monitoring of participants also was associated with large weight losses in the study conducted by Goulis and colleagues (2004). In addition to monthly clinic visits, these participants submitted information by telephone every 3 days about their blood pressure, weight, and adherence to the diet, and they achieved a weight loss of 12.4 kg at 6 months. There are many possible clinical applications of these findings. For instance, patients who wish to lose weight might be encouraged to regularly visit their physician's office to be weighed and to briefly report their behavior change progress to a staff member. Further research is needed to determine the effectiveness of this approach, because not all studies provide support for it (e.g., Hellerstedt & Jeffery, 1997).

In addition to increasing contact with staff, it may help to provide participants with a structured diet plan. For example, the weight losses achieved in Foster and colleagues' (2003) low-carbohydrate diet intervention were superior to those achieved in the low-fat diet intervention at 3 months and at 6 months, perhaps because a low-carbohydrate diet provides greater structure for food choices. Similarly, the use of meal replacements, a highly structured approach, produces large weight losses that are well maintained over time (Heber et al., 1994; Rothacker, 2000). Large weight losses were also achieved by participants in the study conducted by Miller and colleagues (1993), which provided a more structured intervention than traditional bibliotherapy: Participants were instructed to use a scoring system through which they monitored specific weight-control behaviors each day. Although minimally intensive interventions that provide frequent contact and increase the structure of the diet do not all produce substantial weight losses, the pattern of results from these studies is promising and suggests that more research on this area should be conducted.

Many questions about self-guided dieting remain unanswered. Few observational studies on this group of dieters have been conducted, and no precise definition of self-guided dieting has been agreed on in the field. It is difficult to accurately determine how many individuals are likely to be successful with a self-guided program. It is possible that self-help dieters truly do better long-term than those who enroll in organized programs but that this difference is due to the former having less entrenched weight-control problems than the latter. Conversely, it is possible that self-guided dieters may have less success long term, perhaps because they do not learn effective strategies for weight control and do not have any opportunity for continued supportive contact.

There are several obstacles to conducting the research that will answer such questions. Self-guided dieters are, by definition, not enrolled in a formal program. Randomization to a self-guided dieting approach may not accurately capture an important self-selection factor, and assessment of weight and other behaviors may reduce the external validity of the approach. Researchers must develop innovative techniques to capture samples of individuals in the general population who are attempting self-guided weight loss and to prospectively monitor their behaviors and weight changes. Long follow-up periods are necessary, particularly because successful weight-loss maintenance often occurs only after several attempts at dieting. It will be important to distinguish those individuals who succeed with this approach from those who do not. Clinical researchers must develop effective, minimally intensive interventions that can be disseminated to individuals who do not wish to enroll in traditional weight-loss programs. Researchers also need to determine the effect of structure and contact on weight loss and to find the best ways to deliver supportive interventions to those who want to lose weight on their own.

REFERENCES

Bish, C. L., Blanck, H. M., Serdula, M. K., Marcus, M., Kohl, H. W., & Khan, L. K. (2005). Diet and physical activity behaviors among Americans trying to lose weight: 2000 Behavioral Risk Factor Surveillance System. *Obesity Research, 13*, 596–607.

Dansinger, M. L., Gleason, J. A., Griffith, J. L., Selker, H. P., & Schaefer, E. J. (2005). Comparison of the Atkins, Ornish, Weight Watchers, and Zone diets for weight loss and heart disease risk reduction: A randomized trial. *Journal of the American Medical Association, 293*, 43–53.

Diabetes Prevention Program Research Group. (2002). Reduction in the incidence of type 2 diabetes with lifestyle intervention or metformin. *New England Journal of Medicine, 346*, 393–403.

Foster, G. D., Wyatt, H. R., Hill, J. O., McGuckin, B. G., Brill, C., Mohammed, B. S., et al. (2003). A randomized trial of a low-carbohydrate diet for obesity. *New England Journal of Medicine, 348*, 2082–2090.

Goulis, D. G., Gialis, G. D., Boren, S. A., Lekka, I., Bontis, E., Balas, E. A., et al. (2004). Effectiveness of home-centered care through telemedicine applications for overweight and obese patients: A randomized controlled trial. *International Journal of Obesity,* *28,* 1391–1398.

Heber, D., Ashley, J. M., Wang, H. J., & Elashoff, R. M. (1994). Clinical evaluation of a minimal intervention meal replacement regimen for weight reduction. *Journal of the American College of Nutrition, 13,* 608–614.

Hellerstedt, W. L., & Jeffery, R. W. (1997). The effects of a telephone-based intervention on weight loss. *American Journal of Health Promotion, 11,* 177–182.

Heshka, S., Anderson, J. W., Atkinson, R. L., Greenway, F. L., Hill, J. O., Phinney, S. D., et al. (2003). Weight loss with a self-help compared with a structured commercial program. *Journal of the American Medical Association, 289,* 1792–1798.

Jeffery, R. W., Adlis, S. A., & Forster, J. L. (1991). Prevalence of dieting among working men and women: The Healthy Worker Project. *Health Psychology, 10,* 274–281.

Kant, A. K. (2002). Weight-loss attempts and reporting of food nutrients, and biomarkers in a national cohort. *International Journal of Obesity, 26,* 1194–1204.

Kayman, S., Bruvold, W., & Stern, J. S. (1990). Maintenance and relapse after weight loss in women: Behavioral aspects. *American Journal of Clinical Nutrition, 52,* 800–807.

Kruger, J., Galuska, D. A., Serdula, M. K., & Jones, D. A. (2004). Attempting to lose weight: Specific practices among U.S. adults. *American Journal of Preventive Medicine, 26,* 402–406.

Levy, A. S., & Heaton, A. W. (1993). Weight control practices of U.S. adults trying to lose weight. *Annals of Internal Medicine, 119,* 661–666.

McGuire, M. T., Wing, R. R., Klem, M. L., & Hill, J. O. (1999). Behavioral strategies of individuals who have maintained long-term weight losses. *Obesity Research, 7,* 334–341.

Miller, W. C., Eggert, K. E., Wallace, J. P., Lindeman, A. K., & Jastremski, C. (1993). Successful weight loss in a self-taught, self-administered program. *International Journal of Sports Medicine, 14,* 401–405.

Paeratakul, S., York-Crowe, E. E., Williamson, D. A., Ryan, D. H., & Bray, G. A. (2002). Americans on diet: Results from the 1994–1996 Continuing Survey of Food Intakes by Individuals. *Journal of the American Dietetic Association, 102,* 1247–1251.

Park, T. L., Perri, M. G., & Rodrigue, J. R. (2003). Minimal intervention programs for weight loss in heart transplant candidates: A preliminary examination. *Progress in Transplantation, 13,* 284–288.

Rothacker, D. Q. (2000). Five-year self-management of weight using meal replacements: Comparison with matched controls in rural Wisconsin. *Nutrition, 16,* 344–348.

Serdula, M. K., Williamson, D. F., Anda, R. F., Levy, A., Heaton, A., & Byers, T. (1994). Weight control practices in adults: Results of a multistate telephone survey. *American Journal of Public Health, 84,* 1821–1824.

Smith, C. F., Burke, L. E., & Wing, R. R. (2000). Vegetarian and weight-loss diets among young adults. *Obesity Research, 8,* 123–129.

Wing, R. R., & Hill, J. O. (2001). Successful weight loss maintenance. *Annual Review of Nutrition, 21,* 323–341.

Wing, R. R., Phelan, S., Butryn, M. L., & Hill, J. O. (2006). *Self-help dieting in the National Weight Control Registry.* Unpublished manuscript.

Wing, R. R., Venditti, E., Jakicic, J. M., Polley, B. A., & Lang, W. (1998). Lifestyle intervention in overweight individuals with a family history of diabetes. *Diabetes Care, 21,* 350–359.

Womble, L. G., Wadden, T. A., McGuckin, B. G., Sargent, S. L., Rothman, R. A., & Krauthamer-Ewing, E. S. (2004). A randomized controlled trial of a commercial Internet weight-loss program. *Obesity Research, 12,* 1011–1018.

2

Popular and Fad Diet Programs
Nutritional Adequacy, Safety, and Efficacy

ALLISON STEVENS, EMILY DIONNE,
and JOHANNA DWYER

This chapter describes the nutritional adequacy, safety, and efficacy of some popular reducing diets. First we introduce the "10-C" method for evaluating popular diets. Then we assess their nutrient content and other characteristics, using several days of menus exactly as prescribed in each currently popular diet book. Most of these reducing diets appeared on the best-seller list in *The New York Times* between August 2003 and August 2005.

USING THE "10-C" METHOD
FOR EVALUATING POPULAR DIETS

The 10-characteristic, or "10-C," method of evaluating each diet is summarized in Table 2.1. It was modified from our earlier work (Dazzi & Dwyer, 1984; Dwyer, 1980, 1985, 1992; Dwyer & Lu, 1993; Konikoff & Dwyer, 2000). These 10 C's describe the key characteristics to focus on when evaluating reducing diets. If the 10 C's are met, health professionals and dieters can be sure that the reducing diet is safe, effective, and nutritionally adequate. All elements are essential for healthy body weight benefits to be realized.

TABLE 2.1. The 10 C's: Critical Characteristics to Assess in Popular Reducing Diets

1. *Calories*: Total caloric intake on the diet minus an estimate of energy needs (using rested energy expenditure and the appropriate activity factor) determines the caloric deficit. A 500-calorie deficit per day results in loss of 1 pound per week.

2. *Composition*: Total and proportional composition of macronutrients (carbohydrate, protein, and fat), as well as the intake of micronutrients (vitamins and minerals), electrolytes, and fluids, must be assessed in order to determine whether needs are being met.

3. *Coping with coexisting health problems*: Recommendations for dealing with co-existing health problems such as hypertension, hyperglycemia, hyperlipidemia, and others need to be addressed.

4. *Continuation provisions for long-term maintenance*: Long-term maintenance of weight loss is vital to ensure good health outcomes; provisions for psychological and social support ensure optimum maintenance.

5. *Contains all the essential components for sound weight management*: These components include a hypocaloric diet coupled with physical activity, sound psychological support, and behavior modification techniques.

6. *Consumer friendliness*: Reasonable procedures and hedonic qualities are necessary for adherence to a reducing diet.

7. *Cost*: The price of the reducing program and of the food itself must be considered, especially if the program requires special foods, bars, supplements, exercise equipment, memberships, physician visits, and so forth.

8. *Comparison with dietary guidelines/My Pyramid recommendations*: Meeting the U.S. Department of Agriculture recommendations ensures nutritional adequacy, which is necessary for a weight-maintenance diet.

9. *Common-sense test*: This evaluates the text and readability of the literature. Overall, the information provided must be sensible and easy to read.

10. *Customization*: Individuals differ in many ways; therefore, the weight-loss plan must be individualized not only for physiological factors (height, weight, age, sex, etc.) but for social and psychological characteristics as well.

Calories

We examine each diet by the weight-loss phase (the hypocaloric phase when weight is being lost) and the maintenance phase (the subsequent phase of weight control and maintenance of the reduced weight), as both are important if a weight-control program is to be successful.

Weight-Loss Phase

The calorie level of a reducing diet and the calorie deficit from usual intake that it creates are both vitally important because they determine how much and how fast weight will be lost. The caloric level of the diet is easy to determine by calculating the calories using food composition tables and a representative set of diet menus from a particular reducing diet. The total calories in reducing diets are important, but the optimal caloric amount varies for each individual. For example, the average male requires more calories than the average female; on a similar reducing diet of 1,200 calories, the male's calorie deficit and subsequent weight loss is likely to be greater than the female's. In addition to sex, both body size (height and weight) and physical activity level need to be taken into account in order to increase precision in estimating energy output needs. (See later sections for how to go about calculating individual caloric requirements.)

Calorie deficit is also important, but knowing the precise caloric deficit a particular individual has brought about is difficult because adherence to the reducing regimen is never perfect. However, rough estimates of the calorie deficit can be obtained with formulas that provide estimates of resting metabolism and include a multiplier to account for the likely level of energy output from physical activity. These two estimates, taken together, give a rough idea of energy output. If the estimate of energy output is appropriate and the reducing diet is perfectly adhered to, the difference between the calculated intake, or energy content of the diet, and the energy output estimate is the energy deficit per day. If that number is multiplied by 7, the weekly energy deficit can be compared with the 3,500 calorie deficit needed to shed a pound of body fat, and the amount of weight lost per week, under ideal circumstances, can be calculated.

In evaluating calorie levels, in addition to total caloric intake and the caloric deficit, the method that is used to achieve these deficits must be considered. The method used to decrease energy intake must be logical, sustainable, safe, and effective. Table 2.2 lists caloric levels commonly used in reducing diets and the pros and cons of each; Table 2.3 describes some of the particular problems with extremely hypocaloric diets. Even for very-low-calorie diets, a minimum of 800 calories per day is recommended (National Task Force on the Prevention and Treatment of Obesity, 1993).

Rate of weight loss is also important. If too much weight is lost too fast, the diet is not safe; therefore, rate of weight loss is another important factor to consider. No more than 10% of body weight should be lost over a period of 6 months. The pattern of loss is also important. It should be slow and steady, no more than 1–2 pounds a week.

Maintenance Phase

Energy deficits for maintaining the reduced weight are less than those that are needed for reducing. Weight loss, once achieved, should be sustained. Even a very large weight loss, if not sustained, does little to decrease the risk of adverse events from the health standpoint. A smaller loss that can be maintained would be more beneficial in producing positive health outcomes and in avoiding adverse health side effects than a larger loss that is regained.

TABLE 2.2. Caloric Levels of Reducing Diets: Pros and Cons of Each

Classification	Calories/day	Pros	Cons
Total fasting/ starvation	0	Not recommended for those trying to lose weight without medical supervision.	• Excessive loss of lean body mass • Adverse metabolic effects include diuresis, kaliuresis, saliuresis, and possible nutrient deficiency • Symptoms: bad taste in mouth, dizziness • Requires vitamin and mineral supplementation • Self-defeating (loss of lean body mass and caloric deficit, decrease in resting metabolic rate, making weight loss more difficult; Garrow, 1995)
Protein-supplemented modified fast	< 300–500 kcal	Preserves lean tissue to a greater extent than total fasting.	• Requires medical supervision, especially for those on multiple medications or with multiple comorbidities • Large (~10-lb) gains in fluid weight in response to refeeding • Needs vitamin and mineral supplementation • May need additional Ca and Fe supplementation
Very-low-calorie diet	< 600 kcal	To be used for individuals who are 30–40% overweight (Position of American Dietetic Association, 1990).	• Decreases resting metabolism, may cause lethargy and fatigue • Requires vitamin supplementation • May need additional Ca and Fe supplementation
Low-calorie diet	800–1200 kcal	Easier to adopt for maintenance.	• Some may overconsume energy • Requires vitamin and mineral supplementation if diet is based on regular foods (not specifically formulated or fortified products)
Balanced-deficit diet	1200+ kcal	Similar to usual eating patterns but lower in energy. Easy to adopt for maintenance.	• Some may overconsume calories

TABLE 2.3. Serious Potential Side Effects Due to Misuses of Very-Low-Calorie Diets

Effect	Starvation/ total fast	VLCD	Periodic fasts
Lean-body-mass decrease	XXX	XX	X
Linear-growth decrease (in children)	XXX	X	X
Possible cardiac changes	XX	XX	X
Dehydration (disordered water balance)	XX	X	X
Ketosis	XX	XX	X
Electrolyte imbalances	X	X	X
Nutrient deficiencies if not supplemented (especially folate, vitamin B_6, magnesium, zinc, vitamins A and C, thiamin, iron, and calcium)	XXX	XX	X

Note. XXX, most pronounced; x, least pronounced. Data from Konikoff and Dwyer (2000).

Composition

Weight-Loss Phase

There is much controversy about the ideal macronutrient distributions in diets for weight loss and maintenance. Few long-term studies are available to assess which of them is "best." In general, during the weight-loss phase, it matters little what the macronutrient composition of the diet is; fat loss tends to be the same on all reducing diets if caloric level is the same (Dansinger, Gleason, Griffith, Selker, & Schaefer, 2005; Schoeller & Buchholz, 2005). However, various diets may differ from each other in terms of initial weight loss due to shifts in water balance. On very-low-carbohydrate or very-low-calorie diets of any sort, relative and temporary dehydration occurs, and this contributes to weight loss (Yang, Wang, Pierson, & Van Itallie, 1977). Also, some macronutrient combinations may be better for achieving short- and long-term adherence to reducing plans for certain people, and for this reason they may lose more weight on one diet than on another (Dansinger et al., 2005). Also, some small differences in macronutrient composition can affect biomarkers associated with disease risk during the weight-loss phase.

The *Dietary Guidelines for Americans* (U.S. Department of Health and Human Services and U.S. Department of Agriculture, 2005) state "it is calories that count—not the proportions of fat, carbohydrates, and protein in the diet." However, they also state that when individuals are losing weight, they should follow a diet that is within the acceptable macronutrient distribution ranges (AMDR), which include calorie distributions of 20–35% fat, 45–65% carbohydrate, and 10–35% protein. Diets that provide very low or very high amounts of protein, carbohydrates, or fat are likely to provide low amounts of other nutrients and are not advisable for long-term use. Although these weight-loss diets have been shown to result in weight reduction, the maintenance of a reduced weight ultimately will depend on a change in lifestyle.

CARBOHYDRATE

Carbohydrate needs are at least 50 grams per day and probably higher. At least 100 grams carbohydrate, and preferably 55% or more of total energy intake, should be provided in diets that include more than 800 calories per day. Any diet that includes less than 50–100 grams carbohydrate is ketogenic and may lead to excessive protein breakdown to maintain blood glucose levels unless protein intakes are increased. When the body must rely on degradation of the carbon skeletons of glucogenic amino acids to preserve blood glucose levels (via gluconeogenesis), the catabolism of the protein is accompanied by loss of water. For every gram of tissue protein (or glycogen) that is broken down, 3 grams of water are released, causing rapid weight loss but also a state of dehydration (Van Itallie, 1980). Relative dehydration caused by ketosis does not decrease adipose tissue, although it may temporarily decrease weight. However, failure to drink adequate fluids is undesirable for health reasons, not the least of which is laxation.

FAT

Even on reducing diets, small amounts (e.g., no more than a few teaspoons at most) of essential fatty acids are necessary, and some fat is also needed for absorption of fat-soluble vitamins. Therefore, these diets must contain fat; however, because it is calorically dense (9 calories per gram), fat is usually decreased on reducing diets to increase bulk and reduce energy.

PROTEIN

Protein must be provided in liberal amounts on reducing diets. The reason is that protein not only is an energy-yielding constituent but also has other essential functions, including maintenance of lean tissues. When energy intake falls below the level needed for energy balance, the requirement for protein rises, because some amino acids that could have been used for other functions are diverted into energy-yielding catabolic pathways. In general, for every 100-calorie deficit, 2.0 to 3.0 grams more of nitrogen (or 12.50–18.75 grams high-quality protein) are required to maintain nitrogen balance, because, in a hypocaloric state, protein is used for energy (Calloway & Spector, 1954). Very-low-calorie diets, particularly if they are low in protein, may deplete lean body mass and have negative effects, such as hair loss. A minimum of 1 gram of protein for each kilogram of ideal body weight per day is recommended on very-low-calorie diets (National Task Force, 1993).

FIBER

The 2005 *Dietary Guidelines for Americans* (USDHHS and USDA, 2005) define fiber as being "composed of nondigestible carbohydrates and lignin intrinsic and intact in plants." They go on to state that diets rich in dietary fiber have been shown to have a number of beneficial effects, including decreased risk of coronary heart disease and improvement in laxation. Fibers that occur naturally in intact plants are called dietary fibers, whereas those that have been extracted from plants and then added to foods with the intent of improving health benefits are called functional fibers. Total fiber is the sum of both dietary fibers and functional fibers. For the weight-loss phase, 25–30 grams per day of fiber is recommended to promote laxation.

MICRONUTRIENTS AND VITAMINS

The lower the diet is in calories, the more likely it is that essential vitamins, minerals, and electrolytes such as potassium, magnesium, vitamin B_6, iron, and calcium are also low. Diets that have less than 1,200 kilocalories per day, unless special formulas or fortificants are used, are likely to require vitamin and mineral supplements in amounts approximating the dietary reference intakes (DRIs). Above 1,200 kcal per day, women in the reproductive-age group may still need iron, calcium, and folic acid supplements (or to include fortified foods rich in these nutrients in the diet plan), as their needs for these nutrients are especially high. Most other nutrient needs can be met by a well-balanced diet that follows the DRIs. For this reason, nutrient-dense, lower calorie foods such as fruits, vegetables, and whole grains with high micronutrient density but relatively low energy density are especially important to include on a reducing diet.

WATER/FLUIDS

Adequate fluid intake is important to avoid dehydration, especially if fluid needs are elevated because of such factors as a ketogenic diet very low in calories, high physical activity, or use in a hot climate. The fatigue that some dieters associate with hypocaloric diets is often due, in part, to dehydration, especially if they have also dramatically increased their physical activity and exercise regimens (Melanson & Dwyer, 2002). Adequate fluids also promote laxation. Losses of body glycogen and protein are accompanied by losses of body water. On reducing diets, intakes of low-calorie or calorie-free fluids, especially water, should be emphasized. Large quantities of beverages containing caffeine and alcohol should be avoided, as they increase diuresis. Body water losses of as little as 2% have been associated with decreased physical and mental performance and impaired thermoregulation (Kleiner, 1999; Gopinathan, Pichan, & Sharma, 1988; Salmon, 1994). The evidence that supports water as an appetite suppressant is weak. However, fluids are important to prevent constipation. At least eight glasses of water daily is reasonable, and a fluid intake plan should be incorporated into every weight-loss regimen.

Maintenance Phase

The effects of composition are more striking during the period of weight maintenance. The effects of diet composition on health outcomes are more pronounced during weight maintenance, and biomarkers of risk factors may also differ markedly from one regimen to another. Aside from calories, reducing and maintenance phases of a diet should be adequate in all other nutrients, including vitamins, minerals, electrolytes, and fluids. During maintenance, diets that are relatively high in complex carbohydrates and fiber and low in fat (especially saturated and trans fats) are probably less likely to be associated with adverse health indicators than other combinations of macronutrients.

CARBOHYDRATE

The percent of total calories from carbohydrates and the type of carbohydrate are both important during weight maintenance. The 2005 *Dietary Guidelines for Americans* emphasize the importance of choosing at least half of grain foods from whole-grain sources. One benefit to consuming whole grains is that they tend to be high in fiber (see the section on fiber).

A recent cross-sectional analysis of American adults (Bowman & Spence, 2001) on self-selected usual diets (not necessarily reducing diets) found that usual intakes high in carbohydrate (above 55% of calories) were lower in energy and in the calories per gram of food they supplied and were associated with lower BMIs than diets lower in carbohydrate. Nutrient density (amount of the nutrient per calorie consumed) was also higher for vitamins A, C, carotene, folate, calcium, magnesium, and iron but lower in vitamin B-12 and zinc than those with lower intakes of carbohydrates. Also, the high-carbohydrate group ate more low-fat foods, grain products, and fruits and also had the lowest sodium intakes of the groups studied (Bowman & Spence, 2001).

The glycemic index (GI), originally developed for the therapy of diabetes, is currently also popular in diets for weight management. Various food products are assigned a score based on the blood glucose response from consumption of a defined amount of carbohydrate (usually 50 grams) relative to the same amount of carbohydrate from a control food (usually white bread; Wolever, Jenkins, Jenkins, & Josse, 1991). The premise is that more moderate blood glucose levels with lower GI scores will sustain satiety and energy balance to a greater extent than will large increases in blood glucose resulting from intake of a higher GI food. Low-GI foods are claimed to help prevent excess weight gain. However, before low-GI diets can be advocated as a weight-loss strategy, more research must be done on their acute effects and long-term efficacy (Roberts, 2000). Also, there may be practical problems in their use, as most ratings are for single food items. However, most foods are not eaten alone but in combination with other foods, which alters the GI rating (see also McIntosh, Jordan, Carter, Latner, & Wallace, Chapter 16, this volume).

FAT

Fat intake, especially during the maintenance phase of a diet, should resemble recommendations of the DRIs, emphasizing mono- and polyunsaturated fats. Dietary fat is not a major determinant of body fat (Willet & Leibel, 2002). But type of fat is important to take into consideration, as high levels of saturated and trans fatty acids can increase risks for coronary artery disease, among other adverse health risks.

PROTEIN

The recommended dietary allowance (RDA) for protein is 0.8 g/kg per day. This amount should be met during the maintenance phase of the diet.

FIBER

An adequate intake for fiber during weight maintenance is 14 grams per 1,000 calories of required energy, but currently there is insufficient evidence to determine an upper level (Institute of Medicine, 2005). The DRIs give an adequate intake (AI) of 25 grams per day for our reference subject, a 40-year-old female with a height of 5′4″ (163cm), a weight of 178 pounds (81kg), and a BMI of 31 (classified as obese). In addition, a diet adequate in fiber-containing foods is also usually rich in micronutrients and non-nutritive ingredients that have additional health benefits (Marlett, McBurney, & Slavin, 2002).

WATER/FLUIDS

There is no DRI set for water; however, the AI for total water intake for young men and women (ages 19–30 years) is 3.7 liters and 2.7 liters per day, respectively (Institute of Medicine, 2005).

Coping with Coexisting Health Problems

Weight-Loss Phase

Some people are particularly likely to have coexisting health problems when they embark on reducing diets. Individuals who are at high risk of health complications from dieting include elderly people, adolescents, children, pregnant or nursing women, those who are already underweight, those at risk for eating disorders, and the morbidly obese (BMI 40), who commonly have multiple comorbidities. Common comorbidities of obesity include type 2 diabetes mellitus, impaired glucose intolerance, hyperinsulinemia, dyslipidemia, cardiovascular disease, hypertension, sleep apnea, gallbladder disease, osteoarthritis, some cancers, reduced fertility, and polycystic ovarian disease (Melanson & Dwyer, 2002). Popular diet books and programs should address and ameliorate the dieter's comorbidities, or at least not exacerbate them. When preexisting comorbidities are present that require treatment, medical supervision during weight reduction is mandatory (Konikoff & Dwyer, 2000; Melanson & Dwyer, 2002; Dwyer & Lu, 1993).

Poorly formulated diets for weight reduction or maintenance have the potential to adversely affect comorbidities and risk factors. For example, low-carbohydrate diets may decrease caloric intake and cause weight loss, but at the same time they might increase intakes of saturated and trans fats, which in turn would increase serum cholesterol. If the increase in serum cholesterol were large, it would have to be medically addressed in order to prevent medical complications later on. This is just one example of how failing to address coexisting health problems could potentially be harmful to those embarking on reducing diets.

Coexisting physical problems (injuries, handicaps, etc.) and psychological problems (depression, mood disorders, etc.) also need to be assessed and monitored during the diet. Those with severe illness should not go on diets of their own devising at all and should seek professional assistance.

For those on chronic medications for any of the conditions listed here, medication dosing often needs to be adjusted due to dietary changes and weight loss.

Maintenance Phase

For weight maintenance, coexisting health problems must continue to be managed, although fewer modifications may be needed because intakes are higher and closer to usual levels.

Continuation Provisions for Long-Term Maintenance

Weight-Loss Phase

As described elsewhere in the chapter, the reducing diet that achieves the best adherence varies from one individual to another. A good weight-control program should offer practical guidance on healthy lifestyle changes that will control weight over the long term. The LEARN program is one example of a reasonable program (Brownell & Wadden, 1999). Although many people are currently on reducing diets, their attempts are often unsuccessful. Within 5 years, most dieters regain the weight they originally lost, and after 5 years they often even exceed their initial weight (Crawford, Jeffery, & French, 2000; National Task Force, 1993). By encouraging long-term adherence, more self-controlled dieting efforts may be successful (Knauper, Cheema, Rabiau, & Borten, 2005).

Maintenance Phase

It is much easier to lose weight initially than to maintain weight loss over the long term. During weight maintenance, energy intake must be lower than it was prior to embarking on the reducing diet in order for weight loss to be maintained. The reason is that some actively metabolizing lean body mass was lost along with the fat mass. As a result, resting metabolic rate (RMR) falls slightly. Also, carrying a lighter body weight requires less energy, so total energy expenditure decreases. This unfortunate reality comes as a shock to many dieters.

Success in maintaining weight is more likely when the dieter is provided with information, tools, social support, and associated lifestyle behaviors to make the long-term changes that are required. These include a reasonable eating pattern and the inclusion of regular physical activity. Social and psychological support, including remotivation, relapse prevention, cognitive restructuring, and behavior modification strategies, are also helpful to many individuals (see also Milsom, Perri, & Rejeski, Chapter 10, and Latner & Wilson, Chapter 11, this volume).

A long-term eating plan for maintenance that conforms to the recent recommendations set forth in the 2005 *Dietary Guidelines for Americans* (USDHHS and USDA, 2005) can be accessed at the website *www.mypyramid.gov*. This site allows for the input of age and activity level and, in turn, gives the appropriate calorie level for weight maintenance. In addition to a recommended calorie level, the recommended daily amounts required from each food group are provided. For those who want additional practical guidance in dieting and nutrition, several good books are available (e.g., Kirby, 2005; Roizen & Oz, 2005; and Duyff, 2002).

Diet Contains All the Essential Components for Sound Weight Management

A sound weight-management program requires much more than a reducing diet. It also requires a maintenance phase, accompanied by education to help the dieter transition to a maintenance diet that is somewhat lower in calories than his or her usual diet before weight reduction. In addition, behavior modification that equally emphasizes coping with social situations and relapse prevention, psychological and social support, and an exercise/physical activity prescription must be included. These must also be addressed in order to safely lose weight and maintain a lowered weight.

Consumer Friendliness

Popular diets should be portrayed honestly. The Federal Trade Commission's *Voluntary Guidelines for Providers of Weight Loss Products or Services* (1999) suggest that providers include information on staff qualifications and major components of the program, information about the risks of obesity, and the benefits of modest weight loss. Also, the provider should discuss risks associated with the program, costs, and outcome information. The complete guidelines are online at *www.ftc.gov/bcp/conline/pubs/buspubs/wtguide.htm*. These regulations are completely voluntary, and monitoring of the safety and honesty of those marketing weight-loss products is sporadic. In the United States there is currently no standard for disclosure of success rate on weight-reduction diets that would ensure that regimens are safe and effective; there is also no mandatory standard for ethical marketing. Some diet books use misleading claims to lure consumers into buying products that are recommended in the books. Making unrealistically high claims, claiming that all persons lose the same amount of weight, or other unethical practices are additional problems that consumers may encounter with weight-reduction programs. In evaluation of any diet, recognition of any false or misleading claims is important.

Costs

The seemingly endless search for the foolproof diet costs a lot of money. Programs such as OPTIFAST that involve a great deal of one-to-one counseling and physician evaluations are usually quite expensive. However, many dieters who turn to less expensive options, such as diet books or commercial weight-loss programs, to avoid the high costs of medical care may find that these can also be expensive. For example, although a book itself may be inexpensive, programs advocated in it may require readers to buy products such as frozen meals, bars, special formulas, dietary supplements, and so forth, which can be expensive. In addition, costs of meetings, along with the expense of the food itself, must also be taken into consideration.

Yet obesity also exacts a cost, and if the reducing diets help to lessen it, they can be worthwhile. The total cost of obesity in America alone has been estimated at $117 billion (this includes a direct cost [including costs of personal healthcare, hospital care, etc.] of $61 billion and an indirect cost [including loss productivity due to morbidity or mortality] of $56 billion; Wolf & Colditz, 1998). This cost is comparable to the economic costs of cigarette smoking. Besides the economic costs, excess body weight is the sixth most important risk factor contributing to the overall burden of disease worldwide. And the number of deaths per year attributable to obesity is roughly 30,000 in the United Kingdom and 10 times that in the United States (Haslam & James, 2005).

Comparison to Dietary Guidelines

Dieters need to keep in mind the U.S. Department of Health and Human Services and U.S. Department of Agriculture's *Dietary Guidelines for Americans* (2005) in order to ensure the nutritional adequacy, balance, and moderation that are necessary both during reducing and in weight maintenance. They are especially important during maintenance, which typically lasts much longer (usually indefinitely) than the weight-loss phase. Details can be found online at *www.healthierus.gov/dietaryguidelines/*.

Commonsense Test

The commonsense test refers to an evaluation of the reducing diet's scientific logic and practicality and the readability and understandability of the text. The information provided must make sense to the reader and be easy to read and understand. It must be presented in a manner such that instructions and guidelines are clear and encourage adherence.

Customization

An important factor for any diet plan is customization or individualization. A diet program needs to take into account the fact that each person who goes on a reducing diet is different in many aspects, including gender, weight, height, activity level, and so forth. Diets must also be tailored to the individual during weight loss and maintenance. Registered dietitians are particularly helpful in individualizing diets.

POPULAR REDUCING DIETS

The Reference Individual

In order to more accurately evaluate the diets in this chapter we chose a 40-year-old female whose height was 5'4" (163 cm); weight, 178 pounds (81 kg); and BMI, 31 (which is classified as obese) as our reference individual. The usual method for calculating energy needs is to estimate resting energy expenditure (REE) at rest, which is multiplied by an "activity factor" to account for physical activity. The result is the individual's usual estimated energy requirement. For example, using our reference subject, a 40-year-old active female, the estimated energy requirement (EER) is 2,403 kcal/day. In order to estimate calorie levels more accurately, as might be necessary for research purposes, the following equation can be used: EER = 354 − 6.91 × age + PA × [9.36 × weight (in kilograms) + 726 × height (in meters)]

PA stands for physical activity and ranges from 1.0 (sedentary) to 1.48 (very active). Using this equation and an activity level of 1.2 (slightly active), the woman would require 2,171 kcals per day. Note that the error in using the abbreviated method is very small, and it is usually used clinically.

From the total EER, the calories necessary to produce loss of fat tissue are subtracted to give the individualized energy prescription for the reducing diet. If the woman had a caloric intake of 1,600–1,700 kcal per day (a 500-kcal-per-day deficit), weight loss of approximately 1 pound per week would be expected.

Standards for Rating Popular Diets

Among the many different ways to go about evaluating weight-reduction and maintenance programs, we chose the "10 C's" method. In order to examine the calorie adequacy and composition with respect to adequacy of other nutrients, we chose 2 representative days within each diet and analyzed the nutrient content of those days using Food Processor SQL, Version 9.6.2 [ESHA Research, Salem, OR]. The nutrient analysis included the distribution of macronutrients and the amount of micronutrients; we then compared each to the DRIs. In addition to the nutrient analysis, we examined the narratives provided in the books to determine whether they were accurate, correct, and reasonable and included all 10 C's as described in the first section of this chapter. Our comments, which follow, represent a combination of these findings. The diets are discussed in roughly ascending order, from lower to higher calorie levels, and by type of book, with reducing diet books first and those with more of an exercise or lifestyle emphasis following.

Examples of Popular Diets

OPTIFAST

OPTIFAST (Novartis Nutrition Corporation, 2005), is a medically supervised weight-loss program that uses a liquid formula and other commercial reducing products. The diet consists of five OPTIFAST products per day, both liquid and solid, depending on the particular OPTIFAST center. Each product provides 160 calories; therefore, five products per day provide 800 calories per day. The program lasts for a total of 18 weeks. Dieters consume only OPTIFAST products for the first 12 weeks, and at week 12, dieters are transitioned to four OPTIFAST products and one regular meal per day, consisting of 4 ounces of meat or a nonmeat protein source and nonstarchy vegetables. At week 15, the regular meal consists of the same components as week 12, with the addition of a starch or fruit. At week 17, either a fruit or starch—whichever was not added to the meal after week 15—is added to the one regular meal per day. OPTIFAST is an 18-week-long, low-calorie diet. Taking our 40-year-old female reference person, who is 5'4" tall and weighs 178 pounds (81kg), the OPTIFAST diet provides a 735-calorie deficit compared with her REE, or 47% of her REE, and only about one-third of her total energy needs. The composition of the 800-calorie OPTIFAST diet includes 52% of calories from carbohydrate (about 100 grams), 29% protein, and 19% fat (see Figure 2.1).

The micronutrient content of the OPTIFAST products meet the RDA for vitamins and minerals if five products per day are consumed (with the exception of sodium and potassium; see Table 2.4). Each product contains 20–30% of the RDA; therefore, consuming five products per day provides dieters with 100% of the RDA (see Table 2.4). For the most part, OPTIFAST does not recommend additional multivitamin/mineral supplementation unless dieters are told to take them by their doctors. The OPTIFAST liquid formulas have no dietary fiber, and the nutrition bars contain only 16% of the RDA for dietary fiber. OPTIFAST recommends using a fiber supplement as needed and suggests specific products such as Fibercon, Benefiber, or Metamucil. In terms of hydration, OPTIFAST recommends that individuals consume at least 2 quarts (eight 8-ounce cups) of calorie-free or very-low-calorie liquids every day. Limiting caffeine intake to two cups of regular coffee, tea, or diet soda is recommended.

The OPTIFAST program utilizes a well-designed multidisciplinary, medically supervised team approach to patient care that integrates the medical, nutritional, and behavioral facets of weight loss therapy. The program is designed for dieters with a BMI of > 30; our sample participant's BMI is 31 and would therefore qualify for enrollment. The program claims that 1 out of 4 participants maintain 75% of their lost weight 2 years after OPTIFAST participation (Novartis Nutrition Corporation, 2005). OPTIFAST also claims a significant reduction in weight: a mean weight loss of 52 pounds in more than 20,000 patients (Novartis Nutrition Corporation, 2005).

As to comorbidities associated with overweight and obesity, OPTIFAST targets Type 2 diabetes, claiming a 29% reduction in blood glucose; hypercholesterolemia, a 15% reduction in total cholesterol; and hypertension, a 10% reduction in blood pressure (Novartis Nutrition Corporation, 2005).

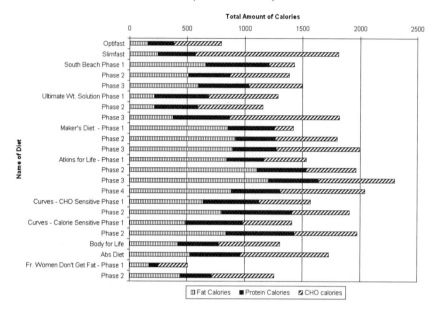

FIGURE 2.1. Caloric composition of various reducing diets.

The active weight-loss phase on OPTIFAST lasts approximately 12 weeks. The purpose of this phase, during which the patient consumes solely five OPTIFAST products, is to remove the cues of food tasting and to limit choices to reduce intake (Novartis Nutrition Corporation, 2005). The transition phase, weeks 12–18, serves to reintroduce self-prepared foods while slowly removing some of the OPTIFAST products from the meal plan. This phase increases calories to a total of 1,250 calories per day by the end of the program.

OPTIFAST program teams include a registered dietitian and a physician, and most include an exercise physiologist. Depending on the particular OPTIFAST center, exercise programs are tailored to meet individual needs and interests. Patients are encouraged to continue with the amount and composition of foods consumed in the final week of the program for long-term weight maintenance, which for our dieter would include an OPTIFAST formula for breakfast and sensible lunches and dinners for a total of 1,250 calories per day. This deficit remains less than our sample participant's REE by 285 calories per day, and therefore would promote continued weight loss for our reference person.

The cost to enroll in the OPTIFAST weight-loss program is dependent on the particular OPTIFAST center, though expenses generally are approximately $550 for the program fee, which includes all of the professional supervision necessary throughout the program, plus an additional $75–$100

TABLE 2.4. Percent Micronutrient Content of Various Reducing Diets Compared with the DRI/AI

	DRI	OPTIFAST	SlimFast	South Beach	Ultimate Weight Solution	Maker's Diet	Atkins for Life	Curves— CHO sensitive	Curves— calorie sensitive	Body for Life	Abs	French Women Don't Get Fat
Sodium[b]	1,500 mg	80%	106%	176%	148%	117%	193%	177%	208%	130%	170%	170%
Potassium[b]	4,700 mg	49%	92%	180%	51%	77%	49%	66%	58%	48%	45%	47%
Iron	18 mg	100%	113%	64%	81%	53%	73%	49%	44%	62%	101%	63%
Calcium	1,000 mg	100%	165%	101%	104%	41%	87%	100%	110%	36%	142%	48%
Vitamin A	700 mcg	100%	84%	106%	156%	168%	108%	100%	52%	19%	71%	59%
Vitamin C	75 mg	100%	689%?	235%	232%	331%	204%	340%	180%	265%	192%	142%
Magnesium	320 mg	100%	149%	62%	65%	69%	66%	70%	57%	60%	97%	68%
Water (amount recommended)	2.7 liters	100%	NS[a]	NS	100%	NS	70%	70%	70%	NS	70%	NS
Multivitamin recommended		No	No	Yes	No	Yes	Yes	Yes	Yes	Yes	Yes	No

Note. These values are derived from an average of the diets' phases; therefore, should a diet provide 100% of the recommended value in Phase 3, this table may underestimate the total amount a person consumes over the long term. **Bolded** values indicates micronutrient values are < Daily Recommended Intake/Adequate Intake (DRI/AI).

[a]Indicates the diet does not provide a recommendation for water.

[b]These micronutrients do not have a DRI, but an adequate intake instead; a value < 100% does not necessarily indicate the diet is "inadequate."

per week for the OPTIFAST products. Therefore, the program costs at least $2,000 for the weight-loss phase.

In summary, for those who can afford the program and related medical expenses, OPTIFAST is a sound medically supervised reducing diet. The program may be less desirable for maintenance.

SlimFast

SlimFast (2005) is a line of shakes, powders, and bars that serve as meal re-placements and/or snacks. SlimFast is available in most grocery stores and drugstores, as well as online. The SlimFast plan is a balanced-deficit diet and includes using a SlimFast shake for breakfast and lunch, balanced with a dinner (recipes and sample menus are provided on their website) and snacks (either SlimFast bars or a piece of fruit) for a total of 1,800 kcals per day, which would be suitable for maintenance for the woman we used as an example. The macronutrient distribution is 13% fat, 18% protein, and 69% carbohydrates, which is slightly low in fat, but otherwise it provides an appropriate distribution. (Refer to Figure 2.1 for a comparison with other diets.) This diet provides the DRI for all micronutrients (see Table 2.4). The monotony and cost of drinking shakes for two meals a day is something to take into consideration before adopting this diet. Using expen-sive shakes for two meals a day may not be a feasible weight-maintenance plan for many people. However, the website does offer plenty of healthy weight-loss techniques, including hints for eating out at various restaurant types. Followers can also opt to sign up to have a weekly e-mail sent as a motivator and can use the interactive website as a tracking tool with links to all types of online support. SlimFast's website includes four "keys to suc-cess in weight control." Nutrition is listed first. Activity, expert advice, counseling and support, and self-monitoring are also included as necessary components for a successful weight-management program.

In summary, for many individuals, SlimFast, which is readily available, would promote weight loss, but energy intake needs to be carefully con-trolled to produce the appropriate deficit. Some may also find the regimen helpful for maintenance.

The South Beach Diet

The South Beach diet (Agatston, 2003) is a regimen described in a book; it comprises three phases. Dieters can purchase various calorie-controlled snacks and meals, which are sold under the South Beach label in a variety of supermarkets. The first phase is followed for 14 days and provides an average of 1,400 calories, approximately 100 calories less than our refer-ence person's estimated REE. This phase of the diet provides 16% of the total calories from carbohydrate, 38% from protein, and 46% from fat (see

Figure 2.1). It provides 0% of the new food guide pyramid's recommendations for servings in the grain food group (see Table 2.5a) and provides just 13 grams of dietary fiber per day, which is 52% of the DRI's recommended dietary allowance for adequate intake (RDA/AI). The author promises that dieters will lose 8–13 pounds after Phase 1, that weight loss will be from the midsection, and that they will notice a difference in the way their clothes fit. No specific claims are made as to how much the dieter will ultimately lose. The total amount of weight loss is contended to vary from individual to individual. Supposedly, cravings for carbohydrates will disappear, and the author claims that "passing up such foods is painless" (Agatston, 2003, p. 4).

Phase 2 of the South Beach diet is to be followed until the dieter has achieved his or her target weight loss. According to our calculations, it provides an average of 1,390 calories per day, about 150 calories less than our reference woman's estimated REE. This phase includes 37% of the total calories from carbohydrate, 26% protein, and 37% fat (see Figure 2.1). Phase 2 allows the reintroduction of some carbohydrate, providing, on average, two servings of the grain food group per day (see Table 2.5b). This phase meets only 76% of the RDA/AI for dietary fiber, providing just 19 grams per day. The book advises the dieter to remain on Phase 2 until the target weight is achieved. It promises dieters that the foods they love and miss can be reintroduced into the diet, such as chocolate—claiming, "If it makes you feel good, then sure, have it" (Agatston, 2003, p. 5).

The third phase is the maintenance phase, which provides an average of 1,500 calories per day, just 35 calories fewer than our sample participants estimated REE. The book recommends that the individual remain on Phase 3 for the rest of his or her life. The composition of the third phase includes 31% of the total calories from carbohydrate, 29% protein, and 40% fat (as shown in Figure 2.1). This final phase provides half of the recommended amount of servings from the grain food group, as shown in Table 2.5c, and meets 100% of the RDA/AI for dietary fiber, providing 25 grams per day. The book claims that this stage of the diet will benefit the cardiovascular system, substantially increasing odds of living long and well (Agatston, 2003). The author of the book is a cardiologist who stresses the importance of the diet and its cardiovascular benefits. He emphasizes how cardiovascular disease is linked to obesity and diabetes and how the diet can both prevent and help treat these conditions.

The South Beach diet does not meet the DRI for iron and magnesium (as shown in Table 2.4). However, the author does recommend a daily multivitamin. Adequate fluid intake is important to prevent dehydration in reducing diets. Although the South Beach diet makes no specific recommendation for fluid intake, it suggests that one "drink when thirsty" (Agatston, 2003, p. 56).

The book recommends that phase 3 be continued for the rest of one's

TABLE 2.5. The New My Pyramid and Popular Diets Compared by Content of Different Food Groups

a. Phase 1 of the various popular diets

	My Pyramid.gov	SlimFast	South Beach (1)	Ultimate Weight Solution (1)	Maker's (1)	Atkins for Life (1)	Curves—calorie sensitive (1)	Curves—CHO sensitive (1)	Body for Life	Abs	French Women (1)
Grains	6 ounces	**2.8**	0	**2.9**	0	3	0.9	0	3	**4.4**	0
Vegetables	2.5 cups	**7.8**	9.5	**6.7**	6.9	4.1	3.5	5.3	2.4	3.6	10.5
Fruits	1.5 cups	**3.1**	1.1	**1.7**	0.6	2	1.3	4.2	4.1	2.8	0.5
Meats	3 cups	**1.3**	5.7	**4.4**	4.8	**2.9**	5.6	5.7	3.4	3.4	1
Milk and dairy	5 ounces	**0.6**	4	**1.7**	0.8	1.2	1.3	1.6	0.6	3.5	0
Fats and oils	5 teaspoons of oils	**2.1**	2.9	**4.8**	6.9	5.1	1.5	2.3	3.4	6.4	1

b. Phase 2

	MyPyramid.gov	South Beach (2)	Ultimate Weight Solution (2)	Maker's (2)	Atkins for Life (2)	Curves—calorie sensitive (2)	Curves—CHO sensitive (2)	French Women (2)
Grains	6 ounces	2	2	0	3.2	0.8	0.8	2.9
Vegetables	2.5 cups	6.4	8.2	12	5.2	6.8	7.1	4.5
Fruits	1.5 cups	3.1	2.9	2.8	1.7	1.1	0.9	3.5
Meats	3 cups	**2.6**	3.7	**2.9**	3.7	6.3	6.8	2.2
Milk and dairy	5 ounces	2.1	1.7	1.1	0.9	1.5	1.1	0.7
Fats and oils	5 teaspoons of oils	5	2.9	8.6	7.6	6	6	4.4

c. Phases 3 and 4

	MyPyramid.gov	South Beach (3)	Ultimate Weight Solution (3)	Maker's (3)	Atkins for Life (3)	Atkins for Life (4)
Grains	6 ounces	**5.8**	1	3.7	5	
Vegetables	2.5 cups	5.6	14	5.1	2.3	
Fruits	1.5 cups	5	3.4	2.3	4.3	
Meats	3 cups	**4.4**	4.2	4	3.6	
Milk and dairy	5 ounces	2	1.1	2.9	0.8	
Fats and oils	5 teaspoons of oils	5.6	5.8	7	6	

Note. **Bolded** values indicate the diet provides < the New My Pyramid's recommendations for a 40-year-old female with an activity level of < 30 minutes per day (My Pyramid based on 1,800 calories).

life in order to maintain the positive health benefits. The author suggests that a dieter who relapses should return to Phase 1 and begin the diet again from the beginning, to prevent complete reversal of the weight lost. However, no specific relapse prevention skills are provided. One chapter, "A Day in the Life," discusses preparing meals in advance in order to prevent relapse but does not specifically teach behavior modification skills.

Exercise is highly recommended—a 30-minute workout that the dieter can perform on a daily basis to help lower blood pressure and cholesterol (Agatston, 2003). Weight training is also suggested, especially for women, to increase bone density and help prevent osteoporosis (Agatston, 2003).

It is not expensive for an individual to follow the South Beach diet. The original price of the hardcover book by Arthur Agatston, MD, is $24.95. The South Beach foods, of course, are an extra expense. Although the meal plan recommends many types of fish and healthy, low-fat cheeses, which can be expensive, all meal plan items can be substituted for others at a lower cost—for example, choosing chicken instead of fish.

In summary, the South Beach diet is relatively rigorous, and dieters may have trouble following it, particularly in the beginning.

The Ultimate Weight Solution

Dr. Phil McGraw's *Ultimate Weight Solution* (McGraw, 2004) is another diet book composed of three diet phases. There are also numerous food products on the market under the Dr. Phil McGraw label, but they are not specifically marketed for use with this diet exclusively. The first phase, titled "The Rapid Start Plan," is a low-calorie phase, providing, on average, 1,300 calories per day, 240 calories fewer than our reference person's REE. Phase 1 is a 14-day plan, and its purpose is to "gear the body up for accelerated weight loss" (McGraw, 2004, p. 28), and to change taste preferences from high-sugar, high-fat foods to healthier choices. Like the author of the South Beach diet, McGraw promises dieters that during Phase 1 they will experience diminished cravings for refined carbohydrates. The caloric distribution of this first phase includes 47% of the total calories from carbohydrate, 36% from protein, and 17% from fat, as shown in Figure 2.1. This phase of the diet also provides 30 grams of dietary fiber per day, 120% of the RDA/AI. McGraw claims that the larger amount of weight lost initially, the greater the chance of long-term weight maintenance.

Phase 2 is titled "The High-Response Cost, High-Yield Weight Loss Plan." It provides an average of 1,100 calories per day, 430 calories fewer than our reference person's REE, and is also a low-calorie-reducing phase. The caloric distribution of this phase includes 49% of the daily calories from carbohydrate, 32% protein, and 19% from fat (shown in Figure 2.1). It provides, on average, 25 grams of dietary fiber per day, 100% of the RDA/AI. McGraw (2004) claims that high-response-cost, high-yield foods are those that take time and effort to prepare, require a great deal of chewing and ingestion energy, cannot be eaten rapidly, suppress hunger, curb cravings, and supply a healthy balance of vitamins, minerals, fiber, and other nutrients. These foods include skinless chicken and turkey breast, seafood, lean meats, eggs, fruits, vegetables, high-fiber whole grains, reduced-fat and fat-free dairy products, and others. According to Dr. Phil, high-response-cost, high-yield foods, such as high-nutrient-density foods, support behavior change.

The purpose of Phase 2 is to exert greater metabolic control so that the body burns calories for energy rather than storing them as fat (McGraw, 2004). This high-response-cost, high-yield plan stresses the importance of consuming complex carbohydrates rather than refined carbohydrates. The book claims that "chaotic, mindless eating will become a thing of the past" (McGraw, 2004, p. 41). Dieters are to remain on this phase until their target weight is achieved.

Phase 3 is referred to as the "Ultimate Maintenance Phase." This phase provides, on average, 1,820 calories, 290 calories greater than our reference person's REE, a sensible deficit. Approximately 52% of the total calories are derived from carbohydrate, 27% from protein, and 21% from fat (see Figure 2.1). On average, this phase of the diet provides 35 grams of dietary fiber per day, 140% of the RDA/AI. The purpose of this phase is to keep weight under control for the remainder of the dieter's life. This phase allows for more servings from the high-response-cost, high-yield foods: three servings of protein, an unlimited amount of nonstarchy vegetables, three to four servings of starchy carbohydrates, three to four servings of fruit, two to three servings of low-fat dairy products, and one to two servings of healthy fats.

On average, over the three phases of the Ultimate Weight Solution, the diet does not meet the DRI for potassium, iron, and magnesium, and the book does not recommend the use of a daily multivitamin with minerals (see Table 2.4). Preventing dehydration is stressed, and all three phases recommend at least 8–10 glasses of pure water per day, 100% of the RDA/AI for fluid intake (also shown in Table 2.4).

The incorporation of exercise into any weight-loss program is very important to both accelerate and maintain weight loss. The Ultimate Weight Solution recommends exercise involving 3–4 hours per week of aerobic activity; in addition to aerobic exercise, weight training is also encouraged to accelerate the individual's metabolism and to help burn fat (McGraw, 2004). McGraw claims that 100% of the weight lost will be fat if weight training is included in the exercise program (McGraw, 2004); this is physiologically impossible.

The chapter titled "No Fail Solutions: The Food Strategies for Success" is devoted to behavioral change and successful weight management, providing strategies to counter mindless eating with mindful eating. It also includes tactics for eating out, vacationing, social situations, dealing with stressful situations, and avoiding overeating. The following chapter is devoted entirely to instructions for using the 557-page food guide. The importance of carbohydrates, protein, fat, fiber, sugar, sodium, and cholesterol is stressed, serving sizes are explained, examples are given, and tips for estimating serving sizes are provided.

It is relatively inexpensive for an individual to follow the *Ultimate Weight Solution Food Guide*. The original price of the book is $7.99, and more sample menus and food choices are provided on www.drphil.com free of charge. However, the foods he advocates cost more money, and these expenses can add up.

In summary, this is a somewhat sensible diet and exercise program, but more stress on portion sizes may be needed to avoid overconsumption, and some of McGraw's claims defy reality.

The Maker's Diet

The Maker's Diet (2004) author Jordan S. Rubin suffered an onslaught of health problems at a young age. The book details the changes he made to his diet and lifestyle that allowed him to live to tell his story (Rubin, 2004). The book claims that this 40-day health plan will completely change the diet and lifestyle of the reader. The plan includes three phases. Phase 1 is very restrictive in carbohydrates, providing only 41 grams per day, which is lower than the recommended minimum of 50 grams. Also the percentage of fat, especially during the initial phase, is too high, with 60% of calories coming from fat. Phase 2 is a slightly less restrictive phase, and the final phase is a maintenance phase that lasts indefinitely. (See Figure 2.1 for a complete breakdown of the macronutrient distribution for the three phases.)

Relapse prevention precautions are addressed. If followers stray off the diet—for example, during the holidays, on a vacation, or at another special event such as an extravagant birthday or anniversary celebration—they are advised to "go back to phase one or two for a week or two to get back into the groove" (Rubin, 2004, p. 222). In addition, mindful eating is addressed, with readers being instructed to take their time to chew food and to avoid eating when angry, sad, scared, or anxious.

The diet is supposed to be appropriate for dieters with any health problem and the target group includes "people hoping to overcome challenging health symptoms" (Rubin, 2004, p. 197). The author implies that following his recommendations may allow the discontinuation of medications (if not right away, then eventually). Although this may occur, it is important that dieters are advised to consult a physician before altering medication dosages. The book is also for readers who are overweight, obese, or have other health problems; these groups in particular are instructed to begin on Phase 1, the most restrictive of the three phases.

Exercise is recommended, but it does not play a major role in this program. Phases 1 and 2 incorporate 10–15 minutes of exercise per day and Phase 3, 15–20 minutes per day. Breathing exercises, which are recommended over straining aerobic exercises, are one form of exercise that can count toward this daily goal. A very specific regimen of vitamins, herbs, and minerals is recommended. Readers choose the level of supplements to take. The basic level provides three core products, the intermediate level adds on two more, and the advanced level recommends a total of nine products. The book has an appendix full of additional supplements and food items, as well as mail-order information for these products. Although foods recommended by the diet are supposed to be unrefined and natural, recommendations for using coconut oil and butter explain the high level of saturated fat in this diet, which is not recommended because high levels of saturated fats in the diet are known to increase serum cholesterol. The extensive list of supplements and other food products that are listed in this book could get rather expensive. The cost of the book itself is $14.00. The supplements are costly, and it is unclear what it is they do or why such branded supplements are needed.

Although this diet has some positive aspects, there are many odd and unsupported recommendations, and therefore it cannot not be recommended.

Atkins for Life

Dr. Robert Atkins, the famous "diet doctor," died a few years ago, but his books go on and on. *Atkins for Life* (Atkins, 2003) is a book that targets dieters who have lost weight on the original Atkins diet and want to successfully maintain that weight, for yo-yo dieters, and for those who are concerned about their health and weight control (Atkins, 2003). The Atkins conglomerate sold a large number of diet products under the Atkins Advantage label until the company fell into financial difficulties last year. Dieters are trained to discover their "ACE"—"Atkins Carbohydrate Equilibrium," or the total amount of "net" carbohydrates he or she can consume without gaining weight. Net carbohydrates are carbohydrates that contribute significant levels of calories to the diet and that consist primarily of sugars and starches, excluding primarily dietary fiber, which provides virtually no caloric value, and the noncaloric portion of sugar alcohols. It should be noted that "net carbohydrates" is not a concept endorsed by the Food and Drug Administration.

Phase 1 is the induction phase, which lasts 2 weeks, the goal being to jump-start the weight-loss program. According to our analysis, Phase 1 provides an average of 1,540 calories per day, a balanced deficit, which is equivalent to our reference person's estimated REE. Approximately 24% of the total calories are derived from carbohydrate, 21% from protein, and

55% from fat, (as shown in Figure 2.1). This phase also provides 25 grams of dietary fiber per day, meeting 100% of the DRI.

Phase 2 is the ongoing weight-loss phase, which encourages high-quality protein and fat. According to our calculations, total calories per day are 1,970, also a balanced deficit. This is an additional 30% of our reference person's estimated REE. It would promote weight maintenance, not weight loss. Carbohydrate makes up 22% of the total calories, protein also provides 22%, and the remaining 56% comes from fat (as shown in Figure 2.1), which is a high percentage of fat. The ongoing weight-loss phase also meets the DRI for dietary fiber, providing approximately 28 grams per day. The purpose of this phase is for the dieter to experiment with the total amount of carbohydrate he or she can consume without gaining any weight. Dieters are told to follow this phase until they are within 5 to 10 pounds of their goal weight.

The third phase is the premaintenance phase. This phase provides 2,310 calories per day, approximately 775 calories more than our sample participant's estimated REE. Carbohydrates contribute 29% of the total calories, protein about 19%, and the remaining 52% comes from fat calories (as shown in Figure 2.1). This phase also provides a sufficient amount of dietary fiber, approximately 32 grams per day. The purpose of this phase is to slow weight loss in order for the dieter's new eating habits to become embedded into their lifestyle. Again, if weight loss stops, the dieter is told to cut back on the amount of carbohydrates consumed by 5 to 10 grams. Dieters are to remain on Phase 3 of the diet until their goal weight is achieved.

The last phase is lifetime maintenance. Dieters start this phase after their target weight goal has been reached. This phase provides about 2,050 calories per day, about 510 calories more than our sample participant's estimated REE. Composition includes 36% of calories from carbohydrate, 20% from protein, and 44% from fat (as shown in Figure 2.1). About 34 grams of dietary fiber per day are included in the lifetime maintenance phase. The book claims this phase is the equilibrium zone in which the dieter will maintain his or her weight effortlessly while consuming a satisfying diet (Atkins, 2003).

On average, the four phases of Atkins for Life do not meet the RDA/AI for potassium, iron, calcium, and magnesium, although the author does recommend a daily multivitamin with minerals, which probably would correct many of these deficits (refer to Table 2.4). The author recommends consumption of 64 ounces (about 2 liters) of water each day, whereas the DRIs suggest about 2.7 liters per day (or 90 ounces), as shown in Table 2.4. Exercise is also encouraged; specifically, the dieter is advised to aim for 1 hour of physical activity per day to reduce the risk factors for disease, as well as to promote the burning of more calories by the body at rest. The book provides relapse prevention tips for the reader, such as how to order out, tips on avoiding overindulging, skills for dinner parties and social events, traveling tips, and more. The cost for dieters to follow Atkins for Life is not substantial. The original cost of the book is $24.95, plus the cost of food, which can be chosen by the individual for the most part. The book does not promote special products or particularly high-priced foods.

In summary, this high-fat (particularly saturated fat), high-calorie reducing diet would prove difficult for many dieters to follow during the weight-loss phase. During maintenance it provides a diet that has atherogenic characteristics, and therefore it cannot be recommended.

Curves

Curves is the largest fitness franchise in the world, with more than 9,000 locations worldwide (Heavin & Colman, 2003). Its target audience is women, and the concept is based on 30-minute workouts three times per week. The workouts consist of a variety of resistance training exercises with weight-lifting machines, as well as some cardiovascular activities. We have noted the trend for diet doctors to develop lines of branded foods. The exercise specialists are also branching out and now are getting into the dieting business. The founder, Gary Heavin, has now developed a diet program, the "Curves diet," to accompany the fitness regimen (Heavin & Colman, 2003). Readers of Curves, the diet book, complete a short quiz to determine whether they are "carbohydrate-sensitive" or "calorie-sensitive"; they then follow the diet that matches their quiz results. The main difference between the two plans is that the plan for those who are "carbohydrate sensitive" is more restrictive in carbohydrates (as shown in Table 2.4), whereas the "calorie-sensitive" plan is slightly lower in calories on Phase 1 (around 1,400 calories) than the carbohydrate-sensitive plan, which has 1,575 calories. The Curves diet does not allow for customization based on factors such as weight, height, and age. Meal plans for both diets consist of six small meals spread throughout the day. Both plans have two phases, beginning with weight loss (Phase 1) and then a less restrictive maintenance period (Phase 2). The transition from Phase 1 to Phase 2 takes place either after 2 weeks or after goal weight is reached. Although our analysis found calorie levels of 1,900–2,000 calories for Phase 2, the author advises that maintenance calorie levels can range from 2,600 all the way up to 3,000 calories per day, quite high for a maintenance phase for women (the target audience). The book emphasizes that the metabolism is "revved up" from following the Curves exercise regimen so that followers require the higher energy intakes. However, using our reference person as an example, she would require around only 2,170 calories a day to maintain weight. For this individual to take in a maintenance calorie level of 2,600–3,000 calories would require more than the 30 minutes of exercise per day prescribed in the book. After completing the first two phases and reaching a desirable weight, readers are told they can "watch what [they] eat for just 2 days of the month and eat without deprivation the other 28 days" (Heavin & Coleman, 2004, p. 3). This is a prescription for disaster for many dieters, especially those who have a tendency toward binges.

The cost of the book is $12.95. Although there are no special food products or supplements endorsed by the author, it will come as no surprise that he does recommend joining a Curves fitness center, which would require a monthly fee that varies from location to location.

One study has been performed to assess the Curves fitness and diet program (Kreider et al., 2004). It consisted of 123 sedentary women who were assigned to participate in a 14-week exercise program coupled with either no diet or with a variation on one of the Curves diet plans. Participants who followed the Curves diet were found to show an average weight loss of 5 pounds over a 10-week period, which is higher than the 1-pound average weight loss experienced by those not put on a version of the Curves diet (all participants were following the exercise program). Although these results seem promising, note that the exercise component was essential to achieving weight loss. Copycat organizations that use principles similar to the Curves concept are starting up. For example, there is a group called Contours in New Zealand that uses many of the same themes.

In summary, this reducing diet places excessive emphasis on the importance of carbohydrates and too little emphasis on energy intakes and portion sizes, and it cannot be recommended.

Body for Life for Women

The *Body for Life for Women* book (Peeke, 2005) is a sister to the original *Body for Life* book by Bill Phillips (Phillips, 1999) and is focused primarily on exercise. Like the original, the cover of this book is adorned with striking before-and-after pictures. The diet prescribed is a low-calorie diet. Our analysis shows that it provides an average of 1,270 calories a day, which is particularly low considering the book focuses on exercise and the fact that this would serve as the maintenance phase for this diet as well. Note that the diet is flexible in allowing slightly more calories once goal weight is reached, but the diet is not split up into phases. Also, our analysis did not take into account the 80/20 rule that the book urges dieters to employ. The diet is based on eating a specific number of carbohydrate and protein servings each day. The meals are frequent and small (5–6 meals/day). Determining servings per day is based on factors such as BMI and activity level. Foods are also divided into "smart foods" and "junk foods" (basically, foods containing refined white flour and/or sugar, such as a piece of cake). A realistic goal of a ratio of at least 80% smart foods to 20% junk foods per day is set.

The book takes into account the different stages of a woman's life, including the reproductive years and menopause, and their effects on diet and exercise. Factors other than diet alone (relapses, mindful eating, relaxation techniques, etc.) that influence adherence are also accounted for. The cost of this book is $17.79. The cost of food and following the prescribed exercises (in which do-at-home versions are given) would not be excessive.

Exercise is a large component of the Body for Life program; followers are instructed to fit in all types of physical activity, including cardio fitness, strength, flexibility, and endurance activities. A 36-page appendix is filled with easy-to-follow exercises. Overall, the flexibility and adaptability of this diet make it a good choice for women of all ages and activity levels.

The Abs Diet

The Abs diet (Zinczenko, 2004) claims that a trimmer midsection is related to better health. There is some research that shows that as abdominal obesity (measured by waist circumference) increases, so does the risk for obesity-related comorbidities (including hypertension, dyslipidemia, and the metabolic syndrome; Janssen, Katzmarzyk, & Ross, 2004). However, some of the claims in this book are overblown.

The diet advocated in this book uses a foundation diet of foods that can be remembered by using the acronym Abs Diet Power 12: almonds and other nuts; beans and legumes; spinach and other green vegetables; dairy (fat-free or low-fat milk, yogurt, cheese, and cottage cheese); instant oatmeal (unsweetened, unflavored); eggs; turkey and other lean meats (lean steak, chicken, fish); peanut butter (all-natural, sugar-free); olive oil; whole-grain breads and cereals; extra-protein (whey) powder; raspberries and other berries (Zinczenko, 2004). The book suggests including two or three of these foods in the three major meals of the day and at least one of them in each of three daily snacks. Other foods can also be included, as long as these 12 "power" foods form the foundation of the diet. This is neither a low-carbohydrate nor a low-fat diet, which helps to keep it from being overly restrictive. Quick and easy recipes are provided (also available is a supplemental book providing a more extensive list of meal plans and recipes). Most of the nutritional advice provided is straightforward and accurate. However, there are no phases in this diet program, and the calorie level of around 1,700 calories per day indicates that it would be more appropriate as a maintenance diet. The macronutrient distribution of calories is 30% fat, 25% protein, and 45% carbohydrates (see Figure 2.1). The diet is adequate in micronutrients (see Table 2.4), except that it meets only 45% of the DRI for potassium (although it could be that we just chose lower potassium foods for the 2-day analysis, as many of the "power 12" foods are good sources of potassium). The primary cost of following this diet would be purchasing the foods, which are specific but not overly expensive. The book costs $15.95.

Exercise also plays a major role in the Abs diet regimen. Detailed explanations and pictures are provided to get the reader started on a workout routine that can be performed either at home or at the gym. In summary, this diet book provides a base for healthful eating habits, but it is more appropriate for weight maintenance than for weight reduction. The "power" foods are good foods but have no special characteristics that make them unique or magical.

French Women Don't Get Fat

This book focuses on lifestyle changes and on the autobiography of the author (Guiliano, 2005). She describes her changes in lifestyle (including weight gain) that occurred when she came to the United States for a student exchange program and her subsequent return to a healthier weight, which she had to work to attain by returning to her prior French eating and lifestyle patterns when she returned to her homeland. She includes some sensible recommendations (e.g., eat small meal portions; take time to savor foods; splurge, but in moderation, etc.) that are her own highly idiosyncratic views about diet. The author recognizes that indulgence is sometimes necessary but warns that it should not be frequent. There are entire chapters dedicated to the subject of both bread and chocolate; the ultimate message is that with these food items, focus on quality, not quantity.

Although there is no strict dietary regimen or list of "power foods," there is a recipe for Magical Leek Soup. As a quick jump start for weight loss, the author suggests eating only this vegetable-based broth soup for an entire weekend, then adding in a few foods to the evening meal on Sunday. Quite aside from being unappetizing, such a regimen would be very low in protein, fat, and calories and is probably not safe without doctor and/or dietitian supervision, as it is close to a total fasting diet. (See Figure 2.1 for the macronutrient distribution of this weekend plan.) Going on this crash magic-soup diet is not recommended for more than the 2-day period suggested.

In addition to the magic leek soup recipe, the author provides a sample day's menu for each of the four seasons. It is from these menus that we derived information for our nutrient analysis that found these menus to provide 1,200–1,300 calories per day. The macronutrient calorie distribution is 35% fat, 22% protein, and 43% carbohydrates (see Figure 2.1). The book also contains recipes throughout.

Although formal exercise is not recommended, the author does emphasize being active through daily activities such as walking to the store and taking the stairs. There are no additional costs required for following the instructions set forth in this book other than the cost of the book itself, $22, and the cost of ingredients for preparing the sample recipes.

In summary, although the author encourages lifestyle changes, the lack of strict diet instruction does not allow recommendation of this diet for weight loss.

CONCLUSIONS

Using a system such as the "10-C" method, nutritional adequacy, safety, and efficacy of popular reducing diets can be evaluated and those found wanting separated out. Many of the latest offerings lack one or more of these characteristics. A few popular diets, such as OPTIFAST; some but not all of the phases of the South Beach diet; and the actual regimens but not all of the rhetoric of the Body for Life for Women diet, the Abs diet, and the SlimFast diet contain some good recommendations. However, until further empirical evidence becomes available, we suggest to those who would use popular diets: *"caveat lector*; a page never rejected ink."

REFERENCES

Agatston, A. (2003) *South Beach diet: The delicious, doctor-designed, foolproof plan for fast and healthy weight loss.* New York: Random House.

American Dietetic Association. (1990). Position of the American Dietetic Association: Very-low-calorie weight loss diets. *Journal of the American Dietetic Association, 90*(5), 722–726.

Atkins, R. C. (2003) *Atkins for life: The complete carb program for permanent weight loss and good health.* New York: St. Martin's Press.

Bowman, S., & Spence, J. T. (2001). A comparison of low-carbohydrate vs. high carbohydrate diets: Energy restriction, nutrient quality and correlation to body mass index. *Journal of the American College of Nutrition, 21,* 268–274.

Brownell, K. D., & Wadden, T. A. (1999). *The LEARN Program for weight control.* Philadelphia: University of Pennsylvania School of Medicine.

Calloway, D. H., & Spector, A. (1954). Nitrogen balance as related to caloric and protein intake in active young men. *American Journal of Clinical Nutrition, 2,* 405–411.

Crawford, D., Jeffery, R. W., & French, S. A. (2000). Can anyone successfully control their weight?: Findings of a three-year community-based study of men and women. *International Journal of Obesity and Related Metabolic Disorders, 24*(9), 1107–1110.

Dansinger, M. L., Gleason, J. A., Griffith, J. L., Selker, H. P., & Schaefer, E. J. (2005). Comparison of the Atkins, Ornish, Weight Watchers, and Zone diets for weight loss and heart disease risk reduction: A randomized trial. *Journal of the American Medical Association, 293*(1), 43–53.

Dazzi, A., & Dwyer, J. T. (1984). Nutritional analyses of popular weight reduction diets in books and magazines. *International Journal of Eating Disorders, 3*(2), 61–79.

Duyff, R. (2002). *Complete food and nutrition guide.* New York: Wiley.

Dwyer, J. (1985). Classifying current popular and fad diets. In J. Hirsch & J. Van Itallie (Eds.), *Recent advances in obesity research* (Vol. 4, pp. 176–191). London: Libbey.

Dwyer, J. T. (1980). Sixteen popular diets: Brief nutritional analyses. In A. J. Stunkard (Ed.), *Obesity* (pp. 249–261). Philadelphia: Saunders.

Dwyer, J. T. (1992). Treatment of obesity: Conventional programs and fad diets. In B. M. Bjorntorp & I. Bradford (Eds.), *Obesity* (pp. 662–676). Philadelphia: Lippincott.

Dwyer, J. T., & Lu, D. (1993). Popular diets for weight loss: From nutritionally hazardous to healthful. In A. J. Stunkard & T. A. Wadden (Eds.), *Obesity: Theory and therapy* (2nd ed., pp. 231–251). New York: Raven Press.

Federal Trade Commission. (1999). *Voluntary guidelines for providers of weight loss products or services*. Retrieved November 10, 2005, from *http://www.ftc.gov/bcp/conline/pubs/buspubs/wgtguide.htm*

Garrow, J. S. (1995). Effect of energy imbalance on energy stores and body weight. In K. D. Brown & C. G. Fairborn (Eds.), *Eating disorders and obesity* (pp. 37–43). New York: Guilford Press.

Gopinathan, P. M., Pichan, G., & Sharma, V. M. (1988). Role of dehydration in heat stress-induced variations in mental performance. *Archives of Environmental Health, 43,* 15–17.

Guiliano, M. (2005). *French women don't get fat*. New York: Knopf.

Haslan, D. W., & Jamet, W. P. (2005). Obesity. *Lancet, 366*(9492), 1197–1209.

Heavin, G., & Colman, C. (2003). *Curves*. New York: Berkeley.

Institute of Medicine. (2005). *Dietary reference intakes for water, potassium, sodium, chloride, and sulfate*. Washington, DC: National Academies Press.

Janssen, I., Katzmarzyk, P. T., & Ross, R. (2004). Waist circumference and not body mass index explains obesity-related health risk. *American Journal of Clinical Nutrition, 79*(3), 379–384.

Kirby, J.(2005). *Dieting For dummies* (2nd ed.). New York: Wiley.

Kleiner, S. M. (1999). Water: An essential but overlooked nutrient. *Journal of American Dietetic Association, 99*(2), 200–206.

Knauper, B., Cheema, S., Rabiau, M., & Borten, O. (2005). Self-set dieting rules: Adherence and prediction of weight loss success. *Appetite, 44*(3), 283–288.

Konikoff, R., & Dwyer, J. (2000). Popular diets and other treatments of obesity. In D. H. Lockwood & T. G. Heffner (Eds.), *Handbook of experimental pharmacology* (pp. 195–236). Berlin, Germany: Springer-Verlag.

Kreider, R., Rasmussen, C., Kerksick, C., Campbell, B., Slonaker, B., Baer, J., et al. (2004). Effects of the Curves fitness and weight loss program on weight loss and resting energy expenditure. *Medicine and Science in Sports and Exercise, 36*(5), 80–81.

Marlett, J. A., McBurney, M. I., & Slavin, J. L. (2002). Position of the American Dietetic Association: Health implications of dietary fiber. *Journal of the American Dietetic Association, 102*(7), 993–1000.

McGraw, P. (2004). *The ultimate weight solution food guide*. New York: Pocket Books.

Melanson, K., & Dwyer, J. (2002). Popular diets for treatment of overweight and obesity. In T. A. Wadden & A. J. Stunkard (Eds.), *Handbook of obesity treatment* (pp. 249–282). New York: Guilford Press.

National Task Force on the Prevention and Treatment of Obesity. (1993). Very low-caloric diets. *Journal of the American Medical Association, 270*, 967–974.

OPTIFAST 800 guidelines. (2005). Minneapolis: Novartis Nutrition Corporation.

Peeke, P. (2005). *Body for life for women*. New York: Rodale.

Phillips, B., & D'Orso, M. (1999). *Body for life*. Scranton, PA: HarperCollins.

Roberts, S. (2000). High–glycemic index foods, hunger, and obesity: Is there a connection? *Nutrition Reviews, 58,* 163–169.

Roizen, M. F., & Oz, M. (2005). *You: The owner's manual: An insider's guide to the body that will make you healthier and younger*. New York: HarperCollins.

Rubin, J. S. (2004). *The maker's diet*. Lake Mary, FL: Siloam Press.

Salmon, P. (1994). Nutrition, cognitive performance, and mental fatigue. *Nutrition, 10,* 427–428.

Schoeller, D. A., & Buchholz, A. C. (2005). Energetics of obesity and weight control: Does diet composition matter? *Journal of American Dietetic Association, 105*(5–1), 24–28.

SlimFast. (2005). *The Slim-Fast Diet*. Retrieved July 21, 2005, from *www.slim-fast.com*.

U.S. Department of Health and Human Services and U.S. Department of Agriculture. (2005). *Dietary guidelines for Americans*. Retrieved December 17, 2005, from *http://www.healthierus.gov/dietaryguidelines/*

Van Itallie, T. (1980). Dietary approaches to the treatment of obesity. In A. Stunkard (Ed.), *Obesity* (pp. 249–261). Philadelphia: Saunders.

Willet, W. C., & Leibel, R. L. (2002). Dietary fat is not a major determinant of body fat. *American Journal of Medicine, 113*(9), 47–59.

Wolever, T., Jenkins, D. J. A., Jenkins, A. L., & Josse, R. G. (1991). The glycemic index: Methodology and clinical implications. *American Journal of Clinical Nutrition, 54*, 846–854.

Wolf, A. M., & Colditz, G. A. (1998). Current estimates of the economic cost of obesity in the United States. *Obesity Research, 6*(2), 97–106.

Yang, M. U., Wang, J., Pierson, R. M., & Van Itallie, T. B. (1977). Estimation of weight loss in man: A comparison of methods. *Journal of Applied Physiology, 43*(2), 331–338.

Zinczenko, D. (2004). *The abs diet*. New York: Rodale.

PART II

PARTIALLY ASSISTED (GUIDED) SELF-HELP

Many individuals can benefit from more assistance than is available with self-guided approaches. Partially assisted self-help, or guided self-help, typically offers periodic contacts with a professional, semiprofessional, or even minimally trained assistant. This contact can help to guide the recipient as he or she works on a specific set of problems, often using a structured manual or program.

The chapters in this section address several different problems that can be treated using guided self-help. The initiation and maintenance of physical activity can be effectively facilitated through self-help interventions, as reviewed in Chapter 3. Chapters 4 and 5 review the evidence and strategies used in guided self-help for two debilitating eating disorders, bulimia nervosa and binge-eating disorder. The efficacy of techniques for the treatment of body image disturbances using self-help is reviewed in Chapter 6.

3

Self-Help Strategies for Promoting and Maintaining Physical Activity

BESS H. MARCUS, DAVID M. WILLIAMS,
and JESSICA A. WHITELEY

RELATIONSHIP OF PHYSICAL ACTIVITY TO OBESITY

Several reviews have been conducted examining the relationship between physical activity and body weight. In a review of cross-sectional studies, a consistent inverse relationship between physical activity and body weight has been found wherein those who are more physically active tend to have lower body weights (DiPietro, 1995). This same review concluded the following regarding the impact of physical activity on weight loss: (1) physical activity promotes fat loss while preserving lean body mass, and (2) increasing the frequency and length of exercise sessions increases weight loss. In addition, increasing physical activity plus improving dietary habits seems to be more effective for weight loss than changing diet alone (Brownell & Stunkard, 1980; Wing & Hill, 2001). Lack of physical activity and the resulting lowering of daily expenditure of calories has been cited as the most likely environmental factor contributing to the current obesity epidemic (Hill & Melanson, 1999). The expending of fewer calories in physical activity is likely due to an increased reliance on technology; this has led to decreased energy expenditure at work and in daily living rather than to leisure-time physical activity, which has remained relatively stable (Hill & Melanson, 1999).

DiPietro (1999) conducted a second review of the literature on longitudinal studies to better understand the causal relationships between physical activity and body weight. This review of 11 prospective and 1 cross-sectional study found that regular participation in physical activity was more effective at minimizing age-related weight gain and preventing weight gain than in aiding in significant weight loss (DiPietro, 1999). Moreover, results from several studies suggested that to prevent the weight gain that occurs with aging, individuals may need to engage in increasing amounts of physical activity as they age (DiPietro, 1999).

OTHER HEALTH BENEFITS OF PHYSICAL ACTIVITY

Physical activity has numerous health benefits that have shown to exist independent of improved body mass index. As reported in *Physical Activity and Health: A Report of the Surgeon General* (U.S. Department of Health and Human Services, 1996), the health benefits of physical activity include reducing the risks of dying prematurely (Lee & Skerrett, 2001), of coronary heart disease (Berlin & Colditz, 1990; Paffenbarger, Wing, & Hyde, 1978), of high blood pressure (Paffenbarger, Jung, Leung, & Hyde, 1991; Paffenbarger & Lee, 1997; Reaven, Barrett-Conner, & Edelstein, 1991), of Type 2 diabetes (Helmrich, Ragland, Leung, & Paffenbarger, 1991; Manson et al., 1991), of osteoporosis (Henderson, White, & Eisman, 1998), and of colon cancer (Colditz, Cannuscio, & Frazier, 1997). In addition, there appears to be an independent effect of physical activity on several obesity-related comorbidities, including insulin resistance, hyperglycemia, and dyslipidemia (Grundy et al., 1999). Finally, physical activity appears to attenuate morbidity and mortality risk in overweight and obese individuals (Grundy et al., 1999).

PREVALENCE OF PHYSICAL ACTIVITY

"Physical activity" is defined as "any bodily movement produced by skeletal muscles that results in energy expenditure," whereas "exercise" is planned, structured physical activity (Caspersen, Powell, & Christenson, 1985). One of the larger epidemiological surveys in the United States, the Behavioral Risk Factor Surveillance System (BRFSS), is a state-based, random-digit-dialed telephone survey. Prior to 2001, the BRFSS collected information on physical activity that more closely falls within the definition of exercise, such as jogging, swimming, or aerobic dance (Macera et al., 2005). In 2001, the BRFSS added in measurements to capture moderate-intensity activities such as yard work, housework, and walking for transportation (Macera et al., 2005). Currently, the Centers for Disease Control

(CDC) and the American College of Sports Medicine (ACSM) recommend at least 30 minutes 5 or more days per week of moderate intensity physical activity or at least 20 minutes 3 or more days per week of vigorous intensity activity (ACSM, 2000; Pate et al., 1995). Results from the 2001 BRFSS survey indicated that 48% of men and 43% of women were active at the levels recommended (Macera, 2005). Specifically, 32% of men and women met the recommendations for moderate intensity activity and 29% of men and 20% of women met the recommendations for vigorous-intensity activity (Macera et al., 2005). The Institute of Medicine (IOM, 2002) issued physical activity recommendations for individuals trying to lose weight in which they recommend that adults should attain a total of at least 1 hour of moderately intense physical activity each day. Unfortunately, if many Americans are having difficulties reaching 30 minutes of activity a day, 60 minutes might pose greater adherence challenges. However, increasing physical activity may be the strategy of choice for public health efforts to prevent obesity (Hill & Melanson, 1999) and to prevent weight regain in those who have lost weight (DiPietro, 1999).

For those people attempting to achieve regular physical activity, research has shown that lack of time is the most consistently reported barrier (Andersen & Jakicic, 2003). Thus, self-help approaches to physical activity promotion make more sense than more time-intensive programs that require participants to attend classes or hold frequent appointments with exercise trainers or counselors. A number of researchers have advocated a lifestyle approach to physical activity that involves incorporating physical activity into everyday life (e.g., Dunn et al., 1997). This approach involves the accumulation of 30 minutes per day of moderate-intensity activity. For example, someone might take the dog for a 5-minute walk each morning, take a 15-minute walk each day after lunch with his or her coworkers, and park in a parking spot that requires a 5-minute walk to and from work. Research has shown that people are just as likely to adhere to a lifestyle approach as to stick to a more structured exercise plan (Dunn et al., 1999). However, even using a lifestyle approach, regular physical activity can be difficult to achieve. Self-help programs can help people to establish and maintain regular physical activity habits. In the sections that follow, we discuss the importance of a theoretical basis for self-help programs, describe a self-help program that we have used successfully in our research, and briefly describe some findings from our studies.

A THEORY-BASED SELF-HELP FRAMEWORK

Self-help strategies have the potential to increase physical activity behavior and therefore may be important in the prevention and management of obesity. In this chapter we define "self-help" as programs that promote a physically active lifestyle without the need for face-to-face contact from a health professional. One important dimension of most successful self-help programs is that they have a theoretical basis. This is important for several reasons. First, programs based in theory are more likely to be supported by empirical evidence for the various components of the program rather than including program components that are created because they "seem to make sense." Second, a theoretical framework specifies how program components interact. Individual program components may have previously been shown to be effective on their own, but they may not have been tested together. A theoretical framework helps to establish how these components may operate within the context of a unified physical activity program. For example, use of "fear tactics" to motivate physical activity behavior have been shown to be effective in raising awareness about the negative outcomes of sedentary behavior, but they may undermine a program in which the goal is to promote physical activity, particularly if the program is grounded in social-cognitive theory (SCT) and focused on increasing participants' self-efficacy for exercising (Bandura, 1997). Third, theory-based programs include established assessment procedures that indicate which program components are effective and which are not, allowing researchers to more easily improve on existing programs (Glanz, Rimer, & Lewis, 2002).

Within the field of physical activity promotion, SCT has been the most widely researched framework (Bandura, 1986, 1997). This theory posits that physical activity behavior is influenced by personal factors, such as thoughts, emotions, and physical characteristics, and by environmental factors, such as social contexts and physical settings. According to SCT, physical activity behavior, personal factors, and environmental factors are mutually influential, such that each set of factors influences the other. For example, an overweight man is more likely to exercise (behavioral factor) if he expects to feel better about himself as a result of exercise (personal factor) and if his family encourages him to begin an exercise program (environmental factor). In turn, beginning an exercise program (behavioral factor) will influence his actual and expected feelings about himself (personal factors), as well as his family's attitude toward his beginning the new exercise program (environmental factor). Moreover, his newfound feelings about himself (personal factor) will likely influence his family's supportiveness concerning his continuation of the program (environmental factor), and his family's reaction to his improved feelings or physical changes (environmental factor) will influence the benefits he expects from continuing exercise (personal factor). In this example, illustrated in Figure 3.1, it can be seen that behavioral, personal, and environmental factors are mutually influential.

SCT posits that self-efficacy and outcome expectancies are two of the most important personal factors that influence our behavior and our envi-

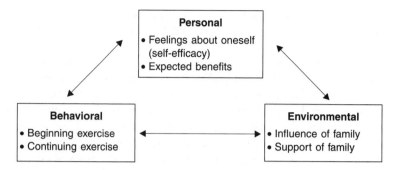

FIGURE 3.1. Examples of the personal, behavioral, and environmental factors that are mutually influential, according to social-cognitive theory.

ronment. *Self-efficacy* is confidence in the ability to carry out the courses of action necessary to produce performance attainments (Bandura, 1997). In the context of physical activity behavior, self-efficacy is not concerned with ability to perform the behavior once. Rather, self-efficacy is part of the process of self-regulation. Self-regulation is the process whereby individuals are able not only to initiate but also to sustain a behavioral change. For example, a woman's confidence in her ability to walk briskly for a single 30-minute session is not likely to predict whether or not she will begin and maintain a regular program of physical activity. However, her confidence that she can carry out a walking program of 30 minutes per day five times per week, despite numerous barriers, such as work and family demands, fatigue, and possible concerns about neighborhood safety, is, according to SCT, likely to predict whether she will begin and maintain the walking program. Numerous studies have shown a strong relationship between self-efficacy and physical activity behavior (for a review, see McAuley & Blissmer, 2000).

Outcome expectancy is another personal factor that may influence physical activity behavior. In the context of physical activity, outcome expectancies refer to the outcomes that one expects will occur as a result of beginning and/or maintaining a program of physical activity. For example, someone might expect that physical activity will lead to positive outcomes such as improved health, appearance, social connections, or weight loss and/or negative outcomes such as sore muscles, sweatiness, and depleted time and financial resources. SCT posits that these expected outcomes affect behavior when they are deemed to be important to the individual. According to SCT, the importance that someone places on each expected outcome is referred to as the outcome value. Decision-making theory (Janis & Mann, 1977) takes this one step further, positing that in deciding whether to adopt a behavior, people weigh the importance of expected positive outcomes of the behavior relative to the expected negative outcomes.

For example, a new parent who expects to lose weight as a result of regular exercise but also thinks that this will not give her enough time to spend with her new child may choose not to exercise if she values spending time with her child more than losing weight. This consideration of the relative importance of positive versus negative expected outcomes is also reflected in the decisional balance construct within the transtheoretical model, which we discuss further later. Although evidence for the impact of outcome expectancy on physical activity behavior has been mixed, some have suggested that we need to assess a broader range of outcomes, including expected affective responses to exercise and expected outcomes of competing sedentary behaviors (Williams, Anderson, & Winett, 2005).

So far we have discussed some personal factors that influence exercise behavior, including self-efficacy and outcome expectancy. According to SCT, a number of environmental factors also influence behavior. *Social support* from family members or friends has been shown to increase the chances of adopting a program of regular exercise (Sallis, Grossman, Pinski, Patterson, & Nader, 1987). Social support may take one of two primary forms. *Instrumental* support occurs when important others do things to help give a person the time and resources to start or continue exercising. For example, someone's friend may agree to pick up his kids after hockey practice so that he can make up for an exercise session that he missed earlier in the week. Social support can also be *emotionally* supportive, such as when someone's spouse encourages her to continue exercising or accompanies her on a brisk walk around the neighborhood.

In addition to social support, SCT also indicates that *physical environmental factors* are important in predicting who will begin a program of physical activity and under what circumstances. Recent research has found that people who live closer to fitness facilities or in neighborhoods that are perceived to be safe and enjoyable to walk in, are more likely to engage in regular physical activity (Owen et al., 2004). Both objectively measured (i.e., proximity of parks) and perceived (i.e., neighborhood safety) environmental factors have been shown to influence physical activity behavior, although there is still debate over which is more important and how strongly these factors influence behavior (Humpel, Owen, & Leslie, 2002).

In addition to having the confidence to adopt a physical activity program, expecting more positive than negative outcomes, and having a supportive social and physical environment, specific behavioral and cognitive skills are necessary to successfully adopt and maintain a program of exercise. The transtheoretical model (TTM) posits 10 behavioral and cognitive *processes of change* that are critical to the successful adoption and maintenance of physical activity. These 10 processes of change were originally developed through examination of the most important change processes across a number of behavior-change theories (Prochaska & DiClemente, 1983), and they have been successfully applied to promoting exercise behavior (Marcus, Rossi, Selby, Niaura, & Abrams, 1992; Marcus & Forsyth, 2003). These processes of change are divided into cognitive and behavioral processes. For a listing of the processes, their definitions, and examples of how these strategies may be utilized, see Table 3.1.

Both cognitive processes and behavioral processes can help people to adopt and maintain a program of physical activity. Using the processes in Table 3.1, "increasing knowledge" may involve reading newspaper or magazine articles about the importance of physical activity in aiding and maintaining weight loss. Someone may use "rewarding yourself" to set up an incentive plan, allowing him- or herself some extra time to watch TV after each physical activity session. Similarly, someone may use "reminding yourself" to put her- or himself in situations that make exercise more likely, such as getting a membership at a health club that is on the route to and from work. Although each of the processes of change can help someone increase their physical activity behavior, it is often difficult to know where to begin. In addition to highlighting important processes of behavior change, the TTM provides stepping-stones to help people to know where they are in the behavior-change process and what strategies are most useful for them at each stage. This concept is commonly known as the "stages of change." There are five "stages of change": (1) *precontemplation,* not thinking about starting exercise; (2) *contemplation,* starting to think about exercise; (3) *preparation,* beginning to engage in exercise, but not regularly; (4) *action,* currently engaging in regular exercise; and (5) *maintenance,* regularly exercising for the past 6 months or more (Marcus, Selby, Niaura, & Rossi, 1992). Questions to determine a person's stage of change, as well as a scoring key for the questions, can be found in Figure 3.2. Although each of the concepts we've discussed is important for promoting exercise behavior, certain strategies and concepts are more important at specific stages. For example, "increasing knowledge" may be more important in the precontemplation stage, whereas "substituting alternatives" may be more important in the preparation or action stages.

In summary, concepts from SCT and the TTM, such as self-efficacy, outcome expectancies, social support, and processes of change, can be used to help people initiate and maintain a program of regular exercise. Some have argued that the TTM's stages of change do not represent a true stage model in that a stage model would necessitate that participants progress through the stages in a linear fashion, which is not always the case with the TTM (Bandura, 1997; Wilson & Schlam, 2004). Nonetheless, intervention research has shown that the TTM can provide a method for understanding where someone is in the change process and what concepts or strategies may be most useful at that time (e.g., Dunn et al., 1997; Marcus, Bock, et al., 1998; Marcus, Emmons, et al., 1998). Taken together, SCT and the TTM provide an excellent self-help framework for physical activity promotion. In the following section we describe exactly how this self-help frame-

TABLE 3.1. Cognitive and Behavioral Processes of Change

Processes of change	Definition	Example
Cognitive processes		
Increasing knowledge	Seeking information about physical activity	Reading fitness magazines, seeking information on the Internet
Being aware of risks	Increasing awareness of the risks of inactivity	Reading brochures from reputable sources, such as the American Heart Association, on the risks of heart disease, diabetes, or osteoporosis
Caring about the consequences to others	Thinking about how inactivity affects those around you	Thinking about how having less energy might lead to less desire to play with children or less time to spend with friends and family
Comprehending benefits	Understanding the personal benefits of being physically active	Creating a list of perceived benefits of physical activity and then prioritizing which may be the most important to you
Increasing healthy opportunities	Increasing awareness of the opportunities to be physically active	Tracking the ways in which time is spent on a typical day, noting times of inactivity and considering these as opportunities for increased physical activity
Behavioral strategies		
Substituting alternatives	Participating in physical activity as a healthy alternative that can improve one's mood better than more sedentary behaviors	Being physically active when tired, stressed, or sad rather then engaging in negative behaviors such as inactivity or overeating
Enlisting social support	Finding someone who is willing to provide support for being active	Asking a coworker to accompany you on a walk, finding a friend or family member who can help with child care
Rewarding yourself	Establishing a reward system for accomplishing physical activity goals	Praising yourself or rewarding yourself by calling a friend you have not spoken to in a while, seeing a movie, or going to a ball game.
Committing yourself	Making promises, plans, and commitments to be active	Planning to walk with a friend, letting others know you have started a physical activity plan
Reminding yourself	Setting up reminders to be active	Keeping walking shoes in the car, putting a gym bag in front of the front door, writing your physical activity plan on the calendar

Note. Adapted from B. H. Marcus and L. H. Forsyth, *Motivating People to Be Physically Active*. © 2003 by Bess H. Marcus and LeighAnn H. Forsyth. Adapted with permission from Human Kinetics (Champaign, IL).

Physical activity or exercise includes activities such as walking briskly, jogging, bicycling, swimming, or any other activity in which the exertion is at least as intense as these activities.

	No	Yes
1. I am currently physically active.	0	1
2. I intend to become more physically active in the next 6 months.	0	1

For activity to be regular, it must add up to a total of 30 minutes or more per day and be done at least 5 days per week. For example, you could take one 30-minute walk or take three 10-minute walks for a daily total of 30 minutes.

	No	Yes
3. I currently engage in regular physical activity.	0	1
4. I have been regularly physically active for the past 6 months.	0	1

Scoring Algorithm

Precontemplation → question 1 = 0 and question 2 = 0
Contemplation → question 1 = 0 and question 2 = 1
Preparation → question 1 = 1 and question 3 = 0
Action → question 1 = 1, question 3 = 1, and question 4 = 0
Maintenance → question 1 = 1, question 3 = 1, and question 4 = 1

FIGURE 3.2. Stage of Change Questionnaire. Adapted from B. H. Marcus and L. H. Forsyth, *Motivating People to Be Physically Active.* © 2003 by Bess H. Marcus and LeighAnn H. Forsyth. Reprinted with permission from Human Kinetics (Champaign, IL).

work can be used to create personalized self-help programs and review some research that has examined the program's efficacy in promoting physical activity.

PUTTING IT ALL TOGETHER: EVIDENCE FOR A THEORY-BASED SELF-HELP PROGRAM

A number of researchers have examined *mediated* interventions for increasing physical activity (Marcus, Owen, et al., 1998). Mediated interventions are delivered through various types of media, such as print, telephone, or the Internet, and thus require little to no face-to-face contact. These interventions typically do not prescribe specific exercises to be done on certain days but, rather, provide a general exercise prescription in terms of volume and intensity and focus on providing motivational messages that help people incorporate physical activity into their daily lives. Therefore, these programs can be considered self-help programs. Although a number of researchers have used mediated programs to help people increase their physical activity (e.g., King, Haskell, Young, Okan, & Stefanik, 1995; Owen, Bauman, Booth, Oldenburg, & Magnus, 1995), we focus here on those programs that follow the theoretical framework outlined earlier in this chapter.

Exercise self-help programs have been created that are *targeted* to particular groups of people. Some programs have been targeted to the individual's stage of change. These programs typically provide print materials that indicate which strategies and techniques, or processes of change, are most important given the individual's particular stage of change (Marshall, Leslie, Bauman, Marcus, & Owen, 2003). For example, for someone in the precontemplation stage, program materials may encourage listing pros and cons of physical activity, whereas someone in the maintenance stage may be encouraged to try various types of physical activity (see Table 3.2). One study showed that motivational-stage-targeted self-help messages were superior to standard self-help materials in promoting physical activity in a workplace setting (e.g., Marcus, Emmons, et al., 1998). These stage-targeted materials have also been shown to increase physical activity when delivered in health care settings and combined with brief physician counseling (Marcus, Goldstein, et al., 1997; Goldstein et al., 1999).

Although stage-targeted interventions can be effective, programs that are *tailored* to a number of individual characteristics are more personalized and thus can be even more effective as the basis for a self-help program. A number of research groups have developed *expert systems*, which provide automated, individualized motivational messages designed to help people begin and maintain exercise programs. These expert systems are built on complex algorithms typically created by a panel of exercise and behavior-change experts and based on both theory and empirical data. For example, Marcus, Bock, and colleagues (1998) designed an exercise-expert-system algorithm in which participants respond to questionnaires that assess their stage of motivational readiness for exercise (i.e., stage of change), self-efficacy, decisional balance, and use of the processes of change; in return they are given a detailed feedback report that reinforces strengths and points out areas for improvement (see Figure 3.2). For example, for a participant who is in the maintenance stage (i.e., who has been regularly active for at least 6 months) and who reports high levels of social support, the feedback report might read:

> "People who are physically active often talk to others and share their experiences about exercise. It's good to know that you have people who are supportive and interested in your active lifestyle. In fact, your responses indicate that you are getting even more support than before. That is great! You have used the support of those around you to maintain your level of physical activity."

This same person may be reporting that he or she does not typically view him- or herself as an "active" person. Although this person is in the maintenance stage and, therefore, has adopted regular activity, this attitude may

TABLE 3.2. Stage-Matched Strategies for Physical Activity Promotion

Stage	Stage goal	Stage-based strategies
Precontemplation	Help to move toward thinking about being physically active.	• List pros (benefits) and cons (barriers) of physical activity. • Encourage seeking information about physical activity (e.g., magazines, the Internet). • Ask someone who is physically active how they were able to become active.
Contemplation	Help to plan how to become active and set a date for starting the activity.	• List pros (benefits) and cons (barriers) of physical activity. • Start to problem-solve solutions for the barriers. • Set a reasonable physical activity goal, such as a 10-minute walk several times per week.
Preparation	Help to develop additional strategies to increase physical activity.	• Identify barriers. • Enlist social support. • Set specific goals for increasing physical activity. • Provide tips for enjoying physical activity.
Action	Help to continue meeting guidelines and determine ways to maintain this level of activity.	• Explore benefits of physical activity not yet realized. • Identify obstacles that might cause relapses. • Discuss negative thoughts that might be getting in the way of being active. Encourage a variety of activities.
Maintenance	Help to consider future obstacles and discuss ways to keep activity enjoyable.	• Work on ways to increase enjoyment. • Encourage a variety of activities. • Seek social support. • Find a race or event in the community to join.

Note. Adapted from B. H. Marcus and L. H. Forsyth, *Motivating People to Be Physically Active.* © 2003 by Bess H. Marcus and LeighAnn H. Forsyth. Adapted with permission from Human Kinetics (Champaign, IL).

put him or her at higher risk for relapse. Therefore, the self-help report might also say:

> "Many individuals who are regularly active view themselves as 'active' people. They think of their activity as part of 'who they are.' You may not be thinking of yourself in this way as much as you have in the past. While you have already been successful in making physical activity a part of your life, thinking of yourself as an active person may help you continue to stay active. Think about how your activity level has changed the way you view yourself."

These examples show how the theory-based self-help materials respond to each participant's stage of change and standing on theoretical constructs. These are just some of the areas that the materials might cover. Therefore, developing these expert-system programs can be resource intensive. However, once the program is developed, it has the potential to reach large numbers of individuals through various media. For example, print-based self-help materials generated through the expert-system approach and combined with stage-targeted manuals have been found to increase physical activity behavior significantly more than do standard self-help materials (Marcus, Bock, et al., 1998). This expert-system approach can also be implemented via telephone. Telephone-assisted programs have the advantage of including a "live" counselor, but their disadvantages include the need to schedule these telephone appointments and the higher cost of the program delivery. However, to the extent that telephone programs are driven by expert-system materials, they may require less training to deliver and thus can be delivered by a broader range of health professionals.

A recent study conducted by Marcus and colleagues (Marcus, Napolitano, et al., 2004) compared individually tailored self-help print materials driven by the expert-system approach with a telephone-based program driven by the same expert-system approach. Thus, although these two programs differed in terms of the mode of delivery (print vs. phone), they were based on identical program content. A third group served as a control group and received non–exercise-related health information. Sedentary participants from the community were randomly assigned to one of the three groups, and their exercise behavior was measured at baseline, 6 months, and 12 months. Results showed significant increases from baseline to 6 months among all three groups; however, the increase among the print and telephone groups (expert-system conditions) was significantly greater than among the control group. At 12 months, the print-condition group continued to increase their physical activity, whereas the telephone-conditioned group leveled off and was not significantly different from the control group. These findings provide further evidence that individually tailored print-based self-help materials can help sedentary individuals become more active. It also provides preliminary evidence that print-based materials may be superior to phone-based programs over time. However, others have used phone-based programs that also include print materials and that are more spontaneous and less driven by the expert system, and they have found significant long-term effects on physical activity behavior (e.g., King et al., 1991).

Yet another medium through which physical activity self-help materials may be delivered is the Internet. As with print materials, the participants can use self-help materials delivered via Internet whenever it is convenient for them. However, unlike print materials, participants in an Internet program can receive individually tailored self-help materials nearly instantaneously after completing the series of questionnaires that drives the expert-system program, whereas participants in a print intervention must wait for printed feedback to be mailed to them. The Internet also has other advantages over print, such as easier storage of previously presented self-help materials and interfaces that allow participants to easily move from one section of the materials to another. Finally, whereas expert-system-driven websites for physical activity interventions can be costly to set up initially, the potential reach is enormous, with little to no incremental cost for each additional user of the program. Indeed, the potential reach of Internet-based individually tailored physical activity programs is limited only by lack of Internet access for certain parts of the population. However, recent surveys reveal that 75% of the population now has Internet access from home and that many who do not have access at home have it at work (Nielsen/NetRatings Enumeration Study, 2004). As with any medium, to maximize behavior change and maintenance, a theoretical framework should drive the development of programs on the Internet. To date, most programs on the Internet are largely informational or do not fully address the theoretical constructs covered in this chapter.

Here we highlight some of the studies that have tested theory-based Internet physical activity promotion programs. Napolitano and colleagues (2003) tested the efficacy of an intervention, which included a website and 12 weekly behaviorally oriented e-mails that contained links to the website, compared with a wait-list control condition among 65 hospital employees. The website was based on SCT and TTM and displayed information and motivational messages targeted to the participant's stage of change. Participants in the Internet intervention group showed significant increases in overall physical activity and walking behavior relative to control participants at 1 month into the intervention. At the completion of the intervention, 3 months after baseline, Internet participants continued to show greater increases in walking behavior than control participants, although differences in overall activity were no longer significant. Although the intervention successfully influenced physical activity behavior change, potential limitations were that few participants visited the website more than once, that most relied heavily on the weekly e-mail tip sheets, and that only a small percentage of employees from the hospital chose to participate (Sciamanna et al., 2002).

Marshall and colleagues (2003) conducted another study that tested a similar theory-based physical activity promotion website and compared it with similar information delivered in print among 665 staff members at an Australian university. As with the Napolitano et al. (2003) study, the website was targeted to stage of change and was combined with email prompts to visit the website. Unlike the Napolitano et al. (2003) study, in this study, the e-mail prompts did not contain detailed behaviorally oriented messages, but only links to the website. In this study, no significant increases were found in physical activity either within groups or between groups. Follow-up analyses revealed that only 46% of the participants in the Internet group visited the site at least once and that only 23% reported seeing all four e-mails that were sent (Leslie, Marshall, Owen, & Bauman, 2005). Although the study did not find significant increases in physical activity and showed a lack of interest in the website, it had a broad reach, enrolling 46% of university staff members who had access to the Internet.

Taken together, these two studies demonstrate that an Internet-based physical activity intervention program that presents theory-based self-help materials can be used to promote initial physical activity change in motivated samples but that lack of interest in the materials may be a problem among larger and more diverse samples. One weakness of both studies was that, although the Web-based intervention was targeted to participants' stage of change, it was not individually tailored. Thus all of the material presented on the website remained unchanged throughout the intervention period.

In an ongoing study, Marcus and colleagues (Marcus & Lewis, 2005) have developed an Internet-based program that delivers individually tailored self-help materials through a website interface. The website content is driven by the same theory-based expert-system approach that was the basis for previously successful print-based physical activity programs (Marcus, Bock, et al., 1998; Marcus et al., 2004). Specifically, participants respond online to a number of theory-based questionnaires and are then given immediate personalized feedback designed to help them to help themselves become more physically active. The website is more dynamic than that used in previous theory-based physical activity Internet studies (e.g., Marshall et al., 2003; Napolitano et al., 2003), with new features added daily, such as a physical activity tip of the day. Although this study is ongoing, preliminary data has shown a significant increase in physical activity among participants in the individually tailored website condition, with mean number of minutes of at least moderate-intensity activity increasing from 20 minutes per week at baseline to 175.74 minutes at month 6 (Marcus, Williams, & Marcus-Blank, 2005).

CONCLUSIONS AND FUTURE DIRECTIONS

Existing research has shown that theory-based mediated approaches delivered through print, phone, or Internet channels can be an effective way to disseminate physical activity promotion self-help materials to large numbers of people (Marcus, Nigg, Riebe, & Forsyth, 2000). These programs are especially beneficial when the self-help messages are individually tailored according to theory-based expert advice (Marcus, Owen, et al., 1998; Marcus et al., 2004). However, many potential avenues of research in this area have yet to be explored. For example, little research has examined whether combinations of message delivery are more effective than a single delivery modality. Perhaps a program that incorporates both print and telephone or Internet and telephone aspects would be even more successful. Internet-based physical activity programs have yet to take full advantage of the capabilities of the Internet, such as use of chat rooms, blogs, and video conferencing. Other technological devices, such as personal data assistants, might be integrated into a tailored physical activity program. New technologies are developing that have the potential to give individualized feedback based on real-time active or sedentary behavior (Intille, 2004).

In addition to further developing the technology of delivery modality, improvements must be made in the content and tailoring of self-help messages. Current theoretical models of behavior change, including SCT and TTM, typically account for only 30% of the variance in behavior change and are even less useful in explaining behavioral maintenance (Baranowski, Anderson, & Carmack, 1998). Therefore, more research is needed to further clarify the variables that cause people to adopt and maintain physical activity and how to incorporate this information into useful behavior-change strategies. It is also critical to understand what personal characteristics and situational circumstances make a person more or less likely to succeed with a given program. Thus uncovering the moderators of treatment success remains an important undertaking.

Finally, a majority of physical activity promotion programs may enroll participants who are already motivated to change their behavior; therefore, much more work needs to be done to reach out to those less motivated individuals who are likely to be the most in need of behavior change. Programs must be designed that can reach even those who are in the precontemplation stage of change, that is, those who are not considering adopting exercise. Moreover, as many individuals are drawn to physical activity programs not only because they are interested in improving their health but also because they want to lose weight, more research is needed on print-, telephone-, and Internet-based approaches to promote healthy eating, along with regular physical activity.

REFERENCES

American College of Sports Medicine. (2000). *ACSM's guidelines for exercise testing and prescription* (6th ed.). Philadelphia: Lippincott Williams & Wilkins.

Andersen, R. E., & Jakicic, J. M. (2003). Physical activity and weight management: Building the case for exercise. *Physician and Sports Medicine, 31*(11), 39–45.

Bandura, A. (1986). *Social foundations of thought and action: A social cognitive theory.* Englewood Cliffs, NJ: Prentice-Hall.

Bandura, A. (1997). *Self-efficacy: The exercise of control.* New York: Freeman.

Baranowski, T., Anderson, C., & Carmack, C. (1998). Mediating variable framework in physical activity interventions: How are we doing? How might we do better? *American Journal of Preventive Medicine, 15,* 266–297.

Berlin, J., & Colditz, G. (1990). A meta-analysis of physical activity in the prevention of coronary heart disease. *American Journal of Epidemiology, 132,* 612–628.

Brownell, K. D., & Stunkard, A. J. (1980). Physical activity in the development and control of obesity. In A. J. Stunkard (Ed.), *Obesity* (pp. 300–324). Philadelphia: Saunders.

Caspersen, C. J., Powell, K. E., & Christenson, G. M. (1985). Physical activity, exercise, and physical fitness: Definitions and distinctions for health-related research. *Public Health Reports, 100,* 126–131.

Colditz, G. A., Cannuscio, C. C., & Frazier, A. L. (1997). Physical activity and reduced risk of colon cancer: Implications for prevention. *Cancer Causes Control, 8,* 649–667.

DiPietro, L. (1995). Physical activity, body weight, and adiposity: An epidemiologic perspective. *Exercise and Sports Science Reviews, 23,* 275–303.

DiPietro, L. (1999). Physical activity in the prevention of obesity: Current evidence and research issues. *Medicine and Science in Sports and Exercise, 31,* S542–S546.

Dunn, A. L., Marcus, B. H., Kampert, J. B., Garcia, M. E., Kohl, H. W., III, & Blair, S. N. (1997). Reduction in cardiovascular disease risk factors: 6-month results from Project Active. *Preventive Medicine, 26,* 883–892.

Dunn, A. L., Marcus, B. H., Kampert, J. B., Garcia, M. E., Kohl, H. W., III, & Blair, S. N. (1999). Project Active: A 24-month randomized trial to compare lifestyle and structured physical activity interventions. *Journal of the American Medical Association, 281,* 327–334.

Glanz, K., Rimer, B. K., & Lewis, F. M. (2002). *Health behavior and education: Theory, research, and practice* (3rd ed.). San Francisco, CA: Jossey-Bass.

Goldstein, M. G., Pinto, B. M., Marcus, B. H., Lynn, H., Jette, A., Rakowski, W., et al. (1999). Physician-based physical activity counseling for middle-aged and older adults: A randomized trial. *Annals of Behavioral Medicine, 21,* 40–47.

Grundy, S. M., Blackburn, G., Higgins, M., Lauer, R., Perri, M. G., & Ryan, D. (1999). Physical activity in the prevention and treatment of obesity and its comorbidities: Round table consensus statement. *Medicine and Science in Sports and Exercise, 31,* S502–S508.

Helmrich, S. P., Ragland, D. R., Leung, R. W., & Paffenbarger, R. S. (1991). Physical activity and reduced occurrence of non-insulin-dependent diabetes mellitus. *New England Journal of Medicine, 325,* 147–152.

Henderson, N. K., White, C. P., & Eisman, J. A. (1998). The role of exercise and fall risk reduction in the prevention of osteoporosis. *Endocrinology and Metabolism Clinics of North America, 27*(2), 369–387.

Hill, J. O., & Melanson, E. L. (1999). Overview of the determinants of overweight and obesity: Current evidence and research issues. *Medicine and Science in Sports and Exercise, 31,* S515–S521.

Humpel, N., Owen, N., & Leslie, E. (2002). Environmental factors associated with adults' participation in physical activity: A review. *American Journal of Preventive Medicine, 22,* 188–199.

Institute of Medicine. (2002). *Dietary reference intakes for energy, carbohydrate, fiber, fat, fatty acids, cholesterol, protein, and amino acids.* Retrieved on November 18, 2005 from *www.iom.edu/report.asp?id=4340*

Intille, S. S. (2004). A new research challenge: Persuasive technology to motivate healthy aging. *IEEE Transactions on Information Technology in Biomedicine, 8,* 235–237.

Janis, I. L., & Mann, L. (1977). *Decision making: A psychological analysis of conflict, choice, and commitment.* New York: Macmillan.

King, A. C., Haskell, W. L., Taylor, C. B., Kraemer, H. C., & DeBusk, R. F. (1991). Group-versus home-based exercise training in healthy older men and women: A community-based clinical trial. *Journal of the American Medical Association, 266,* 1535–1542.

King, A. C., Haskell, W. L., Young, D. R., Oka, R. K., & Stefanick, M. L. (1995). Long-term effects of varying intensities and formats of physical activity on participation rates, fitness, and lipoproteins in men and women aged 50 to 65 years. *Circulation, 91,* 2596–2604.

Lee, I. M., & Skerrett, P. J. (2001). Physical activity and all-cause mortality: What is the dose–response relation? *Medicine and Science in Sports and Exercise, 33,* S459–S471.

Leslie, E., Marshall, A. L., Owen, N., & Bauman, A. (2005). Engagement and retention of participants in a physical activity website. *Preventive Medicine, 40,* 54–59.

Macera, C. A., Ham, S. A., Yore, M. M., Jones, D. A., Ainsworth, B. E., Kimsey, C. D., et al. (2005). Prevalence of physical activity in the United States: Behavioral Risk Factor Surveillance System, 2001. *Prevention and Chronic Disease.* Retrieved November 18, 2005 from *www.cdc.gov/pcd/issues/2005/apr/04_0114.htm*

Manson, J. E., Rimm, E. B., Stampfter, M. J., Colditz, G. A., Willett, W. C., Drolewski, A. S., et al. (1991). Physical activity and incidence of non-insulin-dependen diabetes mellitus. *Lancet, 338,* 774–778.

Marcus, B. H., Bock, B. C., Pinto, B. M., Forsyth, L. H., Roberts, M. B., & Traficante, R. M. (1998). Efficacy of an individualized, motivationally tailored physical activity intervention. *Annals of Behavioral Medicine, 20,* 174–180.

Marcus, B. H., Emmons, K. M., Simkin-Silverman, L. R., Linnan, L. A., Taylor, E. R., Bock, B. C., et al. (1998). Evaluation of motivationally tailored vs. standard self-help physical activity interventions at the workplace. *American Journal of Health Promotion, 12,* 246–253.

Marcus, B. H., & Forsyth, L. A. (2003). *Motivating people to be physically active.* Champaign, IL: Human Kinetics.

Marcus, B. H., Goldstein, M. G., Jette, A., Simkin-Silverman, L., Pinto, B. M., Milan, F., et al. (1997). Training physicians to conduct physical activity counseling. *Preventive Medicine, 26,* 382–388.

Marcus, B. H., & Lewis, B. (2005, April). *Examining the efficacy of a tailored Internet physical activity intervention: Baseline data and preliminary findings.* Paper presented at the meeting of the Society of Behavioral Medicine, Boston.

Marcus, B. H., Napolitano, M., King, A., Albrecht, A., Lewis, B., Parisi, A., et al. (2004, March). *Comparing two innovative channels for physical activity promotion: Project Stride.* Paper presented at the meeting of the Society of Behavioral Medicine, Baltimore.

Marcus, B. H., Nigg, C. R., Riebe, D., & Forsyth, L. H. (2000). Interactive communication strategies: Implications for population-based physical activity promotion. *American Journal of Preventive Medicine, 19*(2), 121–126.

Marcus, B. H., Owen, N., Forsyth, L. H., Cavill, N., & Fridinger, F. (1998). Physical activity interventions using mass media, print media, and information technology. *American Journal of Preventive Medicine, 15,* 362–378.

Marcus, B. H., Rossi, J. S., Selby, V. C., Niaura, R. S., & Abrams, D. B. (1992). The stages and processes of exercise adoption and maintenance in a worksite sample. *Health Psychology, 11,* 386–395.

Marcus, B. H., Selby, V. C., Niaura, R. S., & Rossi, J. S. (1992). Self-efficacy and the stages of exercise behavior change. *Research Quarterly for Exercise and Sport, 63,* 60–66.

Marcus, B. H., Williams, D. M., & Marcus-Blank, B. J. (2005, November). *Using technology to promote physical activity adoption and maintenance.* Paper presented at the New England meeting of the American College of Sports Medicine, Providence, RI.

Marshall, A. L., Leslie, E. R., Bauman, A. E., Marcus, B. H., & Owen, N. (2003). Print versus website physical activity programs: A randomized trial. *American Journal of Preventive Medicine, 25*(2), 88–94.

McAuley, E., & Blissmer, B. (2000). Self-efficacy determinants and consequences of physical activity. *Exercise and Sport Sciences Reviews, 28,* 85–88.

Napolitano, M. A., Fotheringham, M., Tate, D., Sciamanna, C., Leslie, E., Owen, N., et al. (2003). Evaluation of an Internet-based physical activity intervention: A preliminary investigation. *Annals of Behavioral Medicine, 25,* 92–99.

Nielsen//NetRatings Enumeration Study. (2004, February). Retrieved from *www.nielsen-netratings.com/pr/pr_040318.pdf*

Owen, N., Bauman, A., Booth, M., Oldenburg, B., & Magnus, P. (1995). Serial mass-media campaigns to promote physical activity: Reinforcing or redundant? *American Journal of Public Health, 85,* 244–248.

Owen, N., Humpel, N., Leslie, E., Bauman, A., & Sallis, J. F. (2004). Understanding environmental influences on walking: Review and research agenda. *American Journal of Preventive Medicine, 27,* 67–76.

Paffenbarger, R. S., Jr., Jung, D. L., Leung, R. W., & Hyde, R. T. (1991). Physical activity and hypertension: An epidemiological view. *Annals of Medicine, 23,* 319–327.

Paffenbarger, R. S., Jr., & Lee, I. M. (1997). Intensity of physical activity related to incidence of hypertension and all-cause mortality: An epidemiological view. *Blood Pressure Monitoring, 2,* 115–123.

Paffenbarger, R. S., Jr., Wing, A., & Hyde, R. (1978). Physical activity as an index of heart attack risk in college alumni. *American Journal of Epidemiology, 108,* 168–175.

Pate, R. R., Pratt, M., Blair, S. N., Haskell, W. L., Macera, C. A., Bouchard, C., et al. (1995). Physical activity and public health: A recommendation from the Centers for Disease Control and Prevention and the American College of Sports Medicine. *Journal of the American Medical Association, 273,* 402–407.

Prochaska, J. O., & DiClemente, C. C. (1983). The stages and processes of self-change in smoking: Towards an integrative model of change. *Journal of Consulting and Clinical Psychology, 51,* 390–395.

Reaven, P. D., Barrett-Conner, E., & Edelstein, S. (1991). Relation between physical activity and blood pressure in older women. *Circulation, 83,* 559–565.

Sallis, J. F., Grossman, R. M., Pinski, R. B., Patterson, T. L., & Nader, P. R. (1987). The development of scales to measure social support for diet and exercise behaviors. *Preventive Medicine, 16,* 825–836.

Sciamanna, C. N., Lewis, B., Tate, D., Napolitano, M. A., Fotheringham, M., & Marcus, B. H. (2002). User attitudes toward a physical activity promotion website. *Preventive Medicine, 35,* 612–615.

U.S. Department of Health and Human Services, Centers for Disease Control and Prevention, National Center for Chronic Disease Prevention and Health Promotion. (1996). *Physical activity and health: A report of the Surgeon General.* Atlanta, GA: Author.

Williams, D. M., Anderson, E. S., & Winett, R. A. (2005). A review of the outcome expectancy construct in physical activity research. *Annals of Behavioral Medicine 29,* 70–79.

Wilson, G. T., & Schlam, T. R. (2004). The transtheoretical model and motivational interviewing in the treatment of eating and weight disorders. *Clinical Psychology Review, 24*(3), 361–378.

Wing, R. R., & Hill, J. O. (2001). Successful weight loss maintenance. *Annual Review of Nutrition, 21,* 323–341.

4

Guided Self-Help
for Binge-Eating Disorder

CARLOS M. GRILO

This chapter provides an overview of guided self-help (GSH) treatments for binge-eating disorder (BED). To provide the necessary background, we include brief descriptions of BED and an overview of the literature pertaining to traditional therapist-provided treatments for BED. The emerging research literature on GSH is reviewed with a view toward addressing efficacy and effectiveness of such approaches. The findings for guided self-help are briefly contrasted with those for other types of self-help (e.g., pure self-help; PSH) and other therapist-provided psychological therapies. To provide further context and to stimulate future studies, a brief comparison of GSH with the medication treatment literature for BED is offered. Implications of the findings for clinical practice and future research are discussed.

BINGE-EATING DISORDER

BED is an example of an eating disorder not otherwise specified (EDNOS) in the *Diagnostic and Statistical Manual of Mental Disorders* (4th ed., DSM-IV; American Psychiatric Association, 1994) and is also included as a research category in Appendix B, reflecting "criteria sets and axes provided for further study." BED is defined by recurrent binge eating without the inappropriate compensatory weight-control methods that are a defining feature of bulimia nervosa. Binge eating is defined as eating an unusually large quantity of food while experiencing a subjective sense of loss of control.

73

DSM-IV (American Psychiatric Association, 1994) research diagnostic criteria also include several behavioral indicators to help determine loss of control and require that the binge eating is associated with emotional distress, occurs regularly (at least 2 days per week), and is persistent (lasting at least 6 months).

Although debate continues regarding nosology and specifics of the BED diagnosis (Devlin, Goldfein, & Dobrow, 2003; Grilo, 1998; Stunkard & Allison, 2003; Williamson et al., 2002), it is recognized as a prevalent (Striegel-Moore & Franko, 2003) and important clinical problem (Grilo, 1998; Johnson, Spitzer, & Williams, 2001; National Task Force on the Prevention and Treatment of Obesity, 2000; Wilfley, Wilson, & Agras, 2003). Research has generally found that patients with BED often suffer from multiple problems in addition to binge eating—including high levels of eating disorder psychopathology (unhealthy eating patterns, eating concerns, and overvalued ideas regarding weight and shape) and psychological distress (depression and low self-esteem; Allison, Grilo, Masheb, & Stunkard, 2005; Johnson et al., 2001; Grilo, Masheb, & Wilson, 2001a). Research has also documented high rates of psychiatric comorbidity in patients with BED (Grilo, Masheb, & Wilson, 2005; White & Grilo, 2006; Wilfley et al., 2000). BED is associated with obesity; many patients with BED are obese and therefore at increased risk for morbidity and mortality (National Task Force, 2000; Yanovski, 2003). Obese patients with BED have higher rates of psychiatric (Yanovski, Nelson, Dubbert, & Spitzer, 1993) and medical (Johnson et al., 2001) problems than obese persons who do not binge eat. Thus BED signals the need for comprehensive assessment and treatment formulation. Ideally, effective treatments for BED would be able to address the multiple problem areas (Goldfein, Devlin, & Spitzer, 2000).

OVERVIEW OF TREATMENT LITERATURE FOR BED

Recent years have witnessed the development and testing of promising treatments for BED. Cognitive-behavioral therapy (CBT) has demonstrated efficacy for BED in controlled studies using different modes of administration (e.g., Grilo, Masheb, & Wilson, 2005; Wilfley et al., 1993). These controlled trials have reported substantial reductions in binge eating and in most associated problems, except for weight loss, that are significantly superior with groups receiving CBT compared with wait-list controls (Wilfley et al., 1993) and with pharmacotherapy with fluoxetine (Grilo, Masheb, & Wilson, 2005). Moreover, the clinical improvements achieved with CBT are well maintained, at least through 12 months posttreatment (Agras, Telch, Arnow, Eldredge, & Marnell, 1997; Wilfley et al., 2002). Thus CBT is currently regarded as the best established treatment for BED (National Institute for Clinical Excellence [NICE], 2004; Wilson & Shafran, 2005). The association between BED and obesity—and the heightened health risks associated with obesity—highlights the need for treatments that can also reduce weight in these patients. It remains uncertain whether behavioral weight loss (BWL) has efficacy for weight loss in obese patients with BED (Gladis et al., 1998; Goodrick, Poston, Kimball, Reeves, & Foreyt, 1998); this question awaits the completion of two ongoing studies funded by the National Institutes of Health.

Various medications have been tested for BED in randomized placebo-controlled trials. Some (Arnold et al., 2002; Hudson et al., 1998; McElroy et al., 2000, 2003), but not all (e.g., Grilo, Masheb, & Wilson, 2005), controlled trials of antidepressants have reported statistically superior reductions in binge eating and modest or equivocal findings for weight loss relative to controls. Two controlled trials tested antiobesity medications (sibutramine [Appolinario et al., 2003] and d-fenfluramine [Stunkard, Berkowitz, Tanrikut, Reiss, & Young, 1996]), and one trial tested the antiepileptic topiramate (McElroy et al., 2003). Both sibutramine and topiramate resulted in significantly greater reductions in binge eating and weight loss than placebo. Two meta-analyses of the pharmacotherapy literature concluded that limited evidence exists to suggest a clinically significant difference between medication and placebo for either binge eating or weight loss in patients with BED (NICE, 2004; Grilo, 2004).

THE NEED FOR GUIDED
SELF-HELP TREATMENTS FOR BED

The emerging treatment literature for BED, informed by the research literature for both bulimia nervosa (BN) and obesity (Grilo, 1998), has highlighted the utility of certain psychological and cognitive-behavioral treatments and, to a lesser extent, possibly the use of certain pharmacotherapies (Grilo, 2004; NICE, 2004; Wilson & Shafran, 2005). Much of this research has been performed in specialty research clinics. The relevance of such treatments for "real world" clinical settings remains uncertain. First, it is possible that some patients with BED require or respond to less intensive treatments (Wilson, Vitousek, & Loeb, 2000). Second, it is clear that most countries will not have sufficient specialist clinicians or resources to address the full scope of the problem.

It can be argued that pharmacotherapy can probably be reasonably performed in primary care settings by nonspecialists. For example, much of the controlled pharmacotherapy research for obesity has been performed in primary care settings (Davidson et al., 1999; Hauner et al., 2002). A similar argument cannot be made for specialized psychological therapies. Generalist clinicians in busy primary health care settings are unlikely either to receive the necessary training or to have sufficient time with patients to deliver such complex and time-intensive interventions. One obvious potential solution is to develop self-help manuals for patient use based on empirically supported professional therapist manuals and to identify methods by which clinicians can facilitate the use of the manuals. Research has begun to test whether such self-help manuals (primarily CBT-based models) can be effectively delivered. This research, which followed the initial promising results of guided self-help approaches for BN (Grilo, 2000; see also Chapter 5, this volume), has compared different methods of guided self-help for BED in both specialty and generalist clinical settings. A review follows.

GUIDED SELF-HELP TREATMENT STUDIES FOR BED

Peterson and colleagues (Peterson et al., 1998) performed a controlled trial to test the relative efficacy of three methods for administering a specific (Minnesota) form of CBT for BED in a specialty research clinic. Sixty-one women with BED were randomly assigned to one of four 8-week conditions: wait list, therapist-led group CBT, guided-self-help group CBT (CBTgsh), or pure-self-help group CBT (CBTsh). Overall, 84% of randomized patients completed the treatments; completion rates did not differ significantly across conditions and ranged from 73% (CBTsh) to 88% (therapist-led CBT). The three CBT conditions resulted in significantly greater improvements in binge eating than the wait-list condition but did not differ significantly from one another. Peterson and colleagues (2001) evaluated the longer term outcomes of the three methods of delivering CBT. Improvements in various measures of binge-eating and associated symptoms were maintained through the 12-month follow-up, and no significant differences were observed between the treatments at 6- and 12-month follow-ups. At the 12-month follow-up, 17% of the therapist-led CBT group, 46% of the CBTgsh group, and 33% of the CBTsh group reported abstinence from binge eating for the previous week. Diagnostic interviews conducted at the 12-month follow-up revealed that BED was fully absent for 25% of both therapist-led and CBTsh conditions and for 54% of the CBTgsh. This preliminary study suggested that CBT for BED can be effectively delivered (in a specialty clinic) in both guided and pure self-help formats, that the outcomes are comparable to those observed for a professional therapist, and that the outcomes are well maintained for 12 months after treatment.

Loeb and colleagues (Loeb, Wilson, Gilbert, & Labouvie, 2000) performed a randomized controlled trial to test the relative efficacy of CBTgsh and CBTsh for binge-eating problems. Forty women with a range of binge-eating problems (a minimum of once-weekly binge eating; 82.5% met criteria for BED) were randomized to either CBTgsh or CBTsh groups for 12-week treatments that were administered by trained and monitored clinicians at a specialty eating-disorder clinic. Participants were provided with a copy of the

CBT self-help book *Overcoming Binge Eating* (Fairburn, 1995), which is based closely on a specific well-established CBT (Fairburn, Marcus, & Wilson, 1993) for BED. The CBTsh condition involved no further contact until the posttreatment assessment 12 weeks later, although participants were instructed to complete and mail in weekly food and self-monitoring records. The CBTgsh protocol included six brief individual meetings (25 minutes) during the 12-week period. Overall, 67.5% of participants completed the 12-week treatments; the CBTgsh and CBTsh completion rates did not differ significantly (See Sysko & Walsh, Chapter 5, this volume).

Both CBTgsh and CBTsh were associated with significant improvements in binge eating and in associated features of eating disorders and psychological distress; no statistically significant changes in body mass index were observed. Although the CBTgsh and CBTsh differed little on many outcome measures, CBTgsh showed significant superiority over CBTsh for some outcomes (binge frequency, dietary restraint, and interpersonal sensitivity). Participants receiving CBTgsh achieved a 68% reduction in binge-eating frequency, with 50% achieving remission, whereas participants receiving CBTsh reduced their binge eating by 55%, with 30% achieving remission. Participants were followed for 6 months posttreatment, but the low rate of retention (45%), which was biased toward completers, precludes confident analysis. With this important caveat in mind, the authors cautiously noted that for the successfully followed patients, the clinical improvements appeared durable and well maintained at 6 months posttreatment (Fairburn et al., 1993). Collectively, these findings suggest that CBTgsh and CBTsh have utility and are effective methods for delivering CBT at specialized clinics to patients with binge-eating problems.

Palmer and colleagues (Palmer, Birchall, McGrain, & Sullivan, 2002) performed a randomized controlled trial to test the relative efficacy of two methods for delivering CBTgsh (face-to-face vs. telephone guidance) and CBTsh at a specialty clinic. Out of approximately 150 consecutive eligible assessed patients who met criteria for either BED, BN, or subthreshold BN, 121 patients were randomly assigned to one of four treatment conditions: CBTgsh-F (face-to-face therapist contact); CBTgsh-T (telephone contact to provide guidance), CBTsh, or wait list. The treatments were delivered by specialist clinicians over a 16-week period, and participants were reassessed 8 months posttreatment. Participants were provided with a copy of the CBT self-help book *Overcoming Binge Eating* (Fairburn, 1995). The CBTsh condition involved no further contact until the posttreatment assessment 16 weeks later. The two methods for delivering CBTgsh included four brief sessions (30 minutes) during the 16-week period. Following the posttreatment assessment, participants were followed for another 8 months to be reassessed; the majority of participants, however, were offered treatment (full therapy with CBT or interpersonal psychotherapy) based on clinical status (i.e., following a stepped-care model; Wilson et al., 2000).

Palmer et al. (2002) reported that, overall, 75% of participants completed the treatments; the retention rates, which ranged from 81% (wait list) to 78% (CBTsh), did not differ significantly between treatments. Based on findings from the Eating Disorder Examination (Fairburn & Cooper, 1993), overall intent-to-treat findings for "some improvement" were 19% (wait list), 25% (CBTsh), 36% (CBTgsh-T), and 50% (CBTgsh-F). Specific comparisons, or partitioning of the overall findings, revealed that the face-to-face CBTgsh produced a significantly greater proportion of patients who improved than the other conditions, which did not differ significantly from each other. Remission rates, reported only for treatment completers, were as follows: 0% (wait list), 6% (CBTsh), 14% (CBTgsh-T), and 10% (CBTgsh-F). Collectively, these findings suggest that CBTgsh (administered face-to-face) is effective for binge-eating problems, although only a small minority of patients achieved remission. This study did not, however, provide support for CBTsh without guidance, which did not differ from the wait-list condition. Although CBTgsh provided with telephone guidance also did not differ significantly from CBTsh and wait-list conditions, Palmer et al. (2002) noted that the findings, although nonsignificant, show some promise and might suggest using telephone guidance with CBTgsh in instances in which face-to-face contact is not possible.

Grilo and Masheb (2005) performed a randomized controlled trial to test the relative efficacy of CBTgsh and guided self-help behavioral weight loss (BWLgsh) for BED. To control partly for nonspecific influences of attention, this study included a third control (CON) treatment condition that provided the same number of sessions as the CBTgsh and BWLgsh conditions. The CON condition did not provide a treatment manual but required daily self-monitoring (Grilo, Masheb, & Wilson, 2001b, 2001c; Wilson & Vitousek, 1999), as did the other two treatment conditions. Ninety consecutively evaluated patients who met strict DSM-IV (American Psychiatric Association, 1994) research criteria for BED were randomly assigned, using an allocation ratio of 5:5:2, to one of the three treatment conditions for 12 weeks, resulting in the following assignments: CBTgsh (n = 37), BWLgsh (n = 38), and CON (n = 15). This randomization of unequal proportions to the three conditions was used in order to increase efficiency by reducing the number of participants assigned to the control condition (see Woods et al., 1998).

The three 12-week conditions were administered individually by doctoral research clinicians at a specialty clinic following the GSH guidelines of two previous trials with BED (Carter & Fairburn, 1998, described later; Loeb et al., 2000). The CBTgsh therapist manual was adapted from the protocol used previously (Loeb et al., 2000), and a parallel therapist manual was developed for the BWLgsh. The protocol had clinicians focus primarily on maintaining motivation, correcting any misunderstanding of the self-help material, solving difficulties with relevant skill-building exercises, and reinforcing the importance of self-monitoring and record keeping. Participants receiving CBTgsh were provided with a copy of *Overcoming Binge Eating* (Fairburn, 1995), and participants receiving BWLgsh were provided with a copy of the BWL self-help book *The LEARN Program for Weight Management* (Brownell, 2000). This BWL protocol is a widely used manual in obesity treatment studies conducted at university-based clinics (Anderson et al., 1999; Foster et al., 2003) and has also received empirical support as a self-help method for obesity (Womble et al., 2004).

Overall, 78% of participants completed the 12-week treatments. CBTgsh had a significantly higher completion rate (87%) than BWLgsh (66%). The completion rate for CBTgsh is higher than the completion rates reported previously for nonspecialist therapists (76%; Carter & Fairburn, 1998) and specialists (67.5%; Loeb et al., 2000) delivering CBTgsh but is quite similar to the completion rates reported for specialized therapists providing individual CBT (Grilo, Masheb, & Wilson, 2005) and group CBT (Wilfley et al., 1993). The completion rate of 66% for BWLgsh is similar to one specialized group study for obese patients with BED (Devlin et al., 2005) but lower than the 85% rate for group BWL reported in an earlier study for obese patients with binge-eating problems (Goodrick et al., 1998).

Figure 4.1 summarizes the primary treatment outcome findings of "remission" from binge eating, which was defined as zero binge-eating episodes for 28 days. Intent-to-treat using daily self-monitoring assessments revealed the following remission rates: 46% for CBTgsh, 18.4% for BWLgsh, and 13.3% for the control condition. Findings obtained using a second method for assessing binge eating (Eating Disorder Examination—Questionnaire [EDE-Q]; Fairburn & Beglin, 1994) to allow direct comparison with the Carter and Fairburn (1998) study with nonspecialists were: 59.5% for CBTgsh, 23.7% for BWLgsh, and 26.7% for control. Thus these remission rates, based on two assessment methods, are similar to the 50% rate for CBTgsh reported by Carter and Fairburn (1998) for nonspecialist therapists but are slightly lower than those reported for CBT administered by specialized therapists in individual (Grilo, Masheb, & Wilson, 2005) or group (Wilfley et al., 2002) approaches. For context, selected findings for individual CBT are also summarized in Figure 4.1 (right column).

Grilo and Masheb (2005) also reported intent-to-treat analyses for a variety of secondary dimensional outcome variables, revealing that the treatments differed significantly in the frequency of binge eating, in various measures of disordered eating, and in self-esteem; no significant differences were observed for body mass index. Specific pairwise comparisons of the three treatment conditions revealed three significant patterns: CBTgsh was significantly superior to CON, BWLgsh differed little from CON, and CBTgsh was significantly superior to BWLgsh on both measures of binge

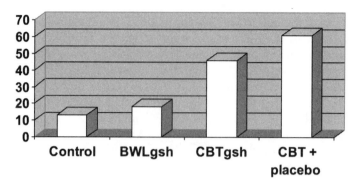

FIGURE 4.1. Comparison of binge-eating remission rates reported in two controlled treatment studies for binge-eating disorder examining cognitive-behavioral therapy (CBT) delivered either through traditional individual sessions (Grilo, Masheb, & Wilson, 2005) or through guided self-help (Grilo & Masheb, 2005). The figure summarizes intent-to-treat (last-observation-carried-forward method) and remission rates (i.e., percentage of participants at the end of treatment who had had no objective bulimic episodes in the preceding 4 weeks) assessed using ongoing daily self-monitoring in both studies. The first three columns summarize findings from Grilo and Masheb (2005) for all partici-pants (*n* = 90) randomized to the treatment conditions: control (*n* = 15), behavioral weight loss—guided self-help (BWLgsh; *n* = 38), and cognitive-behavioral therapy—guided self-help (CBTgsh; *n* = 37). The fourth column summarizes findings from Grilo, Masheb, and Wilson (2005) for participants randomized to CBT plus placebo (*n* = 28).

eating and in reducing hunger, whereas BWLgsh resulted in significantly higher cognitive restraint scores than CBTgsh. In summary, these findings demonstrating the superiority of CBTgsh over BWLgsh—a credible and widely used manualized treatment (Foster et al., 2003) and self-help method (Womble et al., 2004)—and over a second comparison (CON) con-dition (designed to partly control for attention) provide strong support for the specificity of CBTgsh for BED.

CAN GUIDED SELF-HELP CBT FOR BED BE EFFECTIVELY DELIVERED BY NONSPECIALISTS?

Carter and Fairburn (1998) performed a controlled trial to test the effec-tiveness of two methods for administering CBT by nonspecialists ("facilita-tors" without formal clinical training). This study attempted to reproduce some of the conditions that would reflect treatments in primary care or community-based settings without specialists. Seventy-two women with BED (defined using modified criteria of at least once-weekly binge eating over the previous 3 months) were randomly assigned to one of three 12-week conditions (wait list, CBTgsh, or CBTsh) and were followed up for 6 months after treatments. After the 12-week posttreatment assessments, participants (n = 24) from the wait list were then recycled by random allocation to receive either CBTgsh or CBTsh. Thus, with this design, one posttreatment repeated-measures analysis compared the three conditions, and a second repeated-measures analysis compared CBTgsh (n = 34) and CBTsh (n = 35) conditions (with the added recycled patients originally from wait list) at posttreatment and at 3- and 6-month follow-up.

Carter and Fairburn (1998) provided participants with a copy of *Overcoming Binge Eating* (Fairburn, 1995). The CBTsh condition involved no further contact until the posttreatment assessment 12 weeks later. The CBTgsh protocol included six to eight brief individual meetings (25 minutes) during the 12-week period. The therapist manuals provided concrete structure and general guidance about the delivery and pacing of the CBT. Overall, 88% of participants completed treatments; 76% of the participants receiving CBTgsh completed treatments, and all CBTsh were considered completers, as they complied with posttreatment assessments. Both CBTgsh and CBTsh resulted in significantly greater improvements in binge eating and in associated features of eating disorders and psychological functioning than the wait-list condition; no statistically significant changes in body mass index were observed. Overall, in most outcomes, the CBTsh and CBTgsh did not differ significantly from one another, and the improvements were well maintained for 6 months after treatment. Binge-eating remission rates (defined as zero binge episodes for the previous 28 days based on the EDE-Q; Fairburn & Beglin, 1994) were as follows at posttreatment: 8% for wait list, 50% for CBTgsh, and 43% for CBTsh. At the 6-month follow-up, binge remission rates were 50% for CBTgsh and 40% for CBTsh.

The Carter and Fairburn (1998) findings are important in suggesting that both CBTsh and CBTgsh methods are effective for reducing binge eating, even when administered by nonspecialists. Moreover, the findings suggest that the improvements are durable, as they were well maintained at 6 months after treatment. The findings for CBTsh are particularly intriguing because they are especially cost-effective and have potential for secondary prevention, as well as for stepped-care models of treatment (Wilson et al., 2000). However, in contrast to CBTgsh, for which few concerns exist, several issues pertaining to the CBTsh warrant comment and suggest caution in interpreting the outcomes. First, although none of the participants sought additional treatment for their binge eating during the 12-week treatment study, treatment-seeking for weight loss or for other emotional problems, both during and after the 12-week treatment course, was common. Participants receiving CBTsh were much more likely to seek additional forms of treatment than were participants receiving CBTgsh. For example, rates of seeking weight-loss (51%) and psychological (28%) treatments were higher for the CBTsh than for CBTgsh (18% and 14%, respectively). Second, CBTsh appeared less effective than CBTgsh in fostering adherence or compliance with the manual and in addressing dietary restraint. Collectively, this study provides strong support for the effectiveness of CBTgsh and, to a lesser extent, CBTsh, and suggests that it can be delivered by nonspecialists.

Ghaderi and Scott (2003) performed a randomized controlled trial to test the relative efficacy of CBTgsh and CBTsh for diverse binge-eating problems in Sweden. Thirty-one participants with a range of binge-eating problems (BED, BN, and EDNOS) were randomized to either CBTgsh or CBTsh for 16-week treatments that were administered by two specially trained undergraduate psychology students (not therapists). The remaining procedures, including the self-help manuals, essentially followed the Loeb et al. (2000) methodology but used 16 weeks rather than 12 weeks and further broadened the inclusion criteria to include a greater percentage of subthreshold cases of both BN and BED.

In this Swedish study (Ghaderi & Scott, 2003), overall, 58% of participants completed the 16-week treatments; the CBTgsh and CBTsh completion rates did not differ significantly. Intent-to-treat analyses revealed that binge eating was reduced on average by 33% and purging by 17%. Completers had greater improvements in binge eating (58% reduction) and purging (61%). CBTgsh and CBTsh did not differ significantly in outcomes. Six-month follow-up suggested good maintenance.

The findings of the small Ghaderi and Scott (2003) study conducted in Sweden are less impressive (higher attrition and less benefit) than those of the Carter and Fairburn (1998) study in England. The reasons are uncertain. Both studies used nonspecialist nonclinicians (i.e., with no formal clinical credentials) and followed a similar protocol with the same patient self-care manual (Fairburn, 1998). It is possible that the greater diversity of binge-eating participants in the Swedish study (i.e., greater bulimic behaviors) reflects a more difficult patient group than in the Carter and Fairburn (1998) study group. Also, because no details were provided regarding the translation of the Fairburn (1998) manual from English to Swedish, it is not possible to speak to the quality or rigor of the process. Grilo and colleagues (Grilo, Lozano, & Elder, 2005), for example, describe the many complexities that must be overcome in order to produce a conceptually, culturally, and linguistically appropriate translation product. However, although they suggest that CBTsh is comparable to CBTgsh for diverse eating problems, as concluded by Ghaderi and Scott (2003), these findings do raise questions regarding how well nonspecialists can deliver such treatments.

CAN GUIDED SELF-HELP CBT FOR BED BE ENHANCED?

Grilo, Masheb, and Salant (2005) performed a controlled study to test whether adding an obesity medication to CBTgsh facilitates weight loss in patients with BED. This study tested orlistat, a lipase inhibitor, a noncentrally acting FDA-approved obesity medication found to have efficacy for weight loss in obese patients (Davidson et al., 1999). Fifty consecutively evaluated patients who met strict DSM-IV (American Psychiatric Association, 1994) research criteria for BED were randomly assigned to 12-week treatments of either orlistat (120 mg three times daily) plus CBTgsh or placebo plus CBTgsh. The medication was provided in double-blind fashion. The CBTgsh protocol followed the methods of the Grilo and Masheb (2005) study and included giving patients the CBT self-help book *Overcoming Binge Eating* (Fairburn, 1995). Overall, 78% of participants completed the combined treatment conditions without significant differential dropout between orilstat plus CBTgsh (76%) and placebo plus CBTgsh (84%). The double-blind provision of the medication was maintained throughout treatment and was broken after completion of the follow-up assessment, conducted 3 months after discontinuation of the medication and the CBTgsh. During the follow-up assessments, questioning revealed no cases in which orlistat had been restarted (i.e., obtained outside the study protocol) or other treatments had been started.

Figure 4.2 summarizes the Grilo, Masheb, and Salant (2005) findings for two primary treatment outcome variables at three months after completing treatment. The two primary outcomes were "remission" from binge eating (defined as zero binge-eating episodes for 28 days, determined using the Eating Disorder Examination interview [EDE]; Fairburn & Cooper, 1993) and attaining at least a 5% weight loss. A 5% weight loss, although modest, has been found to be associated with improvements in obesity-related medical consequences and has predictive validity for longer term outcomes (Rissanen et al., 2003). Intent-to-treat analyses for all randomized patients using a conservative baseline-carried-forward method were used. At 3 months posttreatment, 52% of participants in both treatment conditions had sustained remissions from binge eating. Participants in the orlistat-plus-CBTgsh group were significantly more likely to achieve a 5% weight loss than participants receiving placebo plus CBTgsh (32% vs. 8%, respectively). These findings provide further support for the robust and durable nature of the clinical improvements associated with CBTgsh and provide preliminary support for the potential benefits of adding orlistat to CBTgsh to facilitate weight loss in obese patients with BED.

CONTEXT

Comparison of CBTgsh and Pharmacotherapy Literatures

To provide a context, this section offers a general comparison of the CBTgsh literature to the pharmacological treatment literature. No studies with BED have directly compared CBTgsh to pharmacotherapy as the case

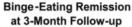

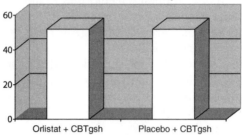

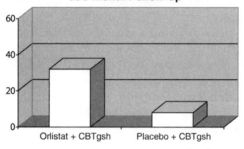

FIGURE 4.2. Summary of a controlled treatment study comparing cognitive-behavioral therapy delivered by guided self-help (CBTgsh) plus either orlistat ($n = 25$) or placebo ($n = 25$) administered in double-blind fashion (Grilo, Masheb, & Salant, 2005). The results shown are for follow-up conducted 3 months posttreatment. The remission rates (left figure) and percentage of patients achieving 5% weight loss from baseline (right figure) shown are for all randomized patients ($n = 50$) in intent-to-treat analyses (using baseline-carried-forward method for missing data). Remission from binge eating is defined as zero binges in preceding month determined using the Eating Disorder Examination (Fairburn & Cooper, 1993) interview.

for BN (e.g., Mitchell et al., 2001; Walsh, Fairburn, Mickley, Sysko, & Parides, 2004), so our comparison cuts across studies and must therefore be viewed cautiously. Overall, treatment completion rates for CBTgsh are comparable to or slightly higher than those reported for some pharmacological trials for BED (e.g., Appolinario et al., 2003; Hudson et al., 1998) but are substantially higher than those reported for most pharmacological trials, despite their shorter durations (Arnold et al., 2002; McElroy et al., 2000; McElroy et al., 2003). The clinical outcomes associated with CBTgsh also compare favorably with those reported in controlled pharmacological trials for BED. Overall, CBTgsh remission rates (requiring 4 weeks of abstinence; e.g., Grilo & Masheb, 2005; Grilo, Masheb, & Salant, 2005) and percentage reductions tend to be higher than those reported for pharmacological studies (Appolinario et al., 2003; Arnold et al., 2002; Hudson et al.,

1998; McElroy et al., 2000), except in one study of topiramate (McElroy et al., 2003). Studies of CBTgsh have suggested that the positive clinical outcomes are well maintained for 3 (Grilo, Masheb, & Salant, 2005) to 12 months (Peterson et al., 2001) after treatment. In contrast, pharmacotherapy studies tend to be of very short duration and fail to provide follow-up data. The few follow-up data available suggest high rates of rapid relapse (Stunkard et al., 1996) and high noncompliance with open-label extended treatments for BED (McElroy et al., 2004).

CBTgsh with Patients with Complex Disorders

The positive findings for CBTgsh for BED cannot be attributed to low severity or to exclusion of patients with poor prognosis due to psychiatric comorbidities. Grilo and colleagues (Grilo & Masheb, 2005; Grilo, Masheb, & Salant, 2005) noted that the characteristics of the patients in the CBTgsh trials were similar to those of patients with BED in recent trials of CBT administered by professional therapists (Grilo et al., 2005; Wilfley et al., 2002). For example, in the Grilo and Masheb (2005) study, 69% of the participants had at least one additional psychiatric disorder (e.g., 46% met criteria for major depressive disorder) and 32% had at least one personality disorder. This rate of major depression disorder is comparable to that of participants in the studies of topiramate (McElroy et al., 2003) and fluoxetine (Arnold et al., 2002), but nearly twice as high as in the studies of sibutramine (Appolinario et al., 2003) and fluvoxamine (Hudson et al., 1998). Thus the participant samples in the CBTgsh studies are complex and are probably reasonably representative of general treatment-seeking patients with BED.

ANOTHER PRESSING CLINICAL NEED

Whereas CBTgsh has clear positive effects on the many of the features associated with BED, it does not produce weight loss. BWLgsh also failed to produce significant weight loss in one study (Grilo & Masheb, 2005). It is possible, but unlikely, that the failure of CBTgsh to produce weight loss is due to the relatively brief duration of the treatments. BWL interventions delivered in typical fashion and over longer periods of time to obese binge eaters also do not necessarily produce weight loss (Goodrick et al., 1998). The few small studies that have directly compared CBT with BWL in obese binge eaters is mixed (Nauta, Hospers, Kok, & Jansen, 2000; Porzelius, Houston, Smith, Arfken, & Fisher, 1995), and reanalyses of obesity studies testing the prognostic significance of binge eating are also mixed (Gladis et al., 1998; Sherwood, Jeffery, & Wing, 1999). Similarly, most medications tested to date for BED have produced limited weight losses (NICE, 2004). Whereas some medication studies have reported statistically significant weight losses, only two have reported potentially clinically meaningful acute weight losses (Appolinario et al., 2003; McElroy et al., 2003). Further research along the lines of Grilo, Masheb, and Salant (2005) testing orlistat plus CBTgsh is needed to determine whether combined or sequential treatment approaches can produce weight loss.

CONCLUSIONS

Although obese persons who binge eat utilize high levels of health care (Johnson et al., 2001), they infrequently receive treatments found to have efficacy in specialized centers (Crow, Peterson, Levine, Thuras, & Mitchell, 2004). There is a gap between the treatment needs and requests for help of obese patients who binge eat and what their primary care clinicians currently offer by way of treatment or referral (Crow et al., 2004).

A recent survey revealed that although obese women were generally satisfied with their general medical care and with their physicians' medical expertise, they were significantly less satisfied with care received for their obesity and with their physicians' knowledge in this specific area (Wadden et al., 2000). Another recent study of 410 consecutive adult patients in two primary care practices found that the vast majority of obese patients wanted substantially more help from their primary care clinicians than they were receiving (Potter, Vu, & Croughan-Minihane, 2001).

The gap between patients' needs and clinicians' services, however, reflects complex factors. Inspection of the findings from the survey conducted by Crow and colleagues (2004) reveals the disconnect between obese patients and clinicians, as well as between basic standards of care versus clinical practice. Body mass index, for example, was rarely or never calculated in roughly 40% of obesity cases. Binge eating received even less attention, with over 40% of clinicians reporting that they never assessed it. Failure to measure a basic physical variable (i.e., BMI to reflect obesity level and health risk) or to identify a behavior (i.e., binge eating to signal risk for greater treatment needs and perhaps specialized treatment) makes it difficult to work effectively with obese patients, either to provide treatment or to offer appropriate referrals. A major challenge confronting health care systems and health research is how to more effectively disseminate information about effective screening and effective interventions.

It does appear, however, that addressing obesity and disordered eating is starting to become an increased priority for general practitioners. Indeed, many of the recent large controlled trials that test the effectiveness of antiobesity medications have been conducted in generalist or primary care settings. Logue and Smucker (2001) have urged family practitioners to change the status quo for obesity-related treatments in primary care. Logue and Smucker (2001) highlight the relevance of evidence-based practice guidelines available from federal sources and urge practitioners to increase their use of psychoeducational materials from reputable sources.

Collectively, these trends highlight the timeliness of research on the "effectiveness" of different forms of treatments in "real world" clinical settings. Although some studies have reported that pure self-help methods of CBT might have utility, careful review of the available evidence suggests an advantage to using some degree of guidance. GSH adaptations of CBT for BED have potential for wider dissemination outside of specialty clinics, but whether such treatments—if suitably adapted—can be effectively delivered in nonspecialist settings remains uncertain. As noted earlier, the study by Carter and Fairburn (1998) reported robust and well-maintained outcomes for CBTgsh administered by nonspecialist clinicians in the community. Replication and extension to general practitioners, however, is needed given the poor findings reported by Ghaderi and Scott (2003) for diverse binge-eating problems and the equivocal research findings regarding CBTgsh for BN. A recent randomized controlled study in England for BN (Durand & King, 2003) found that CBTgsh administered in general practice and CBT administered in specialist eating-disorder clinics both produced substantial improvements that did not differ significantly between settings. In contrast, Walsh and colleagues (2004) reported that CBTgsh appeared ineffective but that pharmacotherapy with fluoxetine was associated with better retention and greater symptomatic improvement than placebo for BN in a general primary care setting. The findings by Walsh and colleagues (2004) for a primary care treatment setting contrast with those reported by Mitchell and colleagues (2001) for a specialized clinic using the same exact design (2-by-2 balanced factorial design testing CBTsh and fluoxetine). The treatment completion rates and clinical outcomes for both CBTsh and fluoxetine were superior in the specialized center (Mitchell et al., 2001) to those in the primary care setting (Walsh et al., 2004). Additionally, in the Mitchell et al. (2001) study, both CBTsh and fluoxetine were found to be effective, and the two treatments had a significant additive effect. Collectively, these mixed findings suggest the need for further research.

ACKNOWLEDGMENT

Preparation of this chapter was supported in part by grant Nos. R01 DK49587 and K24 DK070052 from the National Institutes of Health.

REFERENCES

Agras, W. S., Telch, C. F., Arnow, B., Eldredge, K., & Marnell, M. (1997). One-year follow-up of cognitive-behavioral therapy for obese individuals with binge-eating disorder. *Journal of Consulting and Clinical Psychology, 65*, 343–347.

Allison, K. C., Grilo, C. M., Masheb, R. M., & Stunkard, A. J. (2005). Binge eating disorder and night eating syndrome: A comparative study of disordered eating. *Journal of Consulting and Clinical Psychology, 73*, 1107–1115.

American Psychiatric Association. (1994). *Diagnostic and statistical manual of mental disorders* (4th ed.). Washington, DC: Author.

Appolinario, J. C., Bacaltchuk, J., Sichieri, R., Claudino, A. M., Gody-Matos, A., Morgan, C., et al. (2003). A randomized, double-blind, placebo-controlled study of sibutramine in the treatment of binge-eating disorder. *Archives of General Psychiatry, 60,* 1109–1116.

Arnold, L. M., McElroy, S. L., Hudson, J. I., Welge, J. A., Bennett, A. J., & Keck, P. E. (2002). A placebo-controlled, randomized trial of fluoxetine in the treatment of binge-eating disorder. *Journal of Clinical Psychiatry, 63,* 1028–1033.

Brownell, K. D. (2000). *The LEARN program for weight management 2000.* Dallas, TX: American Health.

Carter, J. C., & Fairburn, C. G. (1998). Cognitive-behavioral self-help for binge-eating disorder: A controlled effectiveness study. *Journal of Consulting and Clinical Psychology, 66,* 616–623.

Crow, S. J., Peterson, C. B., Levine, A. S., Thuras, P., & Mitchell, J. E. (2004). A survey of binge-eating and obesity treatment practices among primary care providers. *International Journal of Eating Disorders, 35,* 348–353.

Davidson, M. H., Hauptman, J., DiGirolamo, M., Foreyt, J. P., Halsted, C. H., Heber, D., et al. (1999). Weight control and risk factor reduction in obese subjects treated for 2 years with orlistat: A randomized controlled trial. *Journal of the American Medical Association, 281,* 235–242.

Devlin, M. J., Goldfein, J. A., & Dobrow, I. (2003). What is this thing called BED? Current status of binge-eating disorder nosology. *International Journal of Eating Disorders, S34,* S2–S18.

Devlin, M. J., Goldfein, J. A., Petkova, E., Jiang, H., Raizman, P. S., Wolk, S., et al. (2005). Cognitive behavioral therapy and fluoxetine as adjuncts to group behavioral therapy for binge-eating disorder. *Obesity Research, 13,* 1077–1088.

Durand, M. A., & King, M. (2003). Specialist treatment versus self-help for bulimia nervosa: A randomized controlled trial in general practice. *British Journal of General Practice, 53,* 371–377.

Fairburn, C. G. (1995). *Overcoming binge eating.* New York: Guilford Press.

Fairburn, C. G., & Beglin, S. J. (1994). Assessment of eating disorders: Interview or self-report questionnaire? *International Journal of Eating Disorders, 16,* 363–370.

Fairburn, C. G., & Cooper, Z. (1993). The Eating Disorder Examination (12th ed.). In C. G. Fairburn & G. T. Wilson (Eds.), *Binge eating: Nature, assessment, and treatment* (pp. 317–360). New York: Guilford Press.

Fairburn, C. G., Marcus, M. D., & Wilson, G. T. (1993). Cognitive behavioral therapy for binge eating and bulimia nervosa: A comprehensive treatment manual. In C. G. Fairburn & G. T. Wilson (Eds.), *Binge eating: Nature, assessment, and treatment* (pp. 361–404). New York: Guilford Press.

Foster, G. D., Wyatt, H. R., Hill, J. O., McGuckin, B. G., Brill, C., Mohammed, B. S., et al. (2003). A randomized trial of a low-carbohydrate diet for obesity. *New England Journal of Medicine, 348,* 2082–2090.

Ghaderi, A., & Scott, B. (2003). Pure and guided self-help for full and sub-threshold bulimia nervosa and binge-eating disorder. *British Journal of Clinical Psychology, 42,* 257–269.

Gladis, M. M., Wadden, T. A., Vogt, R., Foster, G., Kuehl, R. H., & Bartlett, S. J. (1998). Behavioral treatment of obese binge eaters: Do they need different care? *Journal of Psychosomatic Research, 44,* 375–384.

Goldfein, J. A., Devlin, M. J., & Spitzer, R. L. (2000). Cognitive behavioral therapy for the treatment of binge-eating disorder: What constitutes success? *American Journal of Psychiatry, 157,* 1051–1056.

Goodrick, K. G., Poston, W. S. C., Kimball, K. T., Reeves, R. S., & Foreyt, J. P. (1998).

Nondieting versus dieting treatment for overweight binge-eating women. *Journal of Consulting and Clinical Psychology, 66,* 363–368.

Grilo, C. M. (1998). The assessment and treatment of binge-eating disorder. *Journal of Practical Psychiatry and Behavioral Health, 4,* 191–201.

Grilo, C. M. (2000). Self-help and guided self-help treatments for bulimia nervosa and binge-eating disorder. *Journal of Psychiatric Practice, 6,* 18–26.

Grilo, C. M. (2004). *Pharmacotherapy for binge-eating disorder.* Paper presented at the annual meeting of North American Association Study of Obesity, Las Vegas, NV.

Grilo, C. M., Lozano, C., & Elder, K. A. (2005). Interrater and test–retest reliability of the Spanish language version of the Eating Disorder Examination interview: Clinical and research implications. *Journal of Psychiatric Practice, 11,* 231–240.

Grilo, C. M., & Masheb, R. M. (2005). A randomized controlled comparison of guided self-help cognitive behavioral therapy and behavioral weight loss for binge-eating disorder. *Behaviour Research and Therapy, 43,* 1509–1525.

Grilo, C. M., Masheb, R. M., & Salant, S. L. (2005). Cognitive-behavioral therapy, guided self-help and orlistat for the treatment of binge-eating disorder: A randomized, double-blind, placebo-controlled trial. *Biological Psychiatry, 57,* 1193–1201.

Grilo, C. M., Masheb, R. M., & Wilson, G. T. (2001a). Subtyping binge-eating disorder. *Journal of Consulting and Clinical Psychology, 69,* 1066–1072.

Grilo, C. M., Masheb, R. M., & Wilson, G. T. (2001b). A comparison of different methods for assessing the features of eating disorders in patients with binge-eating disorder. *Journal of Consulting and Clinical Psychology, 69,* 317–322.

Grilo, C. M., Masheb, R. M., & Wilson, G. T. (2001c). Different methods for assessing the features of eating disorders in patients with binge-eating disorder: A replication. *Obesity Research, 9,* 418–422.

Grilo, C. M., Masheb, R. M., & Wilson, G. T. (2005). Efficacy of cognitive behavioral therapy and fluoxetine for the treatment of binge-eating disorder: A randomized double-blind placebo-controlled comparison. *Biological Psychiatry, 57,* 301–309.

Hauner, H., Meier, M., Wendlan, G., Kurscheid, T., & Lauterbach, K., for the S.A.T. Group (2002). Weight reduction by sibutramine in obese subjects in primary care medicine: The S.A.T. Study. *Experimental and Clinical Endocrinology and Diabetes, 112,* 201–207.

Hudson, J. I., McElroy, S. L., Raymond, N. C., Crow, S., Keck, P. E., Jr., Carter, W. P., et al. (1998). Fluvoxamine in the treatment of binge-eating disorder: A multicenter placebo-controlled double-blind trial. *American Journal of Psychiatry, 155,* 1756–1762.

Johnson, J. G., Spitzer, R. L., & Williams, J. B. W. (2001). Health problems, impairment and illness associated with bulimia nervosa and binge-eating disorder among primary care and obstetric gynecology patients. *Psychological Medicine, 31,* 1455–1466.

Loeb, K. L., Wilson, G. T., Gilbert, J. S., & Labouvie, E. (2000). Guided and unguided self-help for binge eating. *Behaviour Research and Therapy, 38,* 259–272.

Logue, E. E., & Smucker, W. D. (2001). Obesity management in primary care: Changing the status quo. *Journal of Family Practice, 50,* 520.

McElroy, S. L., Arnold, L. M., Shapira, N. A., Keck, P. E., Rosenthal, N. R., Karim, M. R., et al. (2003). Topiramate in the treatment of binge-eating disorder associated with obesity: A randomized placebo-controlled trial. *American Journal of Psychiatry, 160,* 255–261.

McElroy, S. L., Casuto, L. S., Nelson, E. B., Lake, K. A., Soutullo, C. A., & Keck, P. E. (2000). Placebo-controlled trial of sertraline in the treatment of binge-eating disorder. *American Journal of Psychiatry, 157,* 1004–1006.

McElroy, S. L., Shapiro, N. A., Arnold, L. M., et al. (2004). Topiramate in the long-term treatment of binge-eating disorder associated with obesity. *Journal of Clinical Psychiatry, 65,* 2463–1469.

Mitchell, J. E., Fletcher, L., Hanson, K., Mussell, M. P., Seim, H., Crosby, R., et al. (2001).

The relative efficacy of fluoxetine and manual-based self-help in the treatment of outpatients with bulimia nervosa. *Journal of Clinical Psychopharmacology, 21,* 298–304.

National Institute for Clinical Excellence. (2004). *Eating disorders: Core interventions in the treatment and management of anorexia nervosa, bulimia nervosa, and related eating disorders* (Clinical Guideline No. 9). London: Author.

National Task Force on the Prevention and Treatment of Obesity. (2000). Dieting and the development of eating disorders in overweight and obese adults. *Archives of Internal Medicine, 160,* 2581–2589.

Nauta, H., Hospers, H., Kok, G., & Jansen, A. (2000). A comparison between a cognitive and a behavioral treatment for obese binge eaters and obese non–binge eaters. *Behavior Therapy, 31,* 441–461.

Palmer, R. L., Birchall, H., McGrain, L., & Sullivan, V. (2002). Self-help for bulimic disorders: A randomised controlled trial comparing minimal guidance with face-to-face or telephone guidance. *British Journal of Psychiatry, 181,* 230–235.

Peterson, C. B., Mitchell, J. E., Engbloom, S., Nugent, S., Mussell, M. P., Crow, S. J., et al. (2001). Self-help versus therapist-led group cognitive-behavioral treatment of binge-eating disorder at follow-up. *International Journal of Eating Disorders, 30,* 363–374.

Peterson, C. B., Mitchell, J. E., Engbloom, S., Nugent, S., Mussell, M. P., & Miller, J. P. (1998). Group cognitive-behavioral treatment of binge-eating disorder: A comparison of therapist-led versus self-help formats. *International Journal of Eating Disorders, 24,* 125–136.

Porzelius, L. K., Houston, C., Smith, M., Arfken, C., & Fisher, E. (1995). Comparison of a standard behavioral weight loss treatment and a binge-eating weight-loss treatment. *Behavior Therapy, 26,* 119–134.

Potter, M. B., Vu, J. D., & Croughan-Minihane, M. (2001). Weight management: What patients want from their primary care physicians. *Journal of Family Practice, 50,* 513–518.

Rissanen, A., Lean, M., Rossner, S., Segal, K. R., & Sjastrom, L. (2003). Predictive value of early weight loss in obesity management with orlistat: An evidence-based assessment of prescribing guidelines. *International Journal of Obesity and Related Metabolic Disorders, 27,* 103–109.

Sherwood, N. E., Jeffery, R. W., & Wing, R. R. (1999). Binge status as a predictor of weight loss treatment outcome. *International Journal of Obesity, 23,* 485–493.

Striegel-Moore, R. H., & Franko, D. L. (2003). Epidemiology of binge-eating disorder. *International Journal of Eating Disorders, S34,* S19–S29.

Stunkard, A. J., & Allison, K. C. (2003). Binge-eating disorder: Disorder or marker? *International Journal of Eating Disorders, S34,* S107–S115.

Stunkard, A. J., Berkowitz, R., Tanrikut, C., Reiss, E., & Young, L. (1996). D-fenfluramine treatment of binge-eating disorder. *American Journal of Psychiatry, 153,* 1455–1459.

Wadden, T. A., Anderson, D. A., Foster, G. D., Bennett, A., Steinberg, C., & Sarwer, D. B. (2000). Obese women's perceptions of their physicians' weight management attitudes and practices. *Archives of Family Medicine, 9,* 854–860.

Walsh, B. T., Fairburn, C. G., Mickley, D., Sysko, R., & Parides, M. K. (2004). Treatment of bulimia nervosa in a primary care setting. *American Journal of Psychiatry, 161,* 556–561.

White, M. A., & Grilo, C. M. (2006). Psychiatric comorbidity in binge-eating disorder as a function of smoking history. *Journal of Clinical Psychiatry, 67,* 594–599.

Wilfley, D. E., Agras, W. S., Telch, C. F., Rossiter, E. M., Schneider, J. A., Cole, A. G., et al. (1993). Group cognitive-behavioral therapy and group interpersonal psychotherapy for the nonpurging bulimic individual: A controlled comparison. *Journal of Consulting and Clinical Psychology, 61,* 296–305.

Wilfley, D. E., Friedman, M. A., Dounchis, J. Z., Stein, R. I., Welch, R. R., & Ball, S. A. (2000). Comorbid psychopathology in binge-eating disorder: Relation to eating disorder severity at baseline and following treatment. *Journal of Consulting and Clinical Psychology, 68*, 641–649.

Wilfley, D. E., Welch, R. R., Stein, R. I., Spurrell, E. B., Cohen, L. R., Saelens, B. E., et al. (2002). A randomized comparison of group cognitive-behavioral therapy and group interpersonal psychotherapy for the treatment of overweight individuals with binge-eating disorder. *Archives of General Psychiatry, 59*, 713–721.

Wilfley, D. E., Wilson, G. T., & Agras, W. S. (2003). The clinical significance of binge-eating disorder. *International Journal of Eating Disorders, 34*, S96–S106.

Williamson, D. A., Womble, L. G., Smeets, M. A., Netemeyer, R. G., Thaw, J. M., Kutlesic, V., et al. (2002). Latent structure of eating disorder symptoms: A factor-analytic and taxometric investigation. *American Journal of Psychiatry, 159*, 412–418.

Wilson, G. T., & Shafran, R. (2005). Eating disorders guidelines from NICE. *Lancet, 365*, 79–81.

Wilson, G. T, & Vitousek, K. M. (1999). Self-monitoring in the assessment of eating disorders. *Psychological Assessment, 11*, 480–489.

Wilson, G. T., Vitousek, K. M., & Loeb, K. L. (2000). Stepped-care treatment for eating disorders. *Journal of Consulting and Clinical Psychology, 68*, 564–572.

Womble, L. G., Wadden, T. A., McGuckin, B. G., Sargent, S. L., Rothman, R. A., & Krauthamer-Ewing, E. S. (2004). A randomized controlled trial of a commercial Internet weight-loss program. *Obesity Research, 12*, 1011–1018.

Woods, S. W., Sholomskas, D. E., Shear, M. K., Gorman, J. M., Barlow, D. H., Goddard, A. W., et al. (1998). Efficient allocation of patients to treatment cells in clinical trials with more than two treatment conditions. *American Journal of Psychiatry, 155*, 1446–1448.

Yanovski, S. Z. (2003). Binge eating and obesity in 2003: could treating an eating disorder have a positive effect on the obesity epidemic? *International Journal of Eating Disorders, S34*, S117–S120.

Yanovski, S. Z., Nelson, J. E., Dubbert, B. K., & Spitzer, R. L. (1993). Association of binge-eating disorder and psychiatric comorbidity in obese subjects. *American Journal of Psychiatry, 150*, 1472–1479.

5

Guided Self-Help
for Bulimia Nervosa

ROBYN SYSKO *and* B. TIMOTHY WALSH

Bulimia nervosa (BN) is a serious psychiatric disorder characterized by binge eating and inappropriate compensatory behaviors, which was first clearly described by Russell (1979). Three years after the initial report of this new disorder, Fairburn (1981) published a description of cognitive-behavioral therapy (CBT) for BN. In the past 20 years, the diagnosis of BN, as most recently described in the text revision of the fourth edition of the *Diagnostic and Statistical Manual of Mental Disorders* (DSM-IV-TR; American Psychiatric Association, 2000), and CBT for BN have evolved significantly.

The main components of CBT for BN are: self-monitoring of eating behavior, developing a regular pattern of eating, acquiring skills for coping with high-risk situations for binge eating and compensatory behaviors (e.g., alternative activities, stimulus control, and problem-solving), modifying dieting behaviors and eliminating forbidden foods, and avoiding relapse after the conclusion of acute treatment (Fairburn, Marcus, & Wilson, 1993). The model underlying CBT for BN emphasizes the critical role of both cognitive and behavioral factors in maintaining bulimic symptoms. The overvaluation of body weight and shape is presumed to produce rigid dietary restriction that, in turn, leads to a psychological and physiological vulnerability to binge-eating episodes. When patients attempt to counteract the effects of binge eating, such as by self-induced vomiting or by the use of other inappropriate compensatory behaviors (e.g., laxative or diuretic abuse), the compensatory behavior is reinforced, as it reduces anxiety about weight gain and disrupts the development of satiety. The pattern of binge eating and compensation causes distress and low self-esteem, which reinforce circumstances that will lead to continued dietary restraint and binge eating (Fairburn, 1997).

CBT is the most studied psychological treatment for BN (Wilson & Fairburn, 2002), and an extensive review of the published studies of CBT by the National Institute of Clinical Excellence (NICE) in the United Kingdom found CBT to be the treatment of choice for BN (Wilson & Shafran, 2005). Between 30 and 50% of patients treated with CBT experience a remission of binge eating and purging symptoms, and binge-eating and purging behaviors are reduced by approximately 80% (Wilson & Fairburn, 2002). Long-term follow-up data suggest that changes in binge eating and purging are well maintained by patients with BN treated with CBT at 1, 6, and even 11 years after the end of treatment (Wilson & Fairburn, 2002).

An enhanced manual-based form of CBT for BN (CBT-E) has recently been described (Fairburn, Cooper, & Shafran, 2003), with a flexible treatment including different treatment modules matched to specific problems maintaining the eating disorder. Clinical trials utilizing CBT-E to treat individuals with eating disorders are ongoing in the United Kingdom, and although the results have not yet been published, initial reports of CBT-E's efficacy have been positive (Fairburn, 2004).

Despite the effectiveness of CBT in the treatment of BN, a number of factors limit the availability of this form of treatment, including the amount of time needed to administer CBT, the difficulties of training and supervising therapists to administer CBT, and a shortage of CBT therapists. If it is to be delivered according the original description (Fairburn et al., 1993), CBT requires twenty 50-minute individual treatment sessions over 4–5 months. In the current health care system in the United States, even patients who have insurance coverage may not be reimbursed for 20 sessions of therapy, and the cost can be prohibitive for patients without insurance. Subsequently, access to CBT in the United States, especially among those with restricted financial means, is quite limited.

Ideally, prior to providing CBT for BN, mental health professionals should obtain specialized training, which may include classes, seminars, or workshops in social learning and behavioral principles, as well as listening to therapy tapes of CBT sessions conducted by a trained therapist. For therapists who have already completed training for an advanced degree (e.g., MSW, PhD, MD) and who are interested in pursuing CBT training, it can be problematic to find time to devote to supervised training in CBT, even if an experienced and available supervisor can be identified. Because of these constraints on training therapists, there is a shortage of qualified CBT therapists, and it seems unlikely that an adequate number of professionals will be available in the foreseeable future.

Thus, although CBT is an efficacious treatment for BN, there are significant barriers to making CBT available to all patients who might benefit from receiving it. Therefore, self-help programs outlining CBT techniques have been developed to disseminate this form of treatment more widely. These programs, which are typically presented in book form, are designed to provide information about eating disorders for patients with BN and also to allow patients to complete cognitive and behavioral exercises to address binge-eating and purging behaviors. In some implementations, a limited number of therapy visits are added to the bibliotherapy; such programs have been called "guided self-help."

Most of the empirical studies of self-help treatments for BN have focused on three programs: *Getting Better Bit(e) by Bit(e)* by Ulrike Schmidt and Janet Treasure (1993); *Bulimia Nervosa and Binge-Eating: A Guide to Recovery* by Peter J. Cooper (Cooper, 1993, 1995), and *Overcoming Binge Eating* by Christopher Fairburn (Fairburn, 1995). In the remainder of this chapter, we describe these three self-help programs, present the data regarding their efficacy, and summarize the current evidence concerning the utility of self-help or guided self-help interventions for patients with BN. In addition, we discuss some practical and clinical considerations, including the sequencing of treatments, and information about the circumstances in which such programs appear to be most useful.

GETTING BETTER BIT(E) BY BIT(E)

Getting Better Bit(e) by Bit(e) (Schmidt & Treasure, 1993) was the first cognitive-behavioral self-help treatment manual to be published. The book consists of fifteen chapters presenting a combination of psychoeducational information and treatment strategies. The chapters are as follows.

Chapter 1. The Way Forward

The first chapter allows the reader to assess the severity of bulimic symptoms using the Bulimic Investigatory Test (BITE; Henderson & Freeman, 1987). Subsequently, the reader evaluates his or her reasons for ceasing binge eating and purging and the potential disadvantages of change. The reader also completes an exercise imagining what life would be like 5 years in the future if the eating disorder is not overcome, which helps to further assess and generate reasons for change.

Chapter 2. Tools for the Journey

The second chapter introduces the "therapeutic diary" for monitoring the antecedents (triggers), behavior, and consequences associated with binge eating and purging. The reader is introduced to problem solving as a coping skill. Problem solving includes these seven steps: (1) defining the problem, (2) identifying all of the possible solutions, (3) examining all the options in detail (e.g., pros and cons of all the options), (4) choosing a solution that feels most appropriate, (5) determining how to put the solution into practice, (6) carrying out the solution, and (7) evaluating the final outcome. At the end of the chapter, the reader is provided with an example of problem solving to illustrate the way in which to use the skill.

Chapter 3. Dieting: A Health Warning

The third chapter focuses on weight and dieting. The book provides a chart of healthy weights, weight fluctuations, the health hazards of dieting, and the effects of starvation on the body and mind. Schmidt and Treasure (1993) recommend that readers eat the majority of their food before the evening, eat small amounts regularly throughout the day, exercise regularly but not excessively, restrict the consumption of fat while consuming appropriate amounts of protein and carbohydrates, and avoid multiple courses at meals.

Chapter 4. Bingeing, Nibbling, and Compulsive Overeating: The Black Hole of the Never-Satisfied Stomach

Chapter 4 provides information about binge eating, including the reasons people may experience uncontrolled episodes of eating (e.g., physiological effects of starvation, emotional antecedents of depression, boredom, or stress). The second portion of the chapter focuses on stopping binge-eating episodes. The remainder of the chapter addresses whether binge eating is a sugar addiction, the psychological aspects of binge eating, and coping with lapses while using the program.

Chapter 5. Vomiting, Laxatives, and Diuretics: Have Your Cake and Eat It—or Not?

This chapter emphasizes that vomiting, laxatives, and diuretics are not effective methods of controlling weight and that these behaviors can have very serious physical consequences. Plans for stopping vomiting and the abuse of laxatives, diuretics, and other medications are described, as are the possible consequences of cutting back or stopping these behaviors.

Chapter 6. Learning to Feel Good about Your Body

Chapter 6 focuses on the extreme dissatisfaction with body shape and weight often reported by individuals with BN. Interventions to increase acceptance of body size include learning about different body shapes (e.g., looking at ideals for body shape in different centuries), becoming familiar with one's own body, tackling difficult situations involving body shape or weight, and taking care of one's body. One specific strategy described in the chapter is progressive muscle relaxation, which is offered as one option for self-care.

Chapter 7. Jack Spratt's Wife: Being Fatter May Be Better

Chapter 7 is especially intended for readers who are overweight or obese. The health risks of being overweight are discussed, and the reader is reminded of the relationship between dieting and binge eating (first described in Chapter 3). Readers are encouraged to exercise and are given strategies for overcoming obstacles to getting started with exercise. Information about incorporating exercise as a lifestyle change (e.g., using the stairs) and exercises that can be done at home is also provided.

Chapter 8. Relapse: Walking in Circles—or Not

This chapter suggests that the reader plan a time to binge eat (e.g., a planned relapse) in order to avoid concerns about when the relapse might occur in the future. Strategies are described to help readers cope with slips, learn from slips, and try to find more balance between their needs and the needs of other people.

Chapter 9. The Wounds of Childhood

Chapter 9 addresses the potential consequences of childhood physical or sexual abuse. Information is provided about what constitutes sexual abuse, understanding why the abuse occurred, feelings that might be associated with past abuse (e.g., anger, guilt, self-blame), and coming to terms with the abuse.

Chapter 10. Food for Thought

This chapter describes different types of self-defeating and automatic thoughts (e.g., perfectionism, need for control, guilt) that are common among individuals with eating disorders. The chapter describes how to counter these thinking errors by examining the evidence for and against the thought and trying to evaluate the thought from another perspective.

Chapter 11. Finding Your Voice

This chapter helps readers to become more assertive, to learn methods for expressing needs and feelings in an appropriate and nonaggressive way, and to begin using assertiveness skills in everyday life.

Chapter 12. The Seduction of Self-Destruction

Chapter 12 is focused on problems that often co-occur among individuals with eating disorders (e.g., alcohol and drug abuse, overuse of caffeine and artificial sweeteners, shoplifting, and overspending). Readers can assess whether their current alcohol consumption is problematic and learn about strategies for moderating drinking.

Chapter 13. The Web of Life: Parents, Partners, Children, and Friends

Chapter 13 focuses on improving interpersonal relationships, such as relationships with parents or friends, that may have been affected by the reader's eating disorder. Sexual relationships are also discussed, as individuals with a history of sexual abuse, problematic relationships, or concerns about body shape and weight may have difficulty with sexual intimacy. Finally, issues relating to fertility, pregnancy, and parenting are addressed.

Chapter 14. Working to Live, Living to Work

This chapter focuses on common problems that individuals with eating disorders might experience with work: not having a job, not being in the right job, and working too much. The reader is encouraged to evaluate the pros and cons of his or her current job to determine whether changes need to be made to his or her employment situation.

Chapter 15. Is This the End of the Journey—or Not?

In the final chapter, Schmidt and Treasure (1993) ask the reader to evaluate their progress in changing bulimic symptoms by following the self-help program and determine why changes may not have occurred.

The program presented in *Getting Better Bit(e) by Bit(e)* (Schmidt & Treasure, 1993) was developed for patients with BN at the Maudsley Hospital in London to condense the information provided in traditional CBT for BN. Schmidt and Treasure (1993) indicate that the program should be completed in about 3 months but are explicit that the manual is not designed as a cure for BN. The first six chapters of *Getting Better Bit(e) by Bit(e)* (Schmidt & Treasure, 1993) are intended to be read together, although they do not need to be read in order. Chapters 8–15 are read subsequent to Chapters 1–6, unless the patient has a problem with alcohol, in which case Chapter 12 ("The Seduction of Self-Destruction") should be read early in the program.

A companion volume (*A Clinician's Guide to* Getting Better Bit(e) by Bit(e): *A survival kit for sufferers of bulimia nervosa and binge eating disorder*; Schmidt & Treasure, 1997) was published to address issues of compliance among patients who were using the self-help program. The authors determined that only 60% of patients who received the book read more than half of its contents; therefore, Schmidt and Treasure (1997) developed the *Clinician's Guide* to focus on motivation, stages of change (Prochaska & DiClemente, 1986), and motivational enhancement therapy strategies (Miller & Rollnick, 1991). Eight possible therapy sessions are outlined in the *Clinician's Guide*, and the sessions are designed to move BN patients from a state of ambivalence about making changes to a commitment to change behavior. Two case studies are provided to help illustrate the use of the motivational enhancement therapy in combination with *Getting Better Bit(e) by Bit(e)* (Schmidt & Treasure, 1993).

Getting Better Bit(e) by Bit(e) (Schmidt & Treasure, 1993) has a number of unique features, in comparison with the other self-help manuals described later. The specific interventions designed to increase body acceptance (Chapter 6), the planned relapse (Chapter 8), the explicit approach to a history of childhood sexual abuse (Chapter 9), the encouragement to increase assertiveness (Chapter 11), and the discussion of balancing work and self-care (Chapter 14) are distinctive among the self-help manuals designed to treat binge eating. The manual (Schmidt & Treasure, 1993) is available in paperback but may be difficult to find; it continues to be carried by online bookstores in the United Kingdom (e.g., *www.amazon.co.uk*). The clinician's manual (*A Clinician's Guide to* Getting Better Bit(e) by Bit(e): *A survival kit for sufferers of bulimia nervosa and binge eating disorder*; Schmidt & Treasure, 1997), which includes the full text of the book, is easier to obtain.

Empirical Studies of *Getting Better Bit(e) by Bit(e)*

Five studies have evaluated the efficacy of *Getting Better Bit(e) by Bit(e)* (Schmidt & Treasure, 1993) for the treatment of BN. The first study, an evaluation of pure self-help conducted by Schmidt, Tiller, and Treasure (1993), enrolled 28 women who met the International Classification of Diseases Version 10 (ICD-10) criteria for either BN or atypical BN. The patients worked through a handbook that emphasized CBT techniques, which would later be published as *Getting Better Bit(e) by Bit(e)* (Schmidt & Treasure, 1993), for 4–6 weeks before their next assessment. Twenty-six (92.9%) patients completed the study, and, at the second assessment, 12 of the 26 completers (46.2%) were considered very much or much improved, 8 (30.8%) were somewhat improved, and 6 (23.1%) were unchanged. Fifteen patients (57.7% of completers) were abstaining from vomiting and laxative abuse at the end of treatment; however 5 patients had been abstaining from these behaviors prior to the initiation of treatment. This study indicated that the use of *Getting Better Bit(e) by Bit(e)* (Schmidt & Treasure, 1993) in a pure self-help format was associated with a significant reduction in bulimic symptoms. However, there was no control for the effect of time alone.

Treasure et al. (1996) described the results of a study of sequential treatment for BN, specifically, self-help followed by CBT. An earlier report (Treasure et al., 1994) presented the outcome from the first 8 weeks of the trial, with 81 patients randomized either to receive pure self-help using *Getting Better Bit(e) by Bit(e)* (Schmidt & Treasure, 1993), to receive cognitive-behavioral therapy, or to a wait list. The later report (Treasure et al., 1996) presented data from the full 16-week trial, in which 110 women who met ICD-10 criteria for BN or atypical BN received either CBT (n = 55) or 8 weeks of self-help followed by 8 weeks of CBT for inadequate responders (sequential treatment; n = 55). Of the original 55 patients assigned to sequential treatment, 25 of 41 (60.98%) patients who were assessed after 8 weeks of initial treatment with the manual had not improved sufficiently and were eligible to receive the eight sessions of CBT. Patients assigned to receive CBT without use of the manual either began CBT soon after randomization (n = 28) or following an 8-week waiting period (n = 27); patients who were assigned to the waiting list were subsequently provided with 16 sessions of CBT. As there were multiple phases of the treatment and different numbers of patients at each time point, the findings of the Treasure et al. (1996) study are difficult to summarize. Median scores for overall bulimic symptoms, as assessed by a clinician-administered interview, decreased in both the sequential-treatment and CBT groups. At the end of treatment, abstinence rates for binge eating and vomiting were 30% for the sequential-treatment group and 30% for the CBT group; however, these rates were not calculated on an intent-to-treat basis. Thus the improvements in bulimic symptoms observed at the end of treatment were similar for the sequential-treatment and CBT groups.

Thiels, Schmidt, Treasure, Garthe, and Troop (1998) conducted a study in which 62 patients who met DSM-III-R (American Psychiatric Association, 1987) criteria for BN received either "guided self-change" using *Getting Better Bit(e) by Bit(e)* (Schmidt & Treasure, 1993) and eight sessions of CBT (n = 31) delivered every other week or 16 weekly sessions of CBT (n = 31). Vomiting decreased from an average of 3.65 episodes per 28 days to 2.57 episodes per 28 days in the guided-self-change group and from an average of 3.79 episodes per 28 days to 2.06 episodes per 28 days in the CBT group (p = 0.77). At the end of treatment assessment, 12.9% of the guided-self-change group and 54.8% of the CBT group were abstinent from binge eating and vomiting, $\chi^2(1)$ = 12.17, p < 0.001. Similar improvements were observed in vomiting for both the guided-self-change and CBT conditions, but the proportion of patients who were abstinent from binge eating and vomiting was greater in the CBT group.

Bell and Newns (2002) investigated whether *Getting Better Bit(e) by Bit(e)* (Schmidt & Treasure, 1993) could be used with patients diagnosed with BN who were "multi-impulsive." Multi-impulsive patients were those who reported both bulimic symptoms and at least one of the following: abuse of alcohol or "street drugs," multiple overdoses, repeated self-harm,

sexual disinhibition, or shoplifting (Bell & Newns, 2002). The study included 46 patients who were binge eating and purging at least twice per
week, 11 of whom were multi-impulsive and 35 who were not. Thirty
patients (65.2%) completed the study. Symptom scores on the BITE (Henderson & Freeman, 1987) decreased from 24.59 to 15.33 among multi-
impulsive BN patients and from 22.91 to 8.35 among nonimpulsive BN
patients. Thus patients with and without multi-impulsivity reported improvements in BITE symptom and severity scales after receiving a guided-
self-help intervention utilizing *Getting Better Bit(e) by Bit(e)*.

The most recent evaluation of *Getting Better Bit(e) by Bit(e)* (Schmidt &
Treasure, 1993) is a study by Bailer et al. (2004). Eighty-one patients with BN
were randomized to receive either guided self-help with *Getting Better Bit(e)
by Bit(e)* (*n* = 40) or group CBT (*n* = 41). A total of 56 patients (69.1%) completed the study, 30 (75%) patients in the GSH condition and 26 (63.4%) patients in the group-CBT condition. At the end of treatment, 7.5% of patients
in the GSH condition and 12.2% in the group-CBT condition had abstained
from binge eating or purging in the previous month, and 40% of the patients
in the GSH condition and 29.3% in the group-CBT condition no longer met
DSM-IV criteria for BN. The proportion of patients who were abstinent from
bulimic symptoms or who no longer met DSM-IV BN criteria was not different between the guided-self-help and CBT groups.

Summary of Empirical Studies of *Getting Better Bit(e) by Bit(e)*

All five studies that evaluated *Getting Better Bit(e) by Bit(e)* (Schmidt & Treasure, 1993) found improvements in binge eating and vomiting subsequent to
an intervention with the manual. However, it is difficult to summarize the
findings across studies and draw conclusions about the efficacy of the manual. The studies utilized different implementations of the manual (pure self-
help, guided self-help, self-help followed by CBT, or self-help combined with
CBT), and different types of study designs (uncontrolled vs. controlled trials),
different comparison groups (no comparison, wait-list, individual CBT,
group CBT), and the range of abstinence rates from bulimic symptoms was
large (7.5%–57.7% for self-help and 12.2%–54.8% for the comparison
CBT). Thus use of the manual is associated with a reduction in binge eating
and purging and abstinence from bulimic symptoms for at least some patients; however, the amount of improvement a clinician should expect when
using *Getting Better Bit(e) by Bit(e)* (Schmidt & Treasure, 1993) is not clear.

BULIMIA NERVOSA: A GUIDE TO RECOVERY

Bulimia Nervosa: A Guide to Recovery (Cooper, 1993) describes a cognitive-
behavioral program for BN. The second edition of the book, titled *Bulimia*

Nervosa and Binge Eating: A Guide to Recovery (Cooper, 1995) is described here. The book is divided into two parts, with the first part providing psychoeducational material and the second section describing the self-help treatment program. The first section comprises the following chapters.

Chapter 1. What Are Binge-Eating and Bulimia Nervosa?

This chapter addresses the definitions of binge eating (e.g., the experience of binge eating, how much food constitutes a binge episode, triggers for binge eating), methods of compensation, and attitudes about shape and weight.

Chapter 2. How Binge-Eating and Bulimia Nervosa Affect People's Lives

Chapter 2 provides information about the effects of binge eating on mood states such as depression, anger, and anxiety and on the social lives of those with binge-eating problems.

Chapter 3. The Physical Complications

The third chapter briefly describes the physical effects of binge eating and of common methods of compensation.

Chapter 4. What Causes Binge-Eating and Bulimia Nervosa?

Chapter 4 describes predisposing factors that make individuals vulnerable to binge eating, such as physical factors (e.g., genetics, depression, body weight), psychological factors (e.g., anorexia nervosa, low self-esteem, sexual abuse, perfectionism, problems with alcohol), and social factors (e.g., gender, culture, families). Precipitating factors, or factors that bring on bulimic symptoms, are also discussed, including physical factors (e.g., weight loss from physical illness), psychological and behavioral factors (e.g., dieting), and social factors (e.g., being told one is fat). Finally, the factors that maintain binge eating are described, along with the CBT model.

Chapter 5. How Can Binge-Eating and Bulimia Nervosa Be Treated?

The fifth chapter focuses on treatments designed to address binge eating and reviews evidence for antidepressant medications, cognitive-behavior therapy, and other forms of psychotherapy. A stepped-care approach to the treatment of BN using a self-help manual is also proposed.

Chapter 6. A Short Technical Note

This chapter describes the defining features of eating disorders, the criteria that define the diagnosis, the prevalence of BN, and how BN relates to other disorders, including binge-eating disorder (BED).

The Treatment Program

The treatment program is described in the second part of *Bulimia Nervosa and Binge Eating: A Guide to Recovery* (Cooper, 1995). The intervention is divided into six steps, which include the major concepts from CBT for BN (Fairburn et al., 1993). The steps are designed to be followed in order from 1 to 6, and the reader is asked to complete a review at each step in the process. A flowchart of the major interventions in each step is provided in the introduction. Cooper (1995) indicates that the manual is designed for the treatment of "classic" BN and that, for individuals experiencing difficulties with binge-eating disorder, *Overcoming Binge Eating* (Fairburn, 1995) may be a better treatment option (see Chapter 4, this volume). The steps of the intervention are as follows.

Introduction

The introduction describes the types of individuals for whom the program is most appropriate. Cooper (1995) indicates that the program may not be appropriate for readers who have entrenched eating patterns, who are socially isolated or demoralized, who have significant medical conditions (e.g., pregnancy or diabetes), or for whom binge eating represents a small part of a larger problem (e.g., problems with alcohol or cutting). The introduction also describes the importance of making change a priority, reasons for change (e.g., psychological, social, and medical reasons), and whether the time is right to change. The CBT model for the maintenance of binge eating and purging behaviors is described, and the range of normal weights and the concept of weekly weighing are discussed.

Step 1. Monitoring Your Eating

Step 1 introduces self-monitoring of eating behavior and describes the purpose of and the guidelines for this process. Cooper (1995) provides a sample self-monitoring form completed by a patient, explains the content for the reader, and indicates that the reader should review 1 week's worth of self-monitoring records to begin to draw conclusions about patterns in his or her eating behavior.

Step 2. Instituting a Meal Plan

This step helps the reader to establish a pattern of eating that includes three planned meals and two or three snacks per day. At this point in the program, the types of foods consumed during meals and snacks are not addressed, but the reader is encouraged to plan in advance what foods will be eaten during the day. Cooper (1995) indicates that the goal is to eat an amount of food that is "enough." When problems occur and meals or snacks are missed, the reader is instructed to try and get back on track as soon as possible. Once regular eating is established, it may not be necessary to address vomiting directly; however, for those individuals who continue to self-induce vomiting after regular meals or snacks, Cooper (1995) encourages consuming foods in meals and snacks that are comfortable for the person and that do not need to be purged.

Step 3. Learning to Intervene to Prevent Binge-Eating

The third step describes strategies for stopping binge eating, including talking to other people (e.g., spending time with friends, calling someone on the phone), planning ahead, using stimulus control techniques or eating mindfully, being sensible with alcohol, and intervening the moment the urge to binge-eat occurs by using alternative activities. Alternative activities are easy, pleasurable activities that can be used when a strong urge to eat is experienced. They may include activities that require use of the hands (e.g., knitting, gardening) or that cannot be accomplished in places such as the kitchen, where eating typically occurs (e.g., walking).

Step 4. Problem Solving

Step 4 outlines an approach to problem solving that involves writing the problem down as clearly as possible, generating all possible solutions to the problem, examining all of the solutions realistically, choosing the best solution and acting on it, and reviewing the solution later to determine how effective the solution was. While monitoring, some problems in addition to binge eating (e.g., depression, problems with relationships, or feeling fat) may be identified, and strategies to approach these other issues are described.

Step 5. Eliminating Dieting

Step 5 addresses three types of dieting: (1) going for long periods of time without eating, (2) trying to eat very little, and (3) not eating foods that are high in calories or might trigger a binge. To assist the reader in determining an appropriate amount of food to consume without eating too little, an example of "normal" eating is provided. Readers are encouraged to test predictions about gaining weight from consuming high-fat or high-calorie foods and to construct a hierarchy of forbidden foods.

Step 6. Changing Your Mind

The last step focuses on decreasing weight and shape concerns. To address the importance of shape and weight, the reader is directed to additional books that may be of assistance, and Cooper (1995) suggests making a list of the attributes that the reader values in others, addressing maladaptive thinking styles, or attending a discussion group. The issue of lapses and slips is also discussed.

At the end of the manual, three appendices provide useful addresses for the reader, information for those helping individuals with BN to complete the program, and views of those who have used the program. *Bulimia Nervosa and Binge Eating: A Guide to Recovery* (Cooper, 1995) is available in paperback and can be ordered through commercial bookstores.

Empirical Studies of *Bulimia Nervosa: A Guide to Recovery*

Four studies have examined the utility of *Bulimia Nervosa: A Guide to Recovery* (Cooper, 1993, 1995) as a self-help treatment for BN. The first evaluation of the 1993 manual (Cooper, Coker, & Fleming, 1994) was an uncontrolled trial with 18 patients with BN. In this small sample, notable decreases in bulimic symptoms were observed after patients had used the manual and received a mode of eight 20- to 30-minute sessions with a nonspecialist social worker. Specifically, patients experienced an average reduction in binge eating of 85% and an 88% reduction in vomiting, and 50% of the patients were abstaining from binge eating and vomiting. Cooper, Coker, and Fleming (1996) enrolled a larger number of participants with BM (*n* = 82) in a study with the same design. Of the 67 (81.7%) patients who completed the study, average reductions of 80% in binge eating and 79% in vomiting were observed, and 26.8% were abstinent from binge eating and vomiting. Thus, in both of the Cooper et al. (1994, 1996) studies, a guided-self-help intervention significantly reduced bulimic symptoms for those patients who followed it.

Durand and King (2003) randomized 68 patients to receive a self-help intervention in one of two service settings. Thirty-four patients were treated in a general medical practice using *Bulimia Nervosa: A Guide to Recovery* (Cooper, 1993), and 34 received usual care in a specialist eating disorder clinic. Data at the 6-month follow-up were available for fewer patients in the general medical practice (*n* = 22, 64.7%) than for the patients who received specialist care (n = 28, 82.4%). On the Eating Disorder Examination (Fairburn & Cooper, 1993), baseline objective bulimic episodes decreased from 19.0 over 28 days (~4.75/week) to 16.4 (~4.10/week) at the 6-month follow-up in the self-help group and from 20.4 over 28 days (~5.10/week) to 12.6 over 28 days (~ 3.15/week) at the 6-month follow-up in the specialist-treatment group. At the 6-month follow-up, the last-observation-carried-forward data indicated that 29.4% (n = 10) of the self-help group and 26.5% (n = 9) of the specialist-treatment group had total scores < 20 on the BITE (Henderson & Freeman, 1987), indicating that they did not meet full diagnostic criteria for BN. And although both the self-help and specialist-treatment groups demonstrated significantly improved BITE scores over time (p < 0.001), the groups did not differ statistically from one another on this or the other main outcome measures.

Banasiak, Paxton, and Hay (2005) described a study of *Bulimia Nervosa and Binge-Eating: A Guide to Recovery* (Cooper, 1995) in primary care. Participants with BN or subthreshold BN (n = 109) were randomly assigned to either a wait-list (n = 55) or a guided-self-help (n = 54) intervention. The guided-self-help intervention consisted of 10 sessions with a general practitioner, with a 30- to 60-minute initial session and nine 20- to 30-minute treatment sessions over 16 weeks. Binge-eating frequency was reduced by 60% in the guided-self-help condition compared with 6% on the wait list, and purging episodes were reduced by 61% in the guided-self-help condition compared with 10% on the wait list. Abstinence rates for binge eating were 46% in the guided-self-help condition in comparison with 13% on the wait list (p < 0.001), and rates of abstinence from purging behaviors were 33% in the self-help condition and 12% on the wait list (p < 0.05) at the end of treatment. Thus participants who received self-help demonstrated significant improvements in binge eating and purging symptoms in comparison with those assigned to the wait list. This study suggests that a guided self-help intervention delivered in a primary care setting reduces bulimic symptoms. However, the general practitioners who were recruited expressed a special interest in eating disorders and devoted substantial time to administering the treatment (3.5–5.5 hours of treatment), suggesting that the findings may not be generalizable.

Summary of Empirical Studies of *Bulimia Nervosa: A Guide to Recovery*

Four studies have examined the efficacy of *Bulimia Nervosa and Binge-Eating: A Guide to Recovery* (Cooper, 1995). When the manual was used in conjunction with assistance from nonspecialist social workers (Cooper et al., 1994, 1996) or a general practitioner (Banasiak et al., 2005; Durand & King, 2003), reductions of between 60 and 85% in binge eating and between 61 and 88% in purging were observed. The treatment described in *Bulimia Nervosa and Binge Eating: A Guide to Recovery* (Cooper, 1995), administered under conditions similar to those described by Cooper and colleagues (1994, 1996), Banasiak and colleagues (2005), and Durand and King (2003) may therefore be helpful for patients with BN. However, two of the studies (Cooper et al., 1994, 1996) were uncontrolled, and the other two studies were conducted within health care systems (England; Durand & King, 2003; Australia; Banasiak et al., 2005) quite different from those of other countries, especially the United States. Additional controlled studies of the treatment described in *Bulimia Nervosa and Binge-Eating: A Guide to Recovery* (Cooper, 1995) are warranted.

OVERCOMING BINGE EATING

Like *Bulimia Nervosa: A Guide to Recovery* (Cooper, 1993, 1995), *Overcoming Binge Eating* (Fairburn, 1995) is a cognitive-behavioral manual with two major sections. The first section is devoted to an overall description of binge eating, including the characteristics of binge eating, the prevalence of binge eating, physical problems associated with binge eating, the suspected etiology of binge eating, the risk and maintaining factors for binge eating, the similarities and differences between binge eating and addictions, and a review of the treatment of binge-eating problems. The section comprises the following eight chapters.

Chapter 1. What Is a Binge?

This chapter describes the definition of binge eating, including the importance of a sense of loss of control, the characteristics of a binge, how and when people binge-eat, different types of binge-eating episodes, and how binge-eating episodes start and end (e.g., triggers for binge eating and emotions after the binge-eating episode).

Chapter 2. Binge Eating, Eating Disorders, and Obesity

In this chapter, Fairburn (1995) addresses determining when binge eating constitutes an "eating disorder" and describes the relationship between binge eating and the diagnoses of BN, BED, and anorexia nervosa (AN).

Chapter 3. Who Binges?

Chapter 3 describes the modern origin of the diagnosis of BN and the prevalence and incidence of binge eating among different groups. In addition,

Fairburn (1995) reviews the data suggesting that binge-eating problems are increasing in the general population.

Chapter 4. Psychological and Social Problems Associated with Binge Eating

The fourth chapter is concerned with the features that commonly accompany binge eating: dieting, concerns about appearance and weight, and disturbances in mood, personality characteristics, and social functioning. Specific types of dieting (e.g., going for long periods of time without eating, avoiding forbidden foods, significant caloric restriction) and the effects of dieting are described. The chapter also addresses inappropriate compensatory behaviors, such as vomiting, laxative and diuretic abuse, diet pill usage, and overexercising and the frequency and effectiveness of these behaviors.

Chapter 5. Physical Problems Associated with Binge Eating

This chapter addresses the physical complications associated with binge eating, including the effects of binge eating, dieting, vomiting, laxatives, and diuretics. Information is also provided about the relationship between binge eating and obesity and the effects of binge eating on fertility and pregnancy.

Chapter 6. Causes of Binge Eating Problems

Chapter 6 describes what is known about the causes of binge eating and the difficulties associated with identifying specific causes. A distinction is made between factors that increase the risk of developing a problem with binge eating (e.g., gender, age, trauma, family history) and the factors that maintain binge-eating problems once they have started (e.g., ongoing dieting, interpersonal relationships, pregnancy).

Chapter 7. Binge Eating and Addiction

Chapter 7 discusses whether binge eating should be classified as an addiction and the relationship between binge eating and problems with substance abuse. Fairburn (1995) argues against the addiction model of binge eating and discusses how the effective treatment of binge-eating problems is hindered by this model.

Chapter 8. Treatment of Binge Eating Problems

This chapter reviews what is known about the treatment of binge-eating problems, including data on antidepressant medications, cognitive-behavioral therapy, and other psychological treatments (e.g., behavior therapy, psychoeducational treatments, focal psychotherapy, group therapy, and combined treatment).

The Treatment Program

The second section of *Overcoming Binge Eating* (Fairburn, 1995) outlines the CBT program designed to address problems with binge eating or purging. Like *Bulimia Nervosa: A Guide to Recovery* (Cooper, 1993, 1995), this section is composed of an introduction to the program followed by a six-step intervention that mirrors the way CBT for BN (Fairburn et al., 1993) is delivered. The steps are additive, and the reader is encouraged to follow the steps from 1 to 6 even if some parts of the program appear not to be applicable to their binge-eating problem. A review of the main concepts is included at the end of each of the six steps, such that the most important tasks of the step are highlighted and the reader can determine whether enough progress has been made to move to the next step in the program.

Introduction

In this section, Fairburn (1995) addresses motivation to change by asking the reader to evaluate the advantages and disadvantages of ceasing binge eating and/or purging. Advice is provided about how to proceed if the program does not result in a cessation of binge eating, including seeking professional help (alone or in combination with self-help) and using other forms of self-help, such as support groups. If the reader is at a low body weight, has a serious medical illness, is pregnant, is significantly depressed or demoralized, or has problems with impulse control, Fairburn (1995) indicates that the self-help program described in *Overcoming Binge Eating* might not be an appropriate treatment option.

Step 1. Getting Started

The first step of the program introduces self-monitoring of eating behavior, which helps the reader identify patterns in the types of food consumed, triggers for binge eating, and the emotions associated with binge eating. In the first week, the reader is encouraged not to try to change his or her binge eating and/or purging but just to gather information. At this step, the program includes weekly weighing, by which the reader obtains his or her weight once per week, no more, no less, on one weekday morning. The reader also completes a summary sheet, which helps to identify when the next step of the program should be undertaken once sufficient progress with the first step has been made.

Step 2. Regular Eating

Step 2 aims to develop a pattern of regular eating. This pattern is three planned meals and two to three planned snacks per day, with no more than 3–4 hours elapsing between planned meals or snacks. No meals or snacks should be skipped, and the reader should not eat between the planned meals or snacks. At this point in the program, the specific foods eaten during planned meals or snacks are not a priority, as the focus is solely on when the reader eats. Readers are encouraged to use the preset plan to determine when to eat, not sensations of hunger or fullness, and to introduce the eating pattern in stages, with the first planned meal or snack eaten during the least chaotic part of the day. Fairburn (1995) provides advice on meals, shopping, and cooking and information about how to address self-induced vomiting and laxative and diuretic misuse.

Step 3. Alternatives to Binge Eating

In this step, the reader is instructed in using alternative activities, or activities that are incompatible with binge eating and preferably pleasurable (e.g., exercising, taking a bath/shower, visiting or calling friends or relatives, or playing music). When the reader has an urge to eat between planned meals or snacks, he or she can use the activity list as a way to pass time until the urge to binge-eat decreases.

Step 4. Problem Solving and Taking Stock

Step 4 presents a method for problem solving in six steps, including: (1) identifying the problem as early as possible, (2) describing the problem accurately, (3) considering as many solutions as possible, (4) thinking through the consequences of each solution, (5) choosing the best solution or combination of solutions, and (6) acting on the solution that was chosen. At this point in the program, Fairburn (1995) also asks the reader to "take stock" to determine whether the manual is helping. Several possible outcomes are specified, and different options are suggested (e.g., if the frequency of binge eating has decreased, the reader should continue with the program).

Step 5. Dieting and Related Forms of Food Avoidance

Step 5 of the program addresses any residual dieting behaviors that may be maintaining binge-eating behaviors. Three main forms of dieting—trying not to eat for long periods of time, trying to restrict the overall amount of food eaten, and trying to avoid certain types of food—are described, and interventions to reduce these behaviors are described. For example, the reader is encouraged to make a list of forbidden foods that she or he avoids and to gradually introduce the foods into his or her diet; the foods should continue to be eaten until it is no longer difficult.

Step 6. What Next?

The last step helps the reader determine how to proceed either if binge eating is still a problem or if the reader has improved or recovered. Techniques for preventing relapse, such as having realistic expectations, distinguishing a lapse from a relapse, knowing how to deal with setbacks, and reducing vulnerability, are described. Finally, Fairburn (1995) provides some suggestions about dealing with other problems, including excessive concerns about shape and weight, problems with depression, anxiety, low self-esteem, or relationships.

At the end of the manual, five appendices are presented that describe the body mass index, how readers who are overweight should use the manual, organizations that can help readers, notes for relatives and friends of the reader, and notes for therapists who may be assisting clients through the self-help program.

Overcoming Binge Eating (Fairburn, 1995) provides patients with a comprehensive cognitive-behavioral self-help approach to BN. This book continues to be available through commercial bookstores (both online and in stores) and should be easily available. *Overcoming Binge Eating* (Fairburn, 1995) is quite similar to *Bulimia Nervosa: A Guide to Recovery* (Cooper, 1995), both in content and organization. Fairburn (1995) indicates that *Overcoming Binge Eating* "represent[s] an extension of Dr. Cooper's work, in both focus and scale" and that *Overcoming Binge Eating* is "designed for all those who binge, including those with bulimia nervosa" (p. 132). *Overcoming Binge Eating* (Fairburn, 1995) differs from *Getting Better Bit(e) by Bit(e)* (Schmidt & Treasure, 1993) in separating the psychoeducational information from the treatment program such that patients can choose to begin the self-help intervention before reading all of the material in Part 1 of the book. *Overcoming Binge Eating* (Fairburn, 1995) is available in paperback.

Empirical Studies of *Overcoming Binge Eating*

Four studies have investigated the use of *Overcoming Binge Eating* (Fairburn, 1995) for the treatment of BN. Palmer, Birchall, McGrain, and Sullivan (2002) enrolled 71 patients with BN, 22 patients with partial BN, and 28 patients with BED. Participants were randomized into four groups: wait list ($n = 31$), self-help + minimal guidance ($n = 32$), self-help + face-to-face-guidance ($n = 30$), or self-help + telephone-guidance ($n = 28$). At the end of treatment, 50% of patients in the self-help + face-to-face guidance condition, 36% in the self-help + telephone-guidance condition, 25% in the self-help + minimal-guidance condition, and 19% of the wait-list group showed some improvement (25–75% improvement), with statistically significant differences in improvement only between the face-to-face treatment condition and all other conditions combined ($x^2 = 5.77$, $df = 1$, $p = .016$). Fourteen percent in the self-help + telephone-guidance condition, 10% in the self-help + face-to-face-guidance condition, 6% in the self-help + minimal-guidance condition, and 0% on the wait list were abstinent from binge eating and vomiting. The self-help + face-to-face-guidance and the self-help + telephone-guidance groups were found to be significantly improved In comparison with the wait-list group ($p < .0.05$); however, the outcome for the self-help + minimal-guidance condition did not differ from that of patients assigned to the wait list. Thus, the findings of Palmer et al. (2001) indicate that in order for *Overcoming Binge Eating* (Fairburn, 1995) to be effective, patients may need additional professional contact.

Carter et al. (2003) randomized 85 patients with BN to one of three treatment conditions: (1) using *Overcoming Binge Eating* ($n = 28$), (2) a form of self-help not directed at eating symptoms using the book *Self-Assertion for Women* (Butler, 1992; $n = 28$), or (3) a wait list ($n = 29$). After 8 weeks, 53.6% of the *Overcoming Binge Eating* self-help group, 50% of the nonspecific self-help group, and 31% of the wait list were classified as responders, or had demonstrated a 50% or greater decrease in binge eating or purging. Although there were larger proportions of responders in the two self-help groups than in the wait-list condition, the differences did not quite reach statistical significance. Therefore, this study failed to demonstrate clear superiority of either *Overcoming Binge Eating* (Fairburn, 1995) or *Self-Assertion for Women* (Butler, 1992) over a wait-list control.

Ghaderi and Scott (2003) investigated whether there were differences in the effectiveness of the *Overcoming Binge Eating* program when it was provided in either a pure-self-help or a guided-self-help format. The study was relatively small, with 9 patients diagnosed with BN, 11 patients with subthreshold BN, and 11 patients with BED. Fifteen patients were randomized to receive pure self-help, and 16 patients received guided self-help, which consisted of an additional six to eight 25-minute sessions. Participants reduced their binge eating an average of 33% and their vomiting by 17%. Both the pure and guided self-help interventions using *Overcoming Binge Eating* produced similar improvements in binge eating and vomiting, but the reductions in bulimic behaviors were less than what has been observed in other studies.

Walsh, Fairburn, Mickley, Sysko, and Parides (2004) extended the use of *Overcoming Binge Eating* to the treatment of individuals with BN in a primary care setting. Ninety-one women with either BN or subthreshold BN were randomized into one of four treatment conditions: (1) guided self-help with *Overcoming Binge Eating* + fluoxetine ($n = 24$); (2) guided self-help with *Overcoming Binge Eating* + placebo ($n = 25$); (3) fluoxetine alone

(n = 20); or (4) placebo alone (n = 22). The dropout rate in the study was substantial, and a total of 28 (30.8%) of the 91 patients completed treatment. Fourteen (28.6%) patients from the self-help groups completed, and 14 (33.3%) patients in the medication-only condition completed (p = ns). Vomiting decreased an average of 25.1% in the placebo-alone group, 44.6% in the guided-self-help + fluoxetine group, and 41.3% in the fluoxetine-alone group; surprisingly, it increased an average of 18.8% in the guided-self-help + placebo group. Abstinence rates were lower than in studies in tertiary care centers, with 1.1% in the guided-self-help + placebo group, 2.2% in the placebo-alone group, 5.5% in the guided-self-help + fluoxetine group, and 2.2% in the fluoxetine-alone group reporting no episodes of binge eating and vomiting in the prior 28 days at the end of treatment (p = ns). Compared with patients receiving placebo, those receiving fluoxetine demonstrated significant reductions in binge eating and vomiting (p = 0.03 and p = 0.002, respectively); however, there were no benefits of guided self-help with *Overcoming Binge Eating* (Fairburn, 1995). Additional information about empirical studies of overcoming binge eating can be found in Grilo, Chapter 4, this volume.

Summary of Empirical Studies of *Overcoming Binge Eating*

The studies of *Overcoming Binge Eating* (Fairburn, 1995) are not consistent in their findings. Palmer et al. (2002) found that self-help combined with face-to-face guidance was superior to a wait list and to conditions with less professional contact (minimal guidance, telephone guidance). However, the study by Carter et al. (2003) did not find the use of *Overcoming Binge Eating* (Fairburn, 1995) to be superior to a wait-list control. Ghaderi and Scott (2003) found some reductions in binge eating (33%) and vomiting (17%) after a pure or guided self-help intervention, whereas Walsh et al. (2004) found no effect of the guided-self-help intervention on bulimic symptoms. As these studies used very different methodologies in different settings, it is difficult to determine the true effectiveness of *Overcoming Binge Eating* (Fairburn, 1995) from the research conducted to date. Additional research using this manual is needed to determine the conditions under which the program described is most helpful for patients with BN.

OTHER SELF-HELP STUDIES

Although most of the research evaluating self-help for the treatment of BN has used one of the three manuals previously described, three studies did not. The first study published regarding self-help for the treatment of BN (Huon, 1985) utilized an "eclectic" seven-component program with 120 patients with BN. Thirty patients were randomized to receive pure self-help with the program, 30 patients received the manual and had contact with a "cured" patient with BN, 30 received the manual and had contact with an "improved" patient with BN, and 30 were assigned to a wait list. All of the participants (100%) completed the study. When all of the self-help groups were combined, 88.8% were classified as improved, whereas only 16.7% on the wait list were similarly classified. Abstinence rates for binge eating and purging were 18.8% for all the pure self-help groups, in comparison with 0% on the wait list. The data indicated that there were significantly greater reductions in binge eating and vomiting in all of the self-help conditions in comparison with the wait list but that there were few differences between the self-help groups.

Mitchell et al. (2001) combined medication treatment and a self-help intervention in the treatment of BN. The manual used in the study incorporated portions of a group CBT program used previously (Mitchell et al., 1990) and was structured as 14 reading and homework assignments, with a focus on menu planning, normalizing meal patterns, behavioral avoidance of binge eating, cognitive restructuring, body image issues, and relapse-prevention techniques. Ninety-one patients were enrolled in the study, with 21 patients receiving self-help + fluoxetine, 22 patients receiving the manual + placebo, 26 patients receiving fluoxetine alone, and 22 receiving placebo alone. Vomiting decreased on average 50.2% in the manual + placebo group, 22.8% in the placebo group, 66.7% in the manual + fluoxetine group, and 52.8% in the fluoxetine-alone group. Abstinence rates were 24% in the manual + placebo group, 26% in the manual + fluoxetine group, and 16% in the fluoxetine-alone group at the end of treatment. There was a significant main effect of medication (fluoxetine vs. placebo) on vomiting ($p = 0.043$) and on two global measures of improvement (Clinical Global Improvement, $p = 0.029$, and Patient Global Improvement, $p = 0.036$), but the self-help manual did not appear to add significantly to the medication treatment ($p = ns$).

Pritchard, Bergin, and Wade (2004) studied 20 patients with BN or subthreshold BN. Patients were provided with guided self-help using portions of *Bulimia Nervosa: A Cognitive Therapy Programme for Clients* (Cooper, Todd, & Wells, 2001), a manual for BN with a cognitive emphasis. This open trial found that 47% of patients were abstinent from binge eating and 27% from vomiting at the end of treatment. This guided-self-help intervention also produced significant reductions in bulimic symptoms and sizeable abstinence rates.

CONSIDERATIONS WHEN USING SELF-HELP INTERVENTIONS FOR THE TREATMENT OF BN

Two of the manuals described previously (Cooper, 1995; Fairburn, 1995) suggest using self-help programs as part of "stepped care," which refers to the idea of starting with the least intensive form of treatment and, if improvement does not occur, "stepping" to a more intensive level of treatment. As some individuals with BN can overcome their problems with binge eating and purging on their own, Fairburn (1995) suggests beginning with pure self-help to determine whether additional help will be required. Step 2 for Fairburn (1995) and Step 1 for Cooper (1995) is guided self-help, or adding guidance from a professional (e.g., primary care doctor, nurse, therapist, etc.). After guided self-help, Fairburn (1995) suggests CBT, whereas Cooper (1995) proposes guided self-help plus an antidepressant medication. After CBT, Fairburn (1995) believes the next step is less clear and suggests that patients could try focal psychotherapy, antidepressant medications, and day or inpatient treatment. Subsequent to guided self-help plus an antidepressant medication, Cooper (1995) indicates that patients should receive CBT and, if CBT fails, try interpersonal psychotherapy, day treatment, or inpatient treatment.

Although the stepped-care model makes sense intuitively, it is clear from the examples of Fairburn (1995) and Cooper (1995) and from the modest amount of research cited earlier that no consensus has yet been achieved about what intervention should be employed at each step. In addition, although stepped care appears to be a helpful option, research studies of this type of treatment show that attrition rates tend to be significant. For example, in the Treasure et al. (1996) study, 14 patients dropped out of the study after receiving the manual, and of the 25 patients who could have received an additional eight sessions of CBT, 9 chose not to participate in any further treatment. Thus the total number of patients who complete all aspects of the stepped-care program tends to be low. Although additional studies are ongoing in this area, it is currently unclear how best to use self-help in a stepped-care model.

In addition, it is uncertain when self-help should be used and by whom. Different results have been found even when these programs are delivered within the same type of clinical setting (e.g., primary care). Such variability may be related to the type of patient presenting for treatment, the individual providing the treatment, or other factors. For example, Banasiak et al. (2005) found benefits from using guided self-help in a primary care setting in Australia, but the primary care physicians who delivered the treatment spent a significant amount of time delivering the treatment and had expressed interest in helping to treat patients with eating disorders; it is likely that these characteristics would not apply to most primary care physicians. When guided self-help delivered by nurses was studied in a primary care setting in the United States, there was a substantial dropout rate (71.4%), and the manual was not found to add significantly to a medication intervention (Walsh et al., 2004).

Other issues of experimental design also make the self-help studies difficult to interpret. Many of the studies have used wait-list controls (Bell & Newns, 2002; Carter et al., 2003; Cooper et al., 1994; Cooper et al., 1996; Ghaderi & Scott, 2003; Schmidt et al., 1993). Most, but not all (Carter et al., 2003), found that self-help was superior to the wait list, that is, to no treatment whatsoever, but they do not address the efficacy of self-help compared with other credible interventions, such as other forms of popular self-help support that does not focus on eating disorders. Several studies (Bailer et al., 2004; Carter et al., 2003; Durand & King, 2003; Treasure et al., 1994) found no difference between the impact of self-help and standard treatments, such as CBT, suggesting that self-help is as effective as much more time-consuming and accepted interventions. However, these studies typically do not have sufficient statistical power to distinguish important differences in outcome and do not include a control group, so that it is impossible to assess to what degree the improvement was due only to the passage of time. The few studies that evaluated the effect of self-help when added to medication or compared CBT-based self-help to another intervention and a wait list suggest that the impact of self-help is not specific.

CONCLUSIONS

Several well-developed self-help manuals articulating the principles and implementation of CBT for BN are available. Controlled studies consistently demonstrate that the use of these manuals is associated with greater improvement than assignment to a waiting list. However, the efficacy of self-help relative to more established interventions is not clear. Similarly, it is not certain whether self-help adds substantially to antidepressant treatment nor how it is best employed in a sequenced-care model of treatment. Self-help books may be most useful in informing potential patients of the nature of BN and the available treatment approaches and in offering a treatment program when no other therapeutic options are available.

ACKNOWLEDGMENT

Preparation in this chapter was supported in part by Grant No. DK53635 from the National Institutes of Health.

REFERENCES

American Psychiatric Association. (1987). *Diagnostic and statistical manual of mental disorders* (3rd ed., rev.). Washington, DC: Author.
American Psychiatric Association. (2000). *Diagnostic and statistical manual of mental disorders* (4th ed., text rev.). Washington, DC: Author.
Bailer, U., de Zwaan, M., Leisch, F., Strnad, A., Lennkh-Wolfsberg, C., El Giamal, N., et al.

(2004). Guided self-help versus cognitive-behavioral group therapy in the treatment of bulimia nervosa. *International Journal of Eating Disorders, 35,* 522–537.

Banasiak, S. J., Paxton, S. J., & Hay, P. (2005). Guided self-help for bulimia nervosa in primary care: A randomized controlled trial. *Psychological Medicine, 35,* 1283–1294.

Bell, L., & Newns, K. (2002). What is multi-impulsive bulimia and can multi-impulsive patients benefit from supervised self-help? *European Eating Disorders Review, 10,* 413–427.

Butler, P. E. (1992). *Self-assertion for women.* New York: HarperCollins.

Carter, J. C., Olmsted, M. P., Kaplan, A. S., McCabe, R. E., Mills, J. S., & Aime, A. (2003). Self-help for bulimia nervosa: A randomized controlled trial. *American Journal of Psychiatry, 160,* 973–978.

Cooper, M., Todd, G., & Wells, A. (2001). *Bulimia nervosa: A cognitive therapy programme for clients.* London: Kingsley.

Cooper, P. J. (1993). *Bulimia nervosa: A guide to recovery.* London: Robinson.

Cooper, P. J. (1995). *Bulimia nervosa and binge eating: A guide to recovery* (2nd ed.). New York: New York University Press.

Cooper, P. J., Coker, S., & Fleming, C. (1994). Self-help for bulimia nervosa: A preliminary report. *International Journal of Eating Disorders, 16,* 401–404.

Cooper, P. J., Coker, S., & Fleming, C. (1996). An evaluation of the efficacy of supervised cognitive behavioral self-help for bulimia nervosa. *Journal of Psychosomatic Research, 40,* 281–287.

Durand, M. A., & King, M. (2003). Specialist treatment versus self-help for bulimia nervosa: A randomised controlled trial in general practice. *British Journal of General Practice, 53,* 371–377.

Fairburn, C. G. (1981). A cognitive behavioural approach to the management of bulimia. *Psychological Medicine, 11,* 707–711.

Fairburn, C. G. (1995). *Overcoming binge eating.* New York: Guilford Press.

Fairburn, C. G. (1997). Eating disorders. In D. M. Clark & C. G. Fairburn (Eds.), *Science and practice of cognitive behaviour therapy* (pp. 209–211). Oxford, UK: Oxford University Press.

Fairburn, C. G. (2004, May). *The relationship between treatment research and clinical practice.* Paper presented at the conference of the Academy for Eating Disorders, Orlando, FL.

Fairburn, C. G., & Cooper, Z. (1993). The Eating Disorder Examination (12th ed.). In C. G. Fairburn & G. T. Wilson (Eds.), *Binge eating: Nature, assessment and treatment* (pp. 333–356). New York: Guilford Press.

Fairburn, C. G., Cooper, Z., & Shafran, R. (2003) Cognitive behaviour therapy for eating disorders: A "transdiagnostic" theory and treatment. *Behaviour Research and Therapy, 41,* 509–528.

Fairburn, C. G., Marcus, M. D., & Wilson, G. T. (1993). Cognitive-behavioral therapy for binge eating and bulimia nervosa: A comprehensive treatment manual. In C. G. Fairburn & G. T. Wilson (Eds.), *Binge eating: Nature, assessment, and treatment* (pp. 361–404). New York: Guilford Press.

Ghaderi, A., & Scott, B. (2003). Pure and guided self-help for full and sub-threshold bulimia nervosa and binge-eating disorder. *British Journal of Clinical Psychology, 42,* 257–269.

Henderson, M., & Freeman, C. P. (1987). A self-rating scale for bulimia: The 'BITE.' *British Journal of Psychiatry, 150,* 18–24.

Huon, G. F. (1985). An initial validation of a self-help program for bulimia. *International Journal of Eating Disorders, 4,* 573–588.

Miller, W. R., & Rollnick, S. (1991). *Motivational interviewing: Preparing people for change.* New York: Guilford Press.

Mitchell, J. E., Fletcher, L., Hanson, K., Mussell, M. P., Seim, H., Crosby, R., et al. (2001).

The relative efficacy of fluoxetine and manual-based self-help in the treatment of outpatients with bulimia nervosa. *Journal of Clinical Psychopharmacology, 21,* 298–304.

Mitchell, J. E., Pyle, R. L., Eckert, E. D., Hatsukami, D., Pomeroy, C., & Zimmerman, R. A. (1990). A comparison study of antidepressants and structured intensive group psychotherapy in the treatment of bulimia nervosa. *Archives of General Psychiatry, 47,* 149–157.

Palmer, R. L., Birchall, H., McGrain, L., & Sullivan, V. (2002). Self-help for bulimic disorders: A randomised controlled trial comparing minimal guidance with face-to-face or telephone guidance. *British Journal of Psychiatry, 181,* 230–235.

Pritchard, B. J., Bergin, J. L., & Wade, T. D. (2004). A case series evaluation of guided self-help for bulimia nervosa using a cognitive manual. *International Journal of Eating Disorders, 36,* 144–156.

Prochaska, J. O., & DiClemente, C. C. (1986). Towards a comprehensive model of change. In W. R. Miller & N. Heather (Eds.), *Treating addictive behaviors: Processes of change* (pp. 3–27). New York: Plenum Press.

Russell, G. F. M. (1979). Bulimia nervosa: An ominous variant of anorexia nervosa. *Psychological Medicine, 9,* 429–448.

Schmidt, U., Tiller, J., & Treasure, J. (1993). Self-treatment of bulimia nervosa: A pilot study. *International Journal of Eating Disorders, 13,* 273–277.

Schmidt, U. H., & Treasure, J. L. (1993). *Getting better bit(e) by bit(e).* London: Erlbaum.

Schmidt, U. H., & Treasure, J. L. (1997). *A clinicians guide to getting better bit(e) by bit(e).* East Sussex, UK: Psychology Press.

Thiels, C., Schmidt, U., Treasure, J., Garthe, R., & Troop, N. (1998). Guided self-change for bulimia nervosa incorporating use of a self-care manual. *American Journal of Psychiatry, 155,* 947–953.

Treasure, J., Schmidt, U., Troop, N., Tiller, J., Todd, G., Keilen, M., et al. (1994). First step in managing bulimia nervosa: Controlled trial of therapeutic manual. *British Medical Journal, 308,* 686–689.

Treasure, J., Schmidt, U., Troop, N., Tiller, J., Todd, G., & Turnbull, S. (1996). Sequential treatment for bulimia nervosa incorporating a self-care manual. *British Journal of Psychiatry, 168,* 94–98.

Walsh, B. T., Fairburn, C. G., Mickley, D., Sysko, R., & Parides, M. K. (2004). Treatment of bulimia nervosa in a primary care setting. *American Journal of Psychiatry, 161,* 556–561.

Wilson, G. T., & Fairburn, C. G. (2002). Treatments for eating disorders. In P. E. Nathan & J. M. Gorman (Eds.), *A guide to treatments that work* (pp. 559–592). New York: Oxford University Press.

Wilson, G. T., & Shafran, R. (2004). Eating disorders guidelines from NICE. *Lancet, 365,* 79–81.

6

Self-Help Treatment for
Body-Image Disturbances

JOSHUA I. HRABOSKY *and* THOMAS F. CASH

Body image is a multidimensional "psychological experience of embodiment," which not only includes perceptions of one's physical appearance but also encompasses attitudes and behaviors that relate to one's appearance (Cash, 2004, p. 2; Cash & Pruzinsky, 2002). Body-image attitudes comprise two components. The first is *self-evaluation* of one's looks, including dissatisfaction–satisfaction. These evaluations are based on the discrepancy between self-perceived and idealized physical attributes. A second component of body-image attitudes is *investment*, or the degree of cognitive, behavioral, and emotional importance placed on one's appearance, including the extent to which one's looks are central in defining an individual's sense of self or self-worth.

The severity of body-image problems can be placed on a continuum, ranging from negligible levels of dissatisfaction with certain physical characteristics that result in casual grooming behaviors (e.g., using makeup to cover a blemish) to anxious preoccupation with appearance that results in extreme, and often dangerous, coping and compensatory behaviors (e.g., restrictive eating, social avoidance, compulsive behaviors). Eating disorders are among the most extreme and maladaptive expressions of body-image dysfunction. According to the *Diagnostic and Statistical Manual of Mental Disorders* (American Psychiatric Association, 2000), body-image disturbance is a primary defining feature of anorexia nervosa and bulimia nervosa. Body dysmorphic disorder (BDD), as well as muscle dysmorphia (considered a variant of BDD), are also primarily characterized by severe body-image preoccupation and distress (APA, 2000; Pope, Phillips, &

Olivardia, 2000). Finally, a negative body image can have other harmful psychosocial consequences, such as depression (Noles, Cash, & Winstead, 1985), social anxiety (Cash & Fleming, 2002a), impaired sexual functioning (Wiederman, 2002), poor self-esteem (Powell & Hendricks, 1999), and diminished quality of life (Cash & Fleming, 2002b). Due to the actual or potential development of such psychosocial problems associated with body-image concerns, especially among females in Western societies (e.g., Cash, 2002b; Cash, Morrow, Hrabosky, & Perry, 2004), body image has received increasing empirical and clinical attention (Cash & Pruzinsky, 1990, 2002; Thompson, Heinberg, Altabe, & Tantleff-Dunn, 1999).

The principal purpose of this chapter is to provide a detailed examination of self-help and guided self-help options for the treatment of body-image difficulties. We first discuss the cognitive-behavioral perspective on the development of body-image disturbances. Next, we describe Cash's cognitive-behavioral therapy (CBT) program for body-image difficulties and disorders (Cash, 1991, 1995, 1996, 1997; Cash & Grant, 1995; Cash & Hrabosky, 2004; Cash & Strachan, 2002), with a brief examination of the empirical support for (guided) self-help body-image CBT. We then propose clinical and practical suggestions for the use of this program in a safe and clinically effective manner and consider predictors of success using self-help body-image CBT. We finally discuss the limitations of extant studies and the future aims of research in this area.

BODY-IMAGE DEVELOPMENT AND PROCESSES

From a cognitive-behavioral perspective, an individual develops her or his body image, whether healthy or maladaptive, through historical and developmental, as well as proximal (recent and concurrent), influences (Cash, 2002a). Historical influences are primarily past events and experiences, as well as developmental processes, that shape people's cognitive, emotional, and behavioral patterns that relate to their physical appearance. Influential historical factors include cultural socialization, interpersonal experiences, actual physical characteristics, and personality attributes that impinge on how the individual construes her or his body. Proximal factors are current life events relevant to one's physical appearance and how they are perceived, processed, and reacted to emotionally and behaviorally. They include any precipitating or maintaining factors concerning one's body-related experiences in everyday life (Cash, 2002a). Yet what is most important is the cognitive framework that an individual brings to various situations. An individual's *self-schema*, as it relates to his or her appearance, is an important construct that is believed to be central to body-image development. Markus (1977) defined self-schemas as "cognitive generalizations about the self, derived from past experiences, that organize and guide the processing of self-related information contained in an individual's social experience" (p. 64).

The individual who is self-schematic for physical appearance will likely process information related to appearance differently than will an individual who is not (Cash, Melnyk, & Hrabosky, 2004). For example, appearance-schematic individuals are likely to attend to, and selectively remember, stimuli that are related to their physical attractiveness. Appearance-related situations or events, therefore, can act as signals for the activation of schematic assumptions or beliefs about one's physical appearance (Cash, 2002a; Veale, 2004; Williamson, Stewart, White, & York-Crowe, 2002). Such an individual also tends to overestimate the size or shape of a particular physical attribute of her or his entire body, as well as have an extreme drive to fix the physical "aberrant" attribute (e.g., a drive to be thin; Williamson et al., 2002). Williamson and his colleagues' information-processing model posits that negative emotion interacts with the individual's body-image schema, potentially increasing the likelihood of certain cognitive biases and disturbed body image. Moreover, body-image reactions can activate negative emotions, in turn activating cognitive biases, resulting in a feedback loop consisting of obsessive rumination.

Cash (Cash, 2002a; Cash, Santos, & Williams, 2005) contends that the individual will participate in a number of adjustive behaviors as a means of coping with the distress experienced from ongoing body-image ruminative thoughts. For example, people may engage in avoidant strategies that include behavioral avoidance of certain situations or people, wearing certain body-concealing attire, or efforts to deny or ignore one's upsetting thoughts and emotions. On the other hand, people may perform appearance-correcting strategies, which include rituals to change the perceived "abnormal" characteristic (e.g., dieting or exercise behavior). Finally, individuals may carry out compensatory strategies that involve attempts to enhance other self-evaluative attributes (i.e., physical, personality, emotional, etc.), such as improving one's hairstyle to compensate for weight-related concerns. The extent to which a person's perceptions of and feelings about her or his appearance influences her or his psychosocial functioning and well-being determines how adaptive and healthy her or his body image is.

CBT FOR BODY IMAGE

Based on the prevalence of body-image disturbances and the potential severity of the aforementioned psychosocial consequences, multicomponent and comprehensive programs have been developed for the treatment of body-image problems (Cash, 1991, 1995, 1997; Rosen, 1997). The following section includes a summary of the elements of Cash's most recent revision of his body-image CBT program (Cash, 1997), *The Body Image Workbook*. Whereas other reviews of this program have expanded on the use of this program in a treatment setting with a clinician (e.g., Cash & Hrabosky, 2004), the following summary outlines the major components of the treatment for the reader's orientation. As is discussed, these components have been used in a self-help approach to body-image change.

Step 1: Body-Image Assessment and Goal-Setting

One of the first steps in any CBT intervention is to facilitate a clearer understanding of the presenting problem, the adaptive and maladaptive cognitive, emotional, and behavioral processes, and coping skills, among other things. The purposes of this comprehensive body-image assessment are (1) to develop a baseline understanding of the person's multidimensional body-image experiences; (2) if in a clinical setting, to provide the client with informative feedback about body-image strengths, excesses, and deficits in relation to her or his body-image experiences; and (3) to aid in the creation of a treatment plan. Based on the interpretations of the assessment results, an individual (with or without a clinician) sets specific goals for change. For extensive reviews of body-image measures, see Stewart and Williamson (2004) and Thompson and van den Berg (2002).

Step 2: Body-Image Psychoeducation and Self-Discoveries

Within this section, the individual is taught principles of CBT and the nature of learning, unlearning, and relearning patterns of cognitions, emotions, and behavior. Most important, this training must be personalized with respect to the origins and elements of her or his own body-image experiences. The individual also receives information to "normalize" her or his body-image concerns based on epidemiological evidence and the cultural context in which many people develop body-image difficulties.

The individual is provided with a framework and specific exercises to understand the components and causes of her or his negative body image, documenting critical events and experiences from early childhood to the present that were significant in her or his own body-image development. One of the most useful of these exercises is the "Body Image Diary," a form of self-monitoring of concurrent "Activators" (precipitating events and situations), "Beliefs" (thoughts, assumptions, perceptions, and interpretations), and "Consequences" (resultant emotions and adjustive behaviors). One is taught how to self-monitor these "ABCs" and uses the daily diaries to identify the predictable unfolding of body-image experiences.

Step 3: Relaxation and Body-Image Desensitization

The aim of this component of therapy is to facilitate individuals' exposure to distressful physical attributes and triggering situations. A goal of this exposure is to assist the person in developing self-efficacy in managing body-image dysphoria. Mind-and-body relaxation training includes an integration of progressive muscle relaxation, diaphragmatic breathing, mental imagery exercises, and self-instructional and autogenic techniques.

After a week of practicing such techniques, the person begins to apply them to distressing body-image situations. The individual is instructed to construct two body-image hierarchies: (1) body areas or attributes associated with varying degrees of discontent, and (2) situations or events that trigger body-image distress. The items on each hierarchy are ranked, from those that cause the least to those that cause the greatest distress. Individuals apply the acquired relaxation skills to manage discomfort as they progressively picture in their minds, as well as look directly at, body areas and contexts from least to most distressing, with the goals of controlling and reducing discomfort. Each item is imagined for increasingly longer durations of time as the individual moves up the hierarchy with reasonable control of distress.

Step 4: Identifying and Challenging Appearance Assumptions

Most people with body-image disturbances are highly appearance-schematic—excessively psychologically invested in their appearance as a criterion of self-worth. This element of treatment targets problematic beliefs or assumptions that people hold about their appearance and their sense of self. The goal, therefore, is to aid the individual in discovering such core assumptions; how they influence dysfunctional body-image thoughts, feelings, and behaviors; and how such beliefs are distorted or unsubstantiated. An initial exercise instructs the individual to write about each assumption and its cognitive, emotional, and behavioral consequences. The individual then writes out any possible exceptions, contradictions, and flaws with each assumption. Without ignoring the function or validity of the assumption, the final goal is to develop new, rational, and balanced perspectives, which the individual rehearses.

Step 5: Identifying and Correcting Cognitive Errors

Logically following the previous step, the next facet of treatment involves identifying specific body-image errors or distortions in thinking and developing strategies to alter them. The individual is given eight common body-image errors, and using her or his body-image diaries, the individual's distortions are identified. The individual is then instructed to recognize such cognitive errors *in vivo*, identifying faulty "Private Body Talk" and the distortions it contains and then disputing each with corrective thinking by writing what her or his "new inner voice" would say. The new inner voice includes the "stop, look, and listen" technique, which refers to (1) *stopping* the negative self-talk, (2) *looking* at activating events and maladaptive private body talk to detect distortions that are producing negative body-image emotional reactions, and (3) *listening* to more rational and accurate self-statements.

Step 6: Changing Self-Defeating Body-Image Behaviors

The goal of this step is to modify maladaptive behaviors associated with a body-image disturbance. The appearance-schematic individual, who typically engages in unhealthy coping strategies (e.g., avoidance, compulsive checking, and appearance fixing), is taught that although these behaviors may offer temporary relief, they perpetuate body-image dissatisfaction and dysphoria. Initially, the person identifies current maladaptive behaviors through self-monitoring. Behavioral hierarchies are then constructed for the purposes of *in vivo* exposure and response prevention (ERP) in an effort to eliminate self-defeating behavioral patterns. The person is instructed to use previously acquired skills, such as corrective thinking and adaptive coping.

Step 7: Enhancing Positive Body Image

Whereas all prior techniques have targeted negative body image, the focus in this stage of treatment is on increasing positive body experiences, with a goal of expanding on the client's desire to "treat the body right." The client is taught to engage in body-related activities to create experiences of mastery and pleasure by first identifying various activities over the past year in which she or he had engaged and the level of mastery and pleasure derived from each. The individual is then instructed to select activities from each of three categories—appearance, health and fitness, and sensate experiences—and then carry out one or two daily, recording the mastery and pleasure experiences of each. Perhaps the most important of these activities is regular physical exercise to enhance fitness rather than to alter appearance (e.g., weight loss).

Step 8: Relapse Prevention and Maintaining Body-Image Changes

In this final step of the program, the person evaluates changes and identifies goals for continued work. The focus in this stage is to develop specific strategies to prevent setbacks, cope with high-risk situations, and maintain body-image changes. If any potentially triggering issues have not been dealt with previously, the individual is instructed to prepare for such high-risk situations by drawing on previously learned cognitive and behavioral strategies. Temporary setbacks are normalized as signals to implement skills learned in the program.

BODY-IMAGE TREATMENT OUTCOME RESEARCH

Outcome research although limited, has supported the effectiveness of CBT in reducing body-image disturbances (Jarry & Berardi, 2004; Jarry & Ip, 2005). Specifically, one of the best empirically supported protocols is Cash's (1991, 1995, 1997) CBT program. Much of the research has been done on the program's utility in self-help or guided self-help modalities. Following are summaries of studies that have examined the effectiveness of Cash's body-image CBT program in self-help modalities with varying degrees of "therapist" contact.

Emerson (1995), using Cash's (1991) audiocassette program, *Body-Image Therapy: A Program for Self-Directed Change*, conducted a randomized controlled study comparing the body-image CBT program delivered in a self-administered format with a waitlist control condition. Participants were 40 undergraduate and graduate women endorsing subclinical bulimia symptomatology. Half of the study's sample was randomly assigned to the treatment condition, in which they received Cash's body-image treatment program for 8 weeks. Participants receiving the treatment were instructed to come weekly to the university's counseling center, where they would listen to the program's audiocassettes and complete subsequent treatment-related materials without any therapist contact.

In this first controlled study of Cash's (1991) body-image CBT program administered as self-help, Emerson (1995) found that the treatment sample reported statistically significant reductions in body-image dissatisfaction and concerns; although participants also reported improvements in eating pathology and other psychological dysfunctions (e.g., depressive affect, anxiety), these latter changes were nonsignificant. The treatment sample, initially consisting of 37 participants, had a 46% dropout rate. Although the author did not formally compare the dropout group with those who completed treatment, Emerson did follow up with individuals who dropped out. Individuals who responded reported that they had had difficulties with sustaining their attention to complete the program and with completing body-image desensitization. In fact, most who dropped out did so after the session involving mirror desensitization was employed. Furthermore, when polling treatment participants, Emerson found that a significant majority reported the most difficulty with this exposure component of treatment.

Grant and Cash (1995) compared body-image CBT (Cash, 1991) delivered in a largely self-directed format with modest therapist contact with the program delivered in a group-therapy modality. The study consisted of a subclinical sample of 23 college women with body dissatisfaction. Although both randomly assigned groups completed the audiocassette program, the modest-contact group met for 15 to 20 minutes weekly with a research assistant, who explained and reviewed homework, reinforced compliance, and facilitated problem solving with the program. Group therapy participants completed 11 weekly 90-minute sessions over 4 months.

Despite the more extensive therapist contact within the therapy group, treatment outcomes for the two modalities were equivalent, with all changes maintained at a 2-month follow-up. Changes included significant improvements in body-image satisfaction, reductions in negative body-image affect, less preoccupation with overweight, and increased congruence between self and ideal body size. Other changes included reductions in schematic investment in appearance, fewer cognitive body-image errors and negative body-image thoughts, and less focus on and avoidance of appearance during sexual relations. Grant and Cash (1995) also found improvements in self-esteem, social-evaluative anxiety, self-consciousness, depression, and disordered eating. Improvements in body image for both conditions were clinically significant.

Cash and Lavallee (1997) subsequently compared Grant and Cash's (1995) data with a similar nonclinical sample reporting significant body-image concerns. Cash's (1995) body-image self-help book *What Do You See When You Look in the Mirror?* was used over 10 weeks without face-to-face professional contact. The 16 participants in this study received assignments via postal mail, and contact consisted of 5- to 10-minute scheduled weekly telephone conversations with a research assistant to discuss compliance with assigned reading and homework activities. Compared with the combined treatment conditions of Grant and Cash (1995), this minimal-contact treatment resulted in equivalent body-image and psychosocial outcomes, as well as equivalent rates of compliance. In addition, Grant and Cash (1995) observed a functional recovery rate of 57% of participants in the modest-contact CBT condition, whereas the rate for the minimal-contact CBT from the current study was 75%.

In another uncontrolled study, Lavallee and Cash (1997) compared Cash's (1995) body-image self-help book with McKay and Fanning's (1992) self-help CBT text for self-esteem improvement. Thirty-seven college women with body dissatisfaction were randomly assigned one of the two books at an initial face-to-face meeting with a research assistant, receiving a schedule for the completion of the sections of each book over a 9-week period. There was no contact with participants beyond the pre- and posttreatment assessments. Despite such minimal contact, both self-help books produced statistically and clinically significant improvements in body-image evaluation, investment, and affect. However, only body-image CBT lowered social anxiety, and only self-esteem CBT reduced depressive symptoms. After controlling for pretest levels, body-image CBT was superior to self-esteem CBT in reducing eating pathology and in producing body-image outcomes that reflected less self-reported severity. Finally, greater procedural compliance was significantly related to better body-image outcomes for both treatment groups.

In 1997, Cash published a refinement of his program titled *The Body Image Workbook: An 8-Step Program for Learning to Like Your Looks*. Two recent studies examined the effectiveness of selected components of this program for improving body image and associated psychosocial functioning. First, Strachan and Cash (2002) randomly supplied a subclinical sample of college women and men with body dissatisfaction with either a combination of psychoeducation and systematic self-monitoring (steps 1 and 2 of the program, as previously described) or a combination of these components plus techniques for identifying and altering dysfunctional body-image cognitions (program steps 4 and 5) over a 6-week period. There was no face-to-face contact with participants, as direct contact was limited to an initial phone conversation and all assessments and self-help materials were distributed and returned by postal mail.

Strachan and Cash (2002) found that both conditions resulted in statistically significant improvements on all measures of body image, except for a measure of body-image behaviors. Clinical significance analyses indicated moderate functional recovery rates. In addition, participants in both conditions reported better social self-esteem, reduced social-evaluative anxiety, and fewer depressive symptoms; changes in eating pathology were not significant. Interestingly, the authors found minimal compliance with the added cognitive-change techniques in the second condition. Despite a high attrition rate (53%) observed in this self-help study, intent-to-treat analyses confirmed the observed changes across both groups.

Given Strachan and Cash's (2002) findings, Cash and Hrabosky (2003) investigated the combined treatment of psychoeducation and systematic self-monitoring under more explicated guided or supervised circumstances. Similar to the previous studies, the sample consisted of subclinical college students with body dissatisfaction who reported a desire to improve their body images through self-help. With weekly face-to-face meetings for instructions, pre- and posttreatment assessments, and exchanging of materials, individuals participated in a 3-week program consisting of 1 week of psychoeducation followed by 2 weeks of daily body-image self-monitoring using the Body Image Diaries described previously. At posttreatment, participants reported significantly enhanced body-image evaluations, significantly less preoccupation with overweight, less cross-situational body-image dysphoria, and reduced investment in appearance as a source of self-evaluation. In addition, only approximately 14% of participants dropped out, and all did so immediately after the initial orientation–pretreatment session. This contrasts with the 53% attrition rate found by Strachan and Cash (2002).

BODY-IMAGE SELF-HELP:
IS THERE NEED FOR A THERAPIST?

Collectively, the aforementioned findings consistently support the efficacy of cognitive-behavioral techniques using self-help and guided self-help approaches in the amelioration of body-image disturbances and related psychosocial problems. More specifically, these results suggest that individuals experiencing subclinical body dissatisfaction and distress who enter a body-image CBT self-help program, regardless of the degree of therapist contact, will experience some improvement in body image at the end of treatment. This is not to say, however, that the types of modalities in which treatment is delivered do not affect individuals' degrees of success. In fact, as the results described here reveal, the contrary is true. Although the significant majority of individuals who received body-image CBT experienced considerable remission in their body-image disturbance and other related problems (e.g., depressive affect, low self-esteem, eating pathology), Jarry and Ip (2005) conducted a meta-analysis of the extant outcome research and found that therapist-assisted treatment programs were more effective than treatments delivered with brief contact from a therapist and those with no therapist contact at all. Based on the combined results from Grant and Cash (1995) and Cash and Lavallee (1997), however, participants from three treatment groups (weekly group therapy, individual face-to-face check-ins, and telephone check-ins) were found to be statistically equivalent in their posttreatment reports of body image and psychosocial functioning.

One argument that has been repeatedly supported is that remission of body-image difficulties can result despite the absence of contact with a therapist; however, this seems to occur if the individuals are reasonably compliant with the treatment protocol. In their literature review, Jarry and Berardi (2004) found that the absence of therapist contact was less effective than the provision of even very minimal contact (e.g., telephone conversations), as the former appears to result in impaired compliance with treatment, which, consequently, hinders change. For example, using a similar protocol, Cash and Hrabosky (2003) found minimal attrition in their sample compared with Strachan and Cash (2002), who had an attrition rate of 53%. Although this difference may be due to the weekly face-to-face contact participants had with a researcher in Cash and Hrabosky's design, Strachan and Cash's treatment program was longer (6 weeks versus 3 weeks). Nonetheless, both Strachan and Cash and Lavallee and Cash (1997) found that, when taking into account dropouts, pure self-help resulted in significant improvements in body-image and other psychosocial problems (despite obvious declines in effect size).

Interestingly, Jarry and Ip's (2005) meta-analysis revealed that the dimension of body image that improved the least after body-image CBT (regardless of treatment modality) was investment. Body-image investment, as earlier discussed, is based on core beliefs, or schematic processes, around the importance of an individual's own physical appearance, especially in defining her or his sense of self. It has been previously contended by cognitive theory (e.g., Beck, 1976) that, through identifying and challenging one's cognitive errors, such maladaptive thinking can be significantly altered. However, more recently, exposure and response prevention techniques have been supported as effective in reducing the frequency and influence of cognitive distortions (Hilbert & Tuschen-Caffier, 2004; Hilbert, Tuschen-Caffier, & Vögele, 2002). Therefore, as investment and schematicity are central components of body image, Jarry and Ip contend that treatment must emphasize not only body-image exposure but also its combination with cognitive restructuring techniques. It is essential to recognize this important component of body-image CBT in this chapter, as the effectiveness of body-image exposure in self-help treatment is fairly negligible. As Emerson (1995) discovered, the majority of participants who dropped out of treatment did so at the time body-image exposures were performed. As researchers and clinicians of anxiety disorders know well, there is great difficulty in exposing oneself to that which one fears or despises to such an extent as to cause avoidant and other maladaptive behaviors. Therefore, the successful implementation of body-image exposure in a purely or even partially guided self-help format is unlikely. Those programs that have experienced success in this important component of treatment have delivered it with the full involvement and support of a therapist (e.g., Delinsky & Wilson, 2006; Hilbert, Tuschen-Caffier, & Vögele, 2002).

Therefore, although many components of body-image CBT, such as psychoeducation and self-monitoring, can be effectively employed through self-help or guided self-help modalities, other techniques, including cognitive restructuring, mirror exposure, and behavioral change strategies, may require more therapist assistance and support. Nonetheless, future research must continue to evaluate body-image CBT delivered in multiple modalities, including therapist-directed (in-session treatment), therapist-guided, self-help with brief contact, and pure self-help.

WHO RESPONDS TO SELF-HELP?

Identifying the best candidates for a (guided) self-help approach to body-image change is a worthwhile endeavor. However, few researchers have pursued this. Of course, most of the handful of studies of body-image self-help had relatively small sample sizes that would have reduced statistical power in the detection of moderators of outcome. Nevertheless, Strachan and Cash (2002) examined this question and found that neither weight status nor self-reported history of eating pathology related to the magnitude of body-image change. Similarly, Cash and Hrabosky (2003) failed to find any relationship between baseline body mass and body-image change. In each study, participants of varying degrees of weight showed comparable changes.

Because change is highly unlikely if persons do not implement the self-help program, with or without some external guidance, we must ask: Who will not comply with the program that they need and have seemingly sought? Of course, some may simply be persons who respond to advertisements about research trials—they are curious but not committed. On many occasions, I (TFC) have been told that my *Body Image Workbook* really does require work. The hope that effortless insight can promote change is not reinforced by the homework of detailed behavioral assignments. Of course, as we discussed previously, once they encounter exposure-based aspects of the program, individuals understandably anticipate discomfort and therefore engage in well-learned resistant, avoidant behaviors.

Another set of variables is worthy of consideration in understanding who might be good candidates for self-help. Psychological self-help requires that persons spend considerable time autonomously reading and thinking about psychologically oriented information and then implementing the procedural advice to change their experiences. Wilson and Cash (2000) investigated attitudes toward psychological self-help books among 264 women and men. People with more favorable attitudes about psychological self-help reading held better attitudes toward reading in general, were more psychologically minded, had stronger self-control orientations, and were more satisfied with their lives. Perhaps those who do not enjoy reading, do not wish to understand themselves psychologically, or are unwilling to take control of their unsatisfying lives are less likely to become engaged in and derive benefit from bibliotherapy-based interventions.

SUGGESTIONS FOR CLINICAL PRACTICE

Body-image CBT programs (Cash, 1997; Rosen, 1997) are often used in psychotherapy. Within both individual and group therapies, clinicians have used Cash's (1991, 1995, 1997) text and audiocassettes in multiple ways, whether as the focal point of treatment or as a supplement. The program may be used in its entirety, or the clinician may choose to select certain components of the curriculum in coordination with other treatment approaches to meet the specific needs of the client. It is important to consider some suggestions, however, about how body-image CBT and its techniques are used in clinical practice.

Based on the aforementioned empirical findings, as well as on our clinical experience with body-image CBT, many of the techniques of this treatment work best when used in the therapeutic context. That is to say, as the

results suggest, body-image CBT provided in a self-help modality is beneficial. However, if the client gains guidance from a professional, commitment
and adherence to the treatment is more likely improved. The clinician's role
in improving adherence is twofold. The first role is as a catalyst. In body-
image CBT, the individual is forced to face and critically examine emotionally difficult thoughts and behaviors. Consequently, her or his commitment
to this treatment may waiver. As a result, the clinician's presence alone,
especially if a solid rapport has been developed, may help in ensuring the
client's persistence in the treatment. It is essential that the clinician regularly
follow up with the client on the status of her or his completion of the treatment protocol—especially if the treatment of body-image disturbance is not
the focal point of treatment and is completed outside of the psychotherapy
sessions. Although numerous client variables may predict noncompliance
with treatment, previous research suggests that the therapist's follow-up
and review of work done outside of the therapy sessions is predictive of increased compliance (Bryant, Simons, & Thase, 1999). The second role of
the clinician, which also influences the client's adherence and success in using a self-help program, is her or his ability to assist the client in problem
solving. Such treatment techniques as cognitive restructuring and body-image exposure are complicated and are often difficult to comprehend and
perform. Many mediating variables become hurdles that a client must face
and overcome, and many clients are unable to do so without the assistance
and support of a clinician. Therefore, the clinician must take not only an
empathic approach in understanding the client's difficulties but also a problem-
solving attitude, in which the clinician helps the client overcome her or his
potentially first inclination (avoidance) and instead helps the client consider
ways to surmount any impediments to success.

Self-help body-image CBT, nonetheless, can be implemented as a supplement to treatment. It is possible, and potentially rewarding to the client,
for the focal points of treatment in the sessions and outside of the sessions
to differ. However, although they may somewhat contrast, they should not
be altogether distinct. That is to say, there should be some overlap, some
association between the two components of treatment. For example, the focus of treatment in sessions may be on restructuring negative automatic
thoughts about needing to be perfect and in control while the client is practicing body-and-mind relaxation techniques in which the theme is "letting
go." Such a link between treatments can be extremely beneficial to the patient. An important consideration, however, is to avoid overwhelming the
client. If the treatments in and outside of sessions are parallel, this may not
be a problem, but if the two treatments become increasingly divergent, a
patient may feel inundated, increasing the likelihood of attrition. Furthermore, as we previously discussed, it is essential that the clinician continue
to actively follow up on the body-image exercises that the client is doing
outside of psychotherapy.

An additional consideration is at what point to begin providing body-image CBT. As body-image disturbance can entail a great deal of distress, one would likely assume that the provision of body-image treatment should come immediately. However, although body image appears to be a strong predictor of maintenance of treatment effects for eating disorders (e.g., Fairburn, Peveler, Jones, Hope, & Doll, 1993), it does not appear to predict outcome following the completion of treatment (Peterson et al., 2004; Wilson et al., 1999). For example, in the treatment of obesity, Cooper and Fairburn (2002) argue that body-image therapy may be more beneficial after weight-control treatment is successfully completed in an effort to enhance long-term weight-loss maintenance. Furthermore, some researchers contend that some body dissatisfaction and distress may motivate healthy behavior change in obese individuals seeking weight loss (Heinberg, Thompson, & Matzon, 2001). Therefore, when treating eating disorders or obesity, it may not be necessary to make reducing body-image distress the primary focus early in treatment, although neglecting its overall importance in treatment would be detrimental.

In general, a clinician must be flexible in providing body-image CBT, especially if it is used as adjunctive treatment. Although the clinician can present the program in a bibliotherapeutic modality, its benefits are likely to be enhanced if she or he offers ample guidance and support.

FUTURE DIRECTIONS
IN SELF-HELP FOR BODY IMAGE

Advances in understanding body image and its dysfunctions have facilitated the development of empirically supported treatments (Cash & Pruzinsky, 2002). Cognitive-behavioral therapy has gained the most attention and support as the treatment of choice for body-image disturbances, and its delivery in a self-help format is gaining increasing substantiation as an effective means of reducing body-image and related psychosocial problems. These results are noteworthy, as the current (and probable future) state of mental health care is considerably influenced by managed care. However, as has been intimated throughout this chapter, there is still much to learn about the use of self-help techniques in treating body-image disturbances.

As Grant and Cash (1995) contend, statistically significant change in body image does not necessarily signify restoration of normal or healthy functioning. Self-help CBT has resulted in statistically significant remission in body-image and psychosocially related problems from pre- to posttreatment; however, some of the aforementioned studies also assessed clinical significance. Clinical significance can be computed in several ways, but, as Jacobson, Roberts, Berns, and McGlinchey (1999) contend, two questions must be answered: (1) Is the size of change statistically reliable? and (2) By the conclusion of treatment, does the client end up within a range comparable to that of normally functioning individuals? Kendall, Marrs-Garcia, Nath, and Sheldrick (1999) add that the latter criterion can be determined through the use of normative comparisons. They contend that, although meta-analyses such as that of Jarry and Ip (2005), may reveal important findings in the effectiveness of a treatment, comparing the posttreatment data of a treated sample with the data of an untreated, randomized sample of normally functioning individuals will determine whether clinical significance was achieved.

Using Jacobson and Truax's (1991) analysis of functional recovery, Cash and his colleagues have found that self-help CBT resulted in clinically significant improvement, with a range of 57% (Grant & Cash, 1995) to 75% (Cash & Lavallee, 1997) of participants falling within 1 standard deviation of the norm at posttreatment. Future outcome studies must continue to perform these analyses of clinical significance to determine whether the change individuals experience from self-help CBT does, in fact, result in normal functioning.

Two additional steps that must be performed in assessing the efficacy of self-help body-image CBT are (1) conducting randomized controlled trials and (2) including long-term follow-up assessments. Only Emerson (1995), in her unpublished dissertation, incorporated a randomized untreated control group in examining the effectiveness of Cash's body-image CBT program in a self-help format. Further randomized controlled trials are necessary, and the inclusion of a sample that receives a supportive treatment would be even more beneficial in determining whether the change that individuals experience vis-à-vis self-help body-image CBT is (1) due to the treatment received and (2) a better treatment than a supportive therapy. Furthermore, of the aforementioned outcome studies, only Grant and Cash (1995) performed a follow-up assessment. And, although the authors found that improvements were maintained at the follow-up assessment, the time that elapsed between posttreatment and follow-up was brief (2 months). Therefore, future research must attempt to replicate body-image self-help findings with longer follow-up periods (e.g., 6–12 months).

With the growing constraints of today's financially managed mental health care system, as well as the presentation of comorbid psychopathology in psychotherapy settings, clinicians are much less likely to implement the entire body-image program in its entirety. Therefore, Cash and colleagues (Cash & Hrabosky, 2003; Strachan & Cash, 2002) have more recently begun to perform dismantling studies to determine the components of Cash's (1997) body-image CBT program that are necessary and sufficient for therapeutic change in a self-help modality. Yet such research is still in its infancy, as neither of these studies performed a long-term follow-up assessment. Strachan and Cash discovered that the use of psychoeducation and self-monitoring resulted in changes that were statistically equivalent to those seen with the two components plus cognitive restructuring techniques. The changes were maintained 2 weeks after posttreatment. However, we do not know whether the lack of outcome differences between the two treatment conditions were sustained much longer after the initial follow-up. Therefore, more comprehensive studies must be performed to identify the components of body-image CBT that are sufficient and facilitative of change.

A contemporary application of body-image CBT is as an Internet-delivered program (Winzelberg, Abascal, & Taylor, 2002; Winzelberg, Luce, & Abascal, 2004). Such an administration may be entirely by self-help, by guided self-help, or therapist-directed. The program may be implemented to include extensive psychoeducational content, assessment feedback, asynchronous postings and support, and synchronous chat-room discussions. To the extent that specific body-image interventions can be tied to the assessment-derived needs of the individual, as opposed to assigning all interventions to all participants, this approach has considerable promise. In Chapter 7 of this volume, Taylor and Jones discuss this application and the empirical evidence concerning its efficacy.

Finally, there is no known research on self-help body-image CBT with persons who have clinical eating disorders or obesity, both characterized by significant body-image problems. Furthermore, within treatment protocols for eating disorders and obesity, reducing body-image disturbance is underemphasized. In their manual for bulimia nervosa (BN), Wilson, Fairburn, and Agras (1997) state that the focus of their CBT program is on modification of maladaptive eating patterns and cognitions, whereas very little focus is on changing body-image attitudes. Garner, Vitousek, and Pike (1997), in their description of CBT for anorexia nervosa (AN), contend that the issue of body image in the treatment of AN is unavoidable, as it affects the motivation of the individual to gain and maintain weight. Nonetheless, little research has been performed to assess the influence of body-image CBT techniques on the outcome of treatment, despite the finding that persistence of body dissatisfaction after treatment is a predictor of relapse in BN (e.g., Fairburn et al., 1993). Yet treatment protocols for eating disorders and obesity that include guided self-help body-image CBT techniques may enhance the efficacy of the overall treatment program. However, pure self-help in the treatment of such an extreme disorder as BDD, in which the entire treatment is focused on body-image attitudes and behaviors, must be used cautiously.

Whether CBT is therapist-directed or administered through guided or pure self-help, it has received the most empirical attention in the treatment of body-image difficulties. Another intervention that is appealing as a (guided) self-help approach is "expressive writing" (Lepore & Smyth, 2002; Pennebaker, 1997). In this intervention, individuals write essays about their deepest thoughts and feelings concerning certain stressful experiences, typically about but not limited to traumatic events. Quantitative reviews point to beneficial outcomes across a range of psychosocial problems (Frisina, Borod, & Lepore, 2004; Smyth, 1998). Little empirical work has examined expressive writing as an intervention for negative body image. Earnhardt, Martz, Ballard, and Curtin (2002) compared writing about body-image issues and writing about trivial issues and, surprisingly, found comparable improvements for the two groups over time in body image, mood, and eating disorder symptoms. Unfortunately, various methodological uncertainties and problems were evident in the study. In her unpublished dissertation, Hayaki (2002) compared body-weight-related expressive writing, topic-of-choice expressive writing, and neutral writing for four 15-minute sessions. Few pre- to posttest changes in body image, self-esteem, or dysfunctional attitudes were found; however, relative to the neutral-writing control group, the body-image writing group reported a reduced importance of physical appearance to their self-esteem. Drawing from Cash and Hrabosky's (2003) findings that suggest benefits of body-image psychoeducation plus recorded self-monitoring of the precipitators and consequences of body-image distress, perhaps providing a conceptual CBT framework for understanding one's body image prior to expressive writing about one's past and current body-image experiences could have therapeutic value. Clearly, more research is necessary to determine whether expressive writing interventions are beneficial for persons with a negative body image.

CONCLUSIONS

Cognitive-behavioral treatment has been the most empirically examined self-help approach to eliminating body-image disturbances. Controlled studies of other approaches, such as psychodynamic, interpersonal, or humanistic/experiential therapies, have not been reported (Cash & Pruzinsky, 2002). Based on empirical findings, body-image CBT has received substantial support as a clinically effective form of body-image improvement. Nonetheless, much more research must be performed to understand the most effective and efficient components of this treatment, the best means of delivering the treatment, the predictors of treatment outcome and maintenance of treatment effects and its ability to produce clinically significant remission of related psychosocial problems.

Of utmost importance, however, is the determination of whether, and in what situations body-image CBT can be successful in pure or guided self-help modalities. With increasing constraints of managed health care systems, the ability to disseminate an efficacious treatment protocol to ameliorate body-image disturbance with as little therapeutic guidance as possible would be extremely advantageous. Consequently, controlled experiments on the effectiveness and efficiency of self-help body-image CBT, as well as clinical research in "usual care" settings (Nye & Cash, 2006), must be conducted. Understanding the utility of self-help for the prevention or treatment of body-image problems is pertinent to many populations—for example, at-risk populations, individuals who are obese or who have eating disturbances or disorders, persons seeking cosmetic surgery, and medical patients with appearance-altering conditions (Cash & Pruzinsky, 2002; Sarwer et al., 2006).

REFERENCES

American Psychiatric Association. (2000). *Diagnostic and statistical manual of mental disorders* (4th ed., Text Revision). Washington, DC: Author.

Beck, A. T. (1976). *Cognitive therapy and the emotional disorders.* New York: International Universities Press.

Bryant, M. J., Simons, A. D., & Thase, M. E. (1999). Therapist skills and patient variables in homework compliance: Controlling an uncontrolled variable in cognitive therapy research. *Cognitive Therapy and Research, 23,* 381–399.

Cash, T. F. (1991). *Body-image therapy: A program for self-directed change.* New York: Guilford Press.

Cash, T. F. (1995). *What do you see when you look in the mirror? Helping yourself to a positive body image.* New York: Bantam.

Cash, T. F. (1996). The treatment of body-image disturbances. In J. K. Thompson (Ed.), *Body image, eating disorders, and obesity: An integrative guide for assessment and treatment* (pp. 83–107). Washington, DC: American Psychological Association.

Cash, T. F. (1997). *The body image workbook: An 8–step program for learning to like your looks.* Oakland, CA: New Harbinger.

Cash, T. F. (2002a). Cognitive behavioral perspectives on body image. In T. F. Cash & T. Pruzinsky (Eds.), *Body image: A handbook of theory, research, and clinical practice* (pp. 38–46). New York: Guilford Press.

Cash, T. F. (2002b). A "negative body image": Evaluating epidemiological evidence. In T. F. Cash & T. Pruzinsky (Eds.), *Body image: A handbook of theory, research, and clinical practice* (pp. 269–276). New York: Guilford Press.

Cash, T. F. (2004). Body image: Past, present, and future. *Body Image: An International Journal of Research, 1,* 1–5.

Cash, T. F., & Fleming, E. C. (2002a). Body images and social relations. In T. F. Cash & T. Pruzinsky (Eds.), *Body image: A handbook of theory, research, and clinical practice* (pp. 277–286). New York: Guilford Press.

Cash, T. F., & Fleming, E. C. (2002b). The impact of body-image experiences: Development of the Body Image Quality of Life Inventory. *International Journal of Eating Disorders, 31,* 455–460.

Cash, T. F., & Grant, J. R. (1995). Cognitive-behavioral treatment of body-image disturbances. In V. B. Van Hasselt & M. Hersen (Eds.), *Sourcebook of psychological treatment manuals for adult disorders* (pp. 567–614). New York: Plenum.

Cash, T. F., & Hrabosky, J. I. (2003). The effects of psychoeducation and self-monitoring in a cognitive-behavioral program for body-image improvement. *Eating Disorders: Journal of Treatment and Prevention, 11,* 255–270.

Cash, T. F., & Hrabosky, J. I. (2004). The treatment of body-image disturbances. In J. K.

Thompson (Ed.), *Handbook of eating disorders and obesity* (pp. 515–541). New York: Wiley.

Cash, T. F., & Lavallee, D. M. (1997). Cognitive-behavioral body-image therapy: Extended evidence of the efficacy of a self-directed program. *Journal of Rational-Emotive and Cognitive-Behavior Therapy, 15,* 281–294.

Cash, T. F., Melnyk, S. E., & Hrabosky, J. I. (2004). The assessment of body investment: An extensive revision of the Appearance Schemas Inventory. *International Journal of Eating Disorders, 35,* 305–316.

Cash, T. F., Morrow, J. A., Hrabosky, J. I., & Perry, A. A. (2004). How has body-image changed? A cross-sectional investigation of college women and men from 1983 to 2001. *Journal of Consulting and Clinical Psychology, 72,* 1081–1089.

Cash, T. F., & Pruzinsky, T. (Eds.). (1990). *Body images: Development, deviance, and change.* New York: Guilford Press.

Cash, T. F., & Pruzinsky, T. (Eds.). (2002). *Body image: A handbook of theory, research, and clinical practice.* New York: Guilford Press.

Cash, T. F., Santos, M. T., & Williams, E. F. (2005). Coping with body-image threats and challenges: Validation of the Body Image Coping Strategies Inventory. *Journal of Psychosomatic Research, 58,* 191–199.

Cash, T. F., & Strachan, M. D. (2002). Cognitive behavioral approaches to changing body image. In T. F. Cash & T. Pruzinsky (Eds.), *Body image: A handbook of theory, research, and clinical practice* (pp. 478–486). New York: Guilford Press.

Cooper, Z., & Fairburn, C. G. (2002). Cognitive-behavioral treatment of obesity. In T. A. Wadden & A. J. Stunkard (Eds.), *Handbook of obesity treatment* (pp. 465–479). New York: Guilford Press.

Delinsky, S. S., & Wilson, G. T. (2006). Mirror exposure for the treatment of body-image disturbance. *International Journal of Eating Disorders, 39,* 108–116.

Earnhardt, J. L., Martz, D. M., Ballard, M. E., & Curtin, L. (2002). A writing intervention for negative body image: Pennebaker fails to surpass the placebo. *Journal of College Student Psychotherapy, 17,* 19–33.

Emerson, E. N. (1995). *The efficacy of a self-administered cognitive behavioral treatment program for body image dissatisfaction in women with subclinical bulimia nervosa.* Unpublished doctoral dissertation, Utah State University, Logan.

Fairburn, C. G., Peveler, R. C., Jones, R., Hope, R. A., & Doll, H. A. (1993). Predictors of 12–month outcome in bulimia nervosa and the influence of attitudes to shape and weight. *Journal of Consulting and Clinical Psychology, 61,* 696–698.

Frisina, P. G., Borod, J. C., & Lepore, S. J. (2004). A meta-analysis of the effects of written emotional disclosure on the health outcomes of clinical populations. *Journal of Nervous and Mental Disorders, 192,* 629–634.

Garner, D. M., Vitousek, K. M., & Pike, K. M. (1997). Cognitive-behavioral therapy for anorexia nervosa. In D. M. Garner & P. E. Garfinkel (Eds.), *Handbook of treatment for eating disorders* (2 nd ed., pp. 94–144). New York: Guilford Press.

Grant, J. R., & Cash, T. F. (1995). Cognitive-behavioral body-image therapy: Comparative efficacy of group and modest-contact treatments. *Behavior Therapy, 26,* 69–84.

Hayaki, J. (2002). The effect of written emotional expression on body image dissatisfaction among women. *Dissertation Abstracts International, 63,* 10B. (UMI No. 3066715)

Heinberg, L. J., Thompson, J. K., & Matzon, J. L. (2001). Body image dissatisfaction as a motivator for healthy lifestyle change: Is some distress beneficial? In R. H. Striegel-Moore & L. Smolak (Eds.) *Eating disorders: Innovative directions in research and practice* (pp. 215–232). Washington, DC: American Psychological Association.

Hilbert, A., & Tuschen-Caffier, B. (2004). Body image interventions in cognitive-behavioural therapy of binge-eating disorder: A component analysis. *Behaviour Research and Therapy, 42,* 1325–1339.

Hilbert, A., Tuschen-Caffier, B., & Vögele, C. (2002). Effects of prolonged and repeated body-image exposure in binge-eating disorder. *Journal of Psychosomatic Research, 52,* 137–144.

Jacobson, N. S., Roberts, L. J., Berns, S. B., & McGlinchey, J. B. (1999). Methods for defining and determining the clinical significance of treatment effects: Description, application, and alternatives. *Journal of Consulting and Clinical Psychology, 67,* 300–307.

Jacobson, N. S., & Truax, P. (1991). Clinical significance: A statistical approach to defining meaningful change in psychotherapy research. *Journal of Consulting and Clinical Psychology, 59,* 12–19.

Jarry, J. L., & Berardi, K. (2004). Characteristics and effectiveness of stand-alone body image treatments: A review of the empirical literature. *Body Image: An International Journal of Research, 1,* 319–333.

Jarry, J. L., & Ip, K. (2005). The effectiveness of stand-alone cognitive-behavioural therapy for body image: A meta-analysis. *Body Image: An International Journal of Research, 2,* 317–331.

Kendall, P. C., Marrs-Garcia, A., Nath, S. R., & Sheldrick, R. C. (1999). Normative comparisons for the evaluation of clinical significance. *Journal of Consulting and Clinical Psychology, 67,* 285–299.

Lavallee, D. M., & Cash, T. F. (1997, November). *The comparative efficacy of two cognitive-behavioral self-help programs for a negative body image.* Poster presented at the meeting of the Association for Advancement of Behavior Therapy, Miami Beach, FL.

Lepore, S. J., & Smyth, J. M. (2002). *The writing cure: How expressive writing promotes health and emotional well-being.* Washington, DC: American Psychological Association.

Markus, H. (1977). Self-schemata and processing information about the self. *Journal of Personality and Social Psychology, 35,* 63–78.

McKay, M., & Fanning, P. (1992). *Self-esteem: A proven program of cognitive techniques for assessing, improving, and maintaining your self-esteem.* Oakland, CA: New Harbinger.

Noles, S. W., Cash, T. F., & Winstead, B. A. (1985). Body image, physical attractiveness, and depression. *Journal of Consulting and Clinical Psychology, 53,* 88–94.

Nye, S., & Cash, T. F. (2006). Outcomes of manualized cognitive-behavioral body image therapy with eating disordered women treated in a private clinical practice. *Eating Disorders: Journal of Treatment and Prevention, 14,* 31–40.

Pennebaker, J. W. (1997). Writing about emotional experiences as a therapeutic process. *Psychological Science, 8,* 162–166.

Peterson, C. B., Wimmer, S., Ackard, D. M., Crosby, R., Cavanagh, L. C., Engbloom, S., et al. (2004). Changes in body image during cognitive-behavioral treatment in women with bulimia nervosa. *Body Image, 1,* 139–153.

Pope, H. G., Jr., Phillips, K. A., & Olivardia, R. (2000). *The Adonis complex: The secret crisis of male body obsession.* New York: The Free Press.

Powell, M. R., & Hendricks, B. (1999). Body schema, gender, and other correlates in nonclinical populations. *Genetic, Social, and General Psychology Monographs, 125,* 333–412.

Rosen, J. C. (1997). Cognitive-behavioral body image therapy. In D. M. Garner & P. E. Garfinkel (Eds.), *Handbook of treatment for eating disorders* (2nd ed., pp. 188–201). New York: Guilford Press.

Sarwer, D. B., Pruzinsky, T., Cash, T. F., Goldwyn, R. M., Persing, J. A., & Whitaker, L. A. (Eds.). (2006). *Psychological aspects of reconstructive and cosmetic plastic surgery: Clinical, empirical, and ethical perspectives.* Philadelphia: Lippincott, Williams & Wilkins.

Smyth, J. M. (1998). Written emotional expression: Effect sizes, outcome types, and moderating variables. *Journal of Consulting and Clinical Psychology, 66,* 174–184.

Stewart, T. M., & Williamson, D. A. (2004). Assessment of body-image disturbances. In J. K. Thompson (Ed.), *Handbook of eating disorders and obesity* (pp. 495–514). Hoboken, NJ: Wiley.

Strachan, M. D., & Cash, T. F. (2002). Self-help for a negative body image: A comparison of components of a cognitive-behavioral program. *Behavior Therapy, 33,* 235–251.

Thompson, J. K., Heinberg, L. J., Altabe, M., & Tantleff-Dunn, S. (1999). *Exacting beauty: Theory, assessment, and treatment of body-image disturbance.* Washington, DC: American Psychological Association.

Thompson, J. K., & van den Berg, P. (2002). Measuring body image attitudes among adolescents and adults. In T. F. Cash & T. Pruzinsky (Eds.), *Body image: A handbook of theory, research, and clinical practice* (pp. 142–154). New York: Guilford Press.

Veale, D. (2004). Advances in a cognitive behavioural model of body dysmorphic disorder. *Body Image: An International Journal of Research, 1,* 113–125.

Wiederman, M. W. (2002). Body image and sexual functioning. In T. F. Cash & T. Pruzinsky (Eds.), *Body image: A handbook of theory, research, and clinical practice* (pp. 287–294). New York: Guilford Press.

Williamson, D. A., Stewart, T. M., White, M. A., & York-Crowe, E. (2002). An information-processing perspective on body image. In T. F. Cash & T. Pruzinsky (Eds.), *Body image: A handbook of theory, research, and clinical practice* (pp. 47–54). New York: Guilford Press.

Wilson, D. M., & Cash, T. F. (2000). Who reads self-help books? Development and validation of the Self-Help Reading Attitudes Survey. *Personality and Individual Differences, 29,* 119–129.

Wilson, G. T., Fairburn, C. G., & Agras, W. S. (1997). Cognitive-behavioral therapy for bulimia nervosa. In D. M. Garner & P. E. Garfinkel (Eds.), *Handbook of treatment for eating disorders* (2nd ed., pp. 67–93). New York: Guilford Press.

Wilson, G. T., Loeb, K. L., Walsh, B. T., Labouvie, E., Petkova, E., Liu, Z., et al. (1999). Psychological versus pharmacological treatments of bulimia nervosa: Predictors and processes of change. *Journal of Consulting and Clinical Psychology, 67,* 451–459.

Winzelberg, A. J., Abascal, L., & Taylor, C. B. (2002). Psychoeducational approaches to the prevention and change of negative body image. In T. F. Cash & T. Pruzinsky (Eds.), *Body image: A handbook of theory, research, and clinical practice* (pp. 487–496). New York: Guilford Press.

Winzelberg, A. J., Luce, K. H., & Abascal, L. B. (2004). Internet-based treatment strategies. In J. K. Thompson (Ed.), *Handbook of eating disorders and obesity* (pp. 279–296). Hoboken, NJ: Wiley.

PART III

COMPUTER-ASSISTED SELF-HELP

An alternative method for guiding self-help is new technology that substitutes interactive computer programs for human contact. This type of self-help has the unique advantage of being able to reach people in all locations, even those too distant to access professional specialty treatment. Human contact can also be a part of computer-assisted treatment, in the form of e-mail, chat-room, or bulletin-board-style conversations. Research has examined the efficacy of computer-assisted self-help for obesity and body dissatisfaction, reviewed in Chapter 7, and for bulimia nervosa and binge eating, reviewed in Chapter 8.

7

Internet-Based Prevention and Treatment of Obesity and Body Dissatisfaction

C. BARR TAYLOR *and* MEGAN JONES

Over the past several decades, the prevalence of overweight and obesity has increased at an alarming rate and is now considered to be one of the leading public health problems facing the United States. The rise in overweight and obesity among children and adolescents is of particular concern. (See also Chapters 13 and 14, this volume.) According to National Center for Health Statistics data, the percentage of overweight children and adolescents has consistently increased over time and at a more accelerated rate since 1980. In 1999–2000, 15.3% of children ages 6–11 years and 15.5% of adolescents ages 12–19 years were defined as overweight (Ogden, Flegal, Carroll, & Johnson, 2002). Based on current trends, it is expected that rates of obesity in the adult population will climb from 21% in 2001 to over 40% in the next 25 years (Kopelman, 2000). More than 65% of U.S. adults are overweight or obese, and 31% are obese (Spiegel & Alving, 2005). Given the magnitude of the problem, interventions with potential impact on large populations delivered at relatively low cost are urgently needed.

At the same time that overweight and obesity are increasing, increased attention has been paid to the need to address the issue of body-image dissatisfaction and also to the potential problem that programs designed to promote weight loss may inadvertently increase body-image dissatisfaction and

141

weight and shape concerns. At least four longitudinal studies have shown that increased weight and shape concerns are risk factors for eating disorders (Killen et al., 1994; Killen et al., 1996; McKnight Investigators, 2003; Taylor et al., 2006). In theory, an increase in weight and shape concerns could lead to increased disordered weight-control behaviors or other adverse effects, such as increasing stigma. Weight-related teasing in childhood often serves to exacerbate body dissatisfaction and increased weight and shape concerns, which typically continue into adulthood. Adults in a behavioral weight-loss program who were strongly dissatisfied with their weight and shape were less likely to lose weight when compared with their body-satisfied peers (Kiernan, King, Kraemer, Stefanick, & Killen, 1998). These findings indicate that body dissatisfaction is an important issue to address in the prevention and treatment of obesity. (See also Chapter 6, this volume.)

In this chapter we discuss Internet-based programs for preventing and treating obesity, interventions for improving body image, and programs that have attempted to address both issues simultaneously.

THE INTERNET: POTENTIAL FOR ADDRESSING OBESITY AND BODY DISSATISFACTION

The U.S. Department of Commerce (2002) estimated that approximately 143 million American adults had Internet access in 2002, and Internet access is likely to be nearly universal in the next few years. In a survey done in 2002, the Pew Foundation estimated that 52 million Americans relied on the Internet to make health care decisions (Fox & Rainie, 2002). This same study found that 6 million Americans seek health information online each day, which suggests that more people receive health information online than by visiting health professionals. Sixty-five percent of these consumers reported seeking information regarding nutrition, exercise, or weight control, and 39% reported seeking mental health information (Fox & Rainie, 2002).

The Pew Foundation (Fox & Rainie, 2002) found that consumers' primary reasons for seeking health information online were anonymity and immediacy of contact. Online interventions have the advantage of being able to serve consumers living in remote areas where community support services are unavailable or difficult to access. The Internet also allows individuals with low mobility—often a concern in cases of morbid obesity—or lack of transportation to receive essential psychological treatment. The anonymity of the Internet makes it a safe space for individuals who are socially isolated because of weight-related shame and gives them the ability to connect with others, to contact providers, and to seek assistance.

Internet-delivered programs can also be easily updated with the most current information, allowing providers to offer cutting-edge treatment. Rather than issuing revised editions of self-help books and treatment manuals, existing programs can be altered with keystrokes. The rapid increase in the accessibility to the Internet and the World Wide Web makes it a viable option for the dissemination of health interventions.

Our research group and others show that portable and desktop computers can effectively deliver manualized treatments (Taylor, Agras, Losch, & Plante, 1991). Due to the rise in Internet technology, any program written for a desktop computer can now be effectively delivered on the Internet. Such programs can also be combined with other beneficial treatment components, including support group participation and accessibility to a wide array of resources easily available on the Internet.

Challenges of Internet-Based Interventions

Internet-based interventions face specific challenges, including demonstrating the credibility of online information and the necessity of providing material at an appropriate reading level. Nearly all health-related websites require high school or greater reading ability (Berland, Elliott, Morales, Algazy, Kravitz, et al., 2001). There is a need for a widely recognized and easily available online clearinghouse for health information and Internet-based interventions.

Online interventions can be difficult in populations with low computer literacy or who are anxious about computer use. However, this problem can be easily addressed through initial instructional sessions and easy-to-navigate, user-friendly online programs. There may also be concern that online weight-loss interventions send conflicting messages by recommending decreasing sedentary activities, such as time spent on the computer, while requiring computer use for treatment delivery. Computer use is negatively associated with physical activity among young adults (Fotheringham, Wonnacott, & Owen, 2000), and Fontaine and Allison (2002) fear that online programs might inadvertently lead participants to inaccurately believe that working on the Internet for hours each day is going to help them to lose weight.

Uses of the Internet

Two main functions of the Internet include delivering information and communication. Online information can be delivered via text, pictures, graphics, audio, video, and animation. Websites can be formatted as a book, with all of the material presented at once on one page, or material can be presented sequentially, with links to different pages that consumers can follow for additional information. Interactive Web-based programs allow consumers to enter information and received tailored feedback. An example of this is the National Heart, Lung, and Blood Institute's Aim for a Healthy Weight website (*www.nhlbi.nih.gov/health/public/heart/obesity/lose_*

wt/index.htm), which includes a program that calculates body mass index for interested consumers. The website also provides education about healthy and unhealthy body mass index ranges, as well as several links to related health information. Additionally, programs can be designed to track consumer input and tailor output. For example, scores from an online survey or questionnaire can be used to selectively display information or feedback for an individual. A program could include a body mass index calculator and provide corresponding information about risks associated with a given body mass index, as well as nutrition and physical activity recommendations. The United States Department of Agriculture Center for Nutrition Policy and Promotion (USDA-CNPP) offers a service, *www.mypyramid. gov*, which allows consumers to track dietary consumption and physical activity online. Users can compare their energy input and output balance sheets and receive tailored feedback about their eating and exercise habits.

The Internet also serves an important communication function by connecting two or more people by public (e.g., electronic mailing lists, bulletin boards, chat rooms, newsgroups) or private (e.g., electronic mail, instant messaging, invitation-only chat groups) mechanisms. Communication via the Internet can also vary in time in that messages can be delivered synchronously (i.e., in real time) or asynchronously.

Online interventions have many commonalities with face-to-face individual and group treatments. Services can be provided on an individualized basis, either synchronously by instant messaging or chat or asynchronously by e-mail. Group-based interventions can be facilitated or group-directed. A moderator can be a professional, a mental health trainee, or a peer (another individual with the same diagnosis). Group facilitation style differs depending on the extent to which the communication among the group is directed. Problem-focused behavioral, psychoeducational, and cognitive-behavioral interventions can be easily provided via the Internet and have the ability to reach large populations who may not otherwise have access to treatment. Internet-based programs can be delivered at all levels of intervention: prevention, treatment, and maintenance.

With these considerations, we first review the use of the Internet for improvement of body image and reduction in weight and shape concerns, then consider it for obesity prevention and treatment, and finally discuss interventions that address both issues simultaneously.

ENHANCEMENT OF BODY IMAGE AND REDUCTION OF WEIGHT AND SHAPE CONCERNS

Body-shape disturbance and weight and shape concerns are very similar constructs. Although some individuals may have body-shape disturbance based on specific aspects of their bodies (such as a large nose or disproportionately short legs), most concerns are related to weight and shape. Over the past decade or so we have developed and evaluated a series of programs, titled Student Bodies (Cooper, Taylor, Cooper, & Fairburn, 1987) that are focused on improving body-shape disturbance and on reducing weight and shape concerns. The latter is particularly important because it represents a significant risk factor for the onset of eating disorders. The body satisfaction improvement section of these programs is based on Cash's body image enhancement program (Cash, 1991; see also Chapter 6, this volume). As a main part of the program, the user keeps a body-image journal, providing a brief assessment and feedback on how she or he perceives her or his body image. Over the course of 8 weeks the user provides information on culture as it affects body image, completes exercises to change cognitions about her or his body, provides information on how to "feel" good about her or his body in various situations, and completes body image enhancement exercises. The Student Bodies program also includes sections related to eating-disorder symptoms and attitudes and healthy weight regulation. Student Bodies was initially developed for a CD-ROM program, which proved successful (Winzelberg et al., 2000). The program was revised and put on the Internet to improve access.

Evaluation of Student Bodies

To evaluate the efficacy of the Internet version of Student Bodies, 60 students at San Diego State University were randomized either to Student Bodies (n = 31) or to a control group (n = 29). Students were evaluated pre- and postintervention and again 3 months later. When the data were analyzed using an intention-to-treat analysis, baseline-to-postintervention and baseline-to-follow-up results were significantly different between intervention and control on the major outcome variables. The baseline-to-postintervention and baseline-to-follow-up effect sizes on the Body Shape Questionnaire (BSQ) (Abascal, Brown, Winzelberg, Dev, & Taylor, 2004; Bruning Brown, Winzelberg, Abascal, & Taylor, 2004; Luce, Osborne, Winzelberg, & Taylor, 2004), the main outcome measure, for the intervention group were 0.4 and 0.7, respectively. The effects were particularly encouraging for the high-risk students. Although these results are promising, the sample size was relatively small, the follow-up short, and adherence was under 50% for the final weeks of the program. This study taught us that Internet-based interventions can be effective in reducing body dissatisfaction and weight and shape concerns.

Comparison of In-Person Class and Internet-Based Psychosocial Intervention

Springer, Winzelberg, Perkins, and Taylor (1999) suggested that a Web-based intervention could have a significant impact on improving body image compared with no intervention and that a class designed to help students explore cultural and media messages and other issues related to body image could produce significant within-group effects. The next study was designed to enhance the outcome of the Web-based intervention by increasing adherence through incentives (class grades) and adding the information presented in the body-image class (Celio et al., 2000). We were also interested in comparing a Web-based program with the aforementioned class. Seventy-two female undergraduate students were recruited primarily through flyers posted on campus that advertised a study to help women improve their body image. After informed consent was obtained, participants were randomly assigned to one of three groups: Student Bodies (Internet program), Body Traps (a psychoeducational class), or wait-list control. Participants were offered two units of nongraded academic credit contingent on completion of program requirements. During the treatment phase (baseline to posttest), significant group differences were found for the main outcome measures, with all post hoc analyses favoring Student Bodies over the wait-list control. Intention-to-treat analyses produced similar results. Significant differences were also found on the BSQ at posttest. Intervention effect sizes (mean difference, treatment–control divided by pooled standard deviation) ranged from 0.28 to 0.76 from baseline to posttest and from 0.21 to 0.76 from baseline to follow-up, depending on the measure.

Gollings and Paxton (2006) also suggest that Internet-based interventions are equally as effective as face-to-face treatments in reducing body dissatisfaction and disordered eating. In their pilot study, Gollings and Paxton (2006) randomly assigned 40 adult women to one of two treatment conditions, face-to-face or Internet-facilitated treatment groups. Both programs were based on a manualized psychotherapeutic group intervention, the Set Your Body Free Body Image Program, which was based on motivational interviewing and cognitive-behavioral therapy approaches. The interventions consisted of eight therapist-facilitated group sessions. Online sessions were conducted in a synchronous format, with participants writing comments and responses throughout the session. The online group was also able to communicate between sessions using a discussion board. The results indicated significant improvements in body image and binge eating at postintervention, with effect sizes equal to 0.5 for both outcome variables. There was no difference between intervention modalities in terms of body dissatisfaction and binge eating; however, the face-to-face condition appeared to be more effective in reducing inappropriate weight-loss behaviors.

Are Moderated Groups Needed for Internet Programs?

A major cost of delivering an online intervention such as Student Bodies involves providing group moderation. To examine this issue, 72 nonsymptomatic undergraduate women (complete data for 61 women) were randomized to a control group ($n = 14$), to an Internet-based prevention program only ($n = 14$), or to the Internet prevention program with a moderated ($n = 14$) or unmoderated ($n = 19$) discussion. Participation in the program resulted in better outcomes across all intervention groups compared with controls, and women in the unmoderated discussion group appeared to have the most reduction in risk (Low et al., 2006). The study raises the issue of whether or not moderation of discussion groups, or even the use of discussion groups at all, is essential for successful outcomes. This important issue needs to be examined with larger, high-risk samples.

What Is the Cross-Cultural Effectiveness of Student Bodies?

To examine the effectiveness of Student Bodies provided in another language and culture, the program was translated and adapted for a German population (Jacobi et al., 2006). The controlled effect sizes for the high-risk group actually exceeded those reported by Celio et al. (2000). The study illustrates another advantage of Internet-based programs; that is, they can be rapidly disseminated across cultures and language with similar effects.

Can an Internet-Based Psychosocial Intervention Prevent the Onset of Eating Disorders?

To answer this question, 480 college-age women with high weight and shape concerns were randomized either to the Student Bodies intervention or to a wait-list control group and followed for up to 3 years (Taylor et al., 2006). There was a significant reduction in weight and shape concerns in the Student Bodies intervention group compared with the control group at postintervention ($p < .001$), at 1 year ($p < .001$) and at 2 years ($p < .001$). The slope for reduction in weight and shape concerns was significantly greater in the treatment group than in the control group ($p = .02$). Although there was no overall significant difference in onset of eating disorders between intervention and control groups, the intervention significantly reduced the onset of eating disorders in two subgroups identified through moderator analyses. No intervention participants with an elevated baseline body mass index (BMI) developed eating disorders, whereas the rate of onset of eating disorders in the comparable BMI control group (based on survival analysis) was 4.7% at 1 year and 11.9% at 2 years (confidence interval [CI] = 2.7%–21.1%). In the BMI 25 subgroup, the cumulative survival incidence was also significantly lower at 2 years for the intervention than for the control group (CI = 0% for intervention; 2.7%–21.1% for control). For the sample with baseline compensatory behaviors, 4% of participants in the intervention group developed eating disorders at 1 year and 14.4% by 2 years. Rates for the comparable control group were 16% and 30.4%, respectively. This study suggests that, among college-age women with high weight and shape concerns, an 8-week Internet-based cognitive-behavioral intervention can significantly reduce weight and shape concerns for up to 2 years and decrease risk for eating disorders, at least in some high-risk groups.

Taken together, these studies suggest that an Internet-based body-image enhancement and weight and shape reduction program can have long-lasting and sustained effects and can even, within some subgroups, reduce the rate of onset of eating disorders. The studies discussed here demonstrate that a targeted intervention can have a significant effect in a high-risk group, yet we also wanted to develop a model in which universal and targeted interventions could be presented without stigmatizing participants. Toward this end, we have conducted a series of studies to develop universal and targeted interventions for school-age students.

Effects of an Internet-Delivered, School-Based Intervention on Body Image

Our first study attempted to demonstrate that an eating disorder program delivered to an entire population would improve body image (Bruning Brown, Winzelberg, Abascal, & Taylor, 2003). One hundred fifty-two 10th-grade females and 69 parents were assigned to either the Internet-delivered intervention group or a wait-list comparison group. Students using the program reported significantly reduced eating restraint and had significantly greater increases in knowledge than did students in the comparison group. However, there were no significant differences at follow-up. Parents significantly decreased their overall critical attitudes toward weight and shape. The program demonstrates the feasibility of providing an integrated program for students and their parents with positive changes in parental attitudes toward weight and shape.

School-Based, Internet-Delivered, Combined Universal and Targeted Interventions

In a step toward the development of population-based interventions to simultaneously prevent eating disorders and excessive weight gain, a computer-based algorithm was developed to sort female high school students into one of four risk groups: (1) no eating-disorder or overweight risk (NR), (2) high eating-disorder risk but no overweight risk (EDR), (3) no eating-disorder risk but high overweight risk (OR), and (4) high eating-disorder and high overweight risk (EDOR). Participants completed an online assessment of their weight and shape concerns and entered their self-reported weight and height. Tailored feedback about risk status for developing an eating disorder and/or obesity and a corresponding recommendation for enrollment in a tailored intervention was given to each student. As part of the students' health curriculum, they completed a universal core program on nutrition, physical activity, appearance concerns, and eating-disorder awareness. The EDR group was invited to also complete a targeted body-image (BI) enhancement curriculum. The OR group was asked to indicate their interest in completing a targeted weight-management (WM) curriculum. The EDOR group was asked to indicate their interest in completing either curricula (BI or WM). The algorithm identified 111 NR, 36 EDR, 16 OR, and 5 EDOR. Fifty-six percent of the EDR and 50% of the OR groups elected to receive the recommended targeted curricula. Among the EDOR group, four (80%) selected both, and one student elected to complete the universal core curriculum only. Significant improvements in weight and shape concerns were observed. This study suggests that it is feasible to apply an Internet-delivered algorithm to a population of young women and to simultaneously provide universal and targeted interventions in a classroom setting.

We were also interested in the effect of the recommendations on potential increases of shameful feelings about weight. A slight increase in "shameful" was observed within the EDR participants' ratings (from $M = 1.42$ to $M = 1.67$) and also in the BI group ("shameful" increased from $M = 1.15$ to $M = 1.40$, with an effect size equal to 0.68). For the 15 participants who received feedback on overweight or risk for overweight and a corresponding recommendation for the targeted WM, participant ratings on "shameful" decreased, with an effect size of 0.12. These data suggest that much more information is needed about how weight and shape messages should be combined and how the messages affect students' mood, body image, sense of shame, and motivation (Luce, Osborne, Winzelberg, & Taylor, 2004).

Does Online Feedback Produce Stigma?

In an unpublished study, we examined the effects of online screening and feedback on perceived stigma. Seventy-four 10th-grade girls completed an online screening and were provided feedback, as in the preceding study. We also revised the algorithm to include recommendations for underweight students. At the end of the intervention period, we asked students questions related to perceived stigma. Three percent of students (3 of 104) reported that they felt that they were judged in a negative way by one or more classmates for participating in the program they had chosen. They also felt that 14% (16 of 107) of students were judged "a little" or "somewhat" in a negative way by their peers for participating in their chosen program. One student felt that her classmates were "very much" judged in a negative way. Furthermore, 10% of students (11 of 106) felt they were "a little" or "somewhat" singled out (in a negative way) or stigmatized by the program they participated in, and 17% (18/106) felt that one or more of their class-mates were singled out (in a negative way) or stigmatized for their partici-pation. This study did not permit us to determine whether these feelings arose from the feedback or from other aspects of the program. The data suggest that, although very few girls experience stigma, it is important to measure the impact of feedback on stigma and to provide information to minimize this phenomenon. An advantage of online programs is the poten-tial to assess the impact of feedback and provide intervention as appropri-ate.

Combined Eighth-Grade Boys' and Girls' Groups

Osborne, Luce, House, and Taylor (submitted) tested the feasibility and ac-ceptance of a population-based Internet-delivered universal and targeted fe-male health curriculum for disordered eating and body-image dissatisfac-tion while simultaneously providing a curriculum appropriate for male students. The females completed an online assessment of weight and shape concerns and were sorted into a low-risk group (n = 41) or a high-risk group (n = 37), based on a previous study that suggested that students might benefit by being in groups with similar levels of weight and shape concerns (Abascal, Brown, Winzelberg, Dev, & Taylor, 2004). Male partici-pants (n = 37) were not stratified by risk; thus all received the universal cur-riculum.

All groups significantly increased their knowledge test scores from pretest to posttest. Weight and shape concern scores in the high-risk group dropped from M = 63.7 (SD = 12.1) to M = 44.5 (SD = 14.2), with an effect size equal to 0.74. There was a significant increase in phys-ical activity across all groups. Pretest scores indicated that 68% met the Centers for Disease Control and Prevention (CDC) guidelines (CDC, 1994), which recommend that adolescents participate in at least 60 min-utes of moderate-intensity physical activity most days of the week. At posttest, 82% of participants met the guidelines. In addition, there was a significant decrease in the amount of hours reported watching television during the school week, M = 2.7 (SD = 1.5) at baseline to M = 2.2 (SD = 1.5) at posttest, $t(99)$ = −4.18, p < .01, with an effect size equal to 0.31. Ninety-seven percent of students said they would recommend Stu-dent Bodies to another eighth-grade class, and 99% said they would rather complete the online program than a traditional classroom format. Of over 1,500 online messages posted during the eight sessions, each read by the moderator, 95% of the high-risk groups' postings were considered relevant to the discussion topic, in comparison with 55% of the low-risk group's postings and only 30% of the males' group postings. The moder-ated group seemed to be more useful for the female students. The study demonstrated that universal and targeted programs can be simultaneously provided in classrooms. Furthermore, this study suggests the possible addition of obesity prevention, in terms of the improvement in physical activity, within an online intervention.

Addressing Obesity Prevention and Improving Body Image Simultaneously

Given its potential to reach large populations, it would seem ideal to provide obesity prevention programs via the Internet. However, to our knowledge, no programs have yet been evaluated. On the other hand, there are a number of Internet-based programs designed to improve diet and promote physical activity, two key components of obesity prevention. Also, a number of school-based obesity prevention programs have been developed that could serve as models for Internet-based programs, despite their limited effectiveness. In our most recent studies (e.g., Osborne et al., 2005) we have attempted to combine BI with obesity prevention and treatment. We are currently evaluating the effectiveness of an Internet-based program designed to reduce binge eating and weight gain in students who engage in binge eating and are at risk of overweight or obesity. Some of our preliminary findings point to critical issues that will need to be addressed, particularly in an adolescent population. In our present study, 9th- and 10th-grade students are randomized to an online 16-week obesity treatment program and then followed for 6 months on completion of the study. All 9th- and 10th-grade students in two high schools (one in northern California and one in Boise, Idaho) were invited to participate in a weight-regulation program. Of approximately 5,450 students, 1,507 expressed interest, of which 246 were eligible. The final sample consisted of 105 students (73 girls and 32 boys). All participants reported very high levels of motivation to participate in the program and provided informed assent and parental consent. We have found that compliance with the program is low (below 40% in terms of weeks of activity out of 16). As is noted later, Celio (2005) also found poor compliance with her Internet-based treatment for overweight children. This preliminary data suggests that the Osborne et al. (2005) model, presented earlier, which combines universal and targeted interventions, is more viable than a solely Internet-based targeted prevention program.

The Internet provides a unique vehicle for addressing both obesity prevention and body-image improvement with the potential to monitor potential harmful effects of weight-, diet-, and exercise-related messages. It is possible to assess potential stigmatization following recommendations for an eating disorder or obesity prevention program, as was done with Luce et al. (2004). It is also possible to provide combined programs, as was done

e et al. (2005), although the focus of that study was not on
ntion. At least one recent study of a school-based program has also
obesity prevention can have a positive effect on eating-disorder
and behaviors (Austin, Field, Wiecha, Peterson, & Gortmaker,
200-,

The Dark Side of the Internet

We have discussed the potential for benefit from Internet programs, but the
technology also permits activities that may increase, rather than decrease,
risk. A number of "proanorexia" websites have appeared in recent years,
providing dangerous weight loss suggestions and supporting eating disorders as a way of life and solution to overweight. These websites have far-
reaching negative consequences and impede progress in prevention and
treatment of eating and weight-related disorders. Although the Internet
may be a useful medium for the delivery of effective and healthy eating-
disorder and obesity prevention programs, this technology has the potential
to be employed in harmful ways.

TREATMENT OF OBESITY

Obesity treatments are notoriously unsuccessful (Kirk, 1999). Multiple barriers can obstruct successful weight loss and weight maintenance, including
negative attitudes toward obese individuals held by society and by some
treating clinicians (Harvey, Glenny, Kirk, & Summerbell, 2002), a lack of
social support (Perri, Sears, & Clark, 1993), and the use of inadequate
weight-loss programs (Glenny, O'Meara, Melville, Sheldon, & Wilson,
1997). Patients have higher rates of success in longer treatment programs
(Perri, Nezu, Patti, & McCann, 1989), suggesting that the treatment of
obesity may be better suited to a chronic-disease model than an acute-care
model that involves little or no follow-up (Perri, Nezu, & Viegener, 1992;
see also Chapter 10, this volume). Yet it is often difficult to provide long-
term care because of the added burden on health care providers, as well as
increased time and money required from patients. Longer treatment is also
complicated by the low adherence rates associated with increased duration
of care (Jeffery, Wing, Thorsen, Burton, Raether, et al., 1993; Wing,
Venditti, Jakicic, Polley, & Lang, 1998).

Group behavioral weight-loss programs are among the most widely
used and most effective treatments, usually inducing between an 8 and
10% reduction in initial weight (Wadden & Butryn, 2003). These programs often incorporate social support from both treating professionals
and peers, which is a key factor in maintaining weight loss. Innumerable
studies over the past 20 years have shown the long-term limitations of

weight-loss programs (Jeffery et al., 2000) and have also identified elements of successful obesity treatment, which include behavioral interventions focused on increasing energy expenditure, social support, and long-term maintenance, all of which can be provided via the Internet. The Internet offers a variety of formats through which behavioral interventions and follow-up care may be delivered. A limited but growing number of randomized controlled trials have examined various modes of employing computer and Internet technology to deliver weight-loss interventions (see Table 7.1).

Computer-Assisted Weight Loss

A number of studies, including some by our group, have demonstrated the effectiveness of computer-assisted weight loss (Burnett, Taylor, & Agras, 1985; Taylor et al., 1991). As mentioned, once a program has been demonstrated to be effective on a computer, it is readily and easily translated to the Internet. Computer-based interventions have an additional advantage of permitting analysis of process measures, as much of the data is collected automatically (Burnett, Taylor, & Agras, 1992; Celio et al., 2000).

E-mail Support

E-mail communication and reminders are often employed by Internet-based weight-loss interventions (see Tables 7.1 and 7.2). E-mail can be used to provide consistency between sessions, to deliver individualized feedback, and to encourage compliance. Yager (2001) used e-mail as an adjunct to face-to-face individual psychotherapy for anorexia nervosa. E-mail contact was used to convey emotional support, monitor dietary intake, and improve continuity of care during the referral process. Patients who communicated several times each week via e-mail reported high levels of satisfaction and increased adherence to treatment.

A study conducted by Sansone (2001) demonstrated the utility of e-mail in reducing social isolation by providing social support. The experimenter initiated e-mail contact between patient dyads who had limited social support. Following the initial introduction, the experimenter had no further e-mail contact with patients and provided no supervision of exchanges between patients. All participants who engaged in e-mail exchanges expressed positive feelings about the program, indicating that individuals may be receptive to e-mail as a vehicle for social support.

Online Support Groups

Several early studies examining online support groups for eating disorders and obesity looked at the use of online bulletin boards. Gleason (1995) ex-

TABLE 7.1. Randomized Controlled Trials of Online Weight Control Programs

Study	Sample	Experimental design	Treatment	Outcome
Celio (2005)	• 61 adolescents • Ages 12–17 • Weight: BMI = 34.1 ± 7.1	RCT	• 4-month trial Internet-delivered cognitive and behavioral intervention for weight-reduction, body-satisfaction, and eating-disorder risk factors. 1. Student Bodies: Two Internet program involving self-monitoring, individualized feedback via e-mail, and online discussion forum. 2. Typical care: physician consultation and self-directed behavior change.	$\underline{\Delta \text{ Weight (lb)}}$ <u>4 months</u> 1 = –0.18 2 = +2.3 <u>BMI z-scores</u> 1 = –0.86 2 = –0.003 Effect size = 0.19
Harvey-Berino et al. (2002)	• 101 adults • Ages 48.4 ± 9.6 • Weight: BMI = 32.2 ± 4.5	RCT	• 1-year trial 6-month in-person behavioral weight loss trial followed by a 12-month behavioral maintenance program. 1. Internet-delivered weight-maintenance program involving self-monitoring, online videos of therapist, therapist and peer e-mail support, and access to an online bulletin board. 2. Same program delivered in-person with (a) frequent in-person support and (b) minimal in-person support	$\underline{\Delta \text{ Weight (kg)}}$ <u>6 months</u> 1 = +2.2 ± 3.8 2 = 0 ± 4 Effect size = 0.56 <u>1 year</u> 1 = –5.7 ± 5.9 2 = –10.4 ± 6.3 Effect size = 0.77
Harvey-Berino, Pintauro, Buzzell, & Casey Gold (2004)	• 255 adults • Age 45.8 ± 8.9 • Weight: BMI = 31.8 ± 4.1	RCT	• 1-year trial 6-month behavioral weight-loss trial conducted over interactive television followed by a 12-month weight maintenance intervention. 1. Internet-delivered weight-maintenance program involving self-monitoring, therapist and peer e-mail support, and access to an online bulletin board and chat room. 2. Biweekly in-person meetings including the same core components of the Internet intervention.	$\underline{\Delta \text{ Weight (kg)}}$ <u>1 year</u> 1 = –7.6 ± 7.3 2 = –5.1 ± 6.5 Effect size = 0.36

(continued)

TABLE 7.1. (*continued*)

Study	Sample	Experimental design	Treatment	Outcome
Tate, Jackvony, & Wing (2003)	• 92 adults • Age 48.5 ± 9.4 • Weight: BMI = 33.1 ± 3.8	RCT	• 1-year trial 1. Core Internet program consisting of psychoeducation, self-monitoring of weight, and access to an online bulletin board, as well as behavioral e-counseling and individualized feedback. 2. Core Internet program alone.	Δ Weight (kg) 6 months 1 = −4.4 ± 6.2 2 = −2.0 ± 5.7 Effect size = 0.4 12 months 1 = −5.2 ± 5.4 2 = −2.5 ± 4.7 Effect size = 0.53
Tate, Wing, & Winett (2001)	• 91 adults • Age 40.9 ± 10.6 • Weight: BMI = 29.0 ± 3.0	RCT	• 6-month trial 1. Internet behavior therapy consisting of self-monitoring, weekly e-mail instruction and individualized feedback, access to an online bulletin board. 2. Internet psychoeducation regarding behavioral weight-loss strategies, caloric restriction, and exercise goals.	Δ Weight (kg) 3 months 1 = −4.0 ± 2.8 2 = −1.7 ± 2.7 Effect size = 0.84 6 months 1 = −4.1 ± 4.5 2 = −1.6 ± 3.3 Effect size = 0.63
White et al. (2004)	57 adolescent African American girls Age 13.19 ± 1.37 Weight: BMI = 36.34 ± 7.89 Obese parents Age 43.19 ± 6.16 Weight: BMI = 38.48 ± 7.18	RCT	• First 6 months of 2-year trial 1. Online behavioral condition incorporating behavior modification techniques, self-monitoring with automated feedback, e-mail-delivered therapist support, goal setting, psychoeducation, and relapse prevention. 2. Online psychoeducation about health eating.	Δ Weight (kg) 6 months Adolescents 1 = 0.55 ± 3.26 2 = 2.4 ± 2.86 Effect size = 0.60 Parents 1 = −2.16 ± 4.95 2 = −0.52 ± 2.55 Effect size = 0.42
Womble et al. (2004)	• 47 women • Age 43.7 ± 10.2 • Weight: BMI = 33.5 ± 3.1	RCT	• 1-year trial 1. eDiets.com (a commercial Internet weight-loss program) consisting of psychoeducation, goal setting, professionally moderated online meetings, access to an online bulletin board, e-mail peer contact and reminders. 2. *LEARN Program for Weight Control 2000* (a weight-loss manual) providing 16 structured cognitive-behavioral lessons.	Δ Weight (kg)16 weeks 1 = −0.7 ± 2.7 2 = −3.0 ± 3.1 Effect size = 0.79 1-year 1 = −0.8 ± 3.6 2 = −3.3 ± 4.1 Effect size = 0.65

Note. RCT, randomized controlled trial.

TABLE 7.2. Summary of Online Commercial Weight-Loss Programs

Website	Corporate host	Target audience	Approach	Components
www.jennycraig.com	Jenny Craig	• Adults • Weight loss	• Behavioral • Psychoeducation	• Psychoeducation • Self-monitoring • Weight-tracking graph • Online chat room • Buddy program
www.weightwatchers.com	Weight Watchers	• Adults • Weight loss	• Behavioral • Psychoeducation	• Psychoeducation • Self-monitoring • Online chat room
www.southbeachdiet.com	South Beach Diet	• Adults • Weight loss	• Behavioral • Psychoeducation	• Psychoeducation • Self-monitoring • Online chat room • Buddy program
www.biggestloserclub.com	The Biggest Loser Club	• Adults • Weight loss	• Behavioral • Psychoeducation	• Psychoeducation • Self-monitoring • Online chat room

amined the use of an electronic bulletin board at a college in Massachusetts by women with body-image and eating concerns. Gleason (1995) found that women who reported binge eating were more likely to use the bulletin board than were women who reported food restriction. Over time, participants disclosed more personal information and used the online contact as a support group.

Online Behavioral Weight-Loss Treatment: Randomized Controlled Trials

Although behavioral weight-loss treatments have been extensively studied in face-to-face settings, only a handful of empirical studies have examined online programs. The limited data available suggest that online weight-loss programs are equally as effective as in-person treatment and are more cost-efficient. The published randomized controlled trials to date are summarized in Table 7.1 and outlined in greater detail in this section.

Tate, Wing, and Winett (2001) compared the efficacy of an Internet-delivered behavioral weight-loss program with that of a psychoeducational website with links to Internet weight-loss resources. The participants in the behavioral treatment group received 24 weekly behavioral lessons via e-mail, weekly individualized feedback about self-monitoring diaries from the therapist, and access to an online bulletin board. Participants in the 6-month Internet behavior therapy program lost significantly more weight than the Internet psychoeducation group (3 months, $d = 0.84$; 6 months, $d = 0.63$).

The authors concluded that the Internet and e-mail are viable methods for the delivery of structured behavioral weight-loss programs.

Tate, Jackvony, and Wing (2003) compared the effects of a 1-year Internet weight-loss program alone with those of the same program with the added component of e-mail behavioral counseling. Participants all received one in-person counseling session and the same core Internet program and submitted their weight weekly. The participants receiving the additional e-mail component also submitted weekly calorie and exercise information and received individualized e-mail counseling and feedback. The authors found that the addition of e-mail counseling to a basic Internet weight-loss intervention significantly improved weight loss in overweight and obese adults (6 months, $d = 0.4$; 12 months, $d = 0.53$).

Family-Based Treatment

White et al. (2004) conducted a family-based weight-loss program to address environmental factors of weight gain and obesity in the home environment. African American adolescent girls and one obese parent participated in the online program. Family pairs were assigned to either a behavioral weight-loss condition involving regular e-mail contact with a therapist or to a psychoeducational control group. The behavioral condition emphasized self-monitoring, goal setting for eating and exercise, problem solving, behavioral contracting, and relapse prevention. Participants submitted daily food records online and were provided with automated tailored feedback, including a generated image of the food guide pyramid indicating the extent to which the individual's food records complied with the recommended guidelines. Participants in the control condition accessed a separate website and received psychoeducational materials about serving sizes, the food guide pyramid, hidden calories, and food labels.

White et al. (2004) reported better adherence in the behavioral group and found that family pairs in the behavioral condition also lost more weight (adolescents, $d = 0.60$; adults, $d = 0.42$) and significantly reduced their overall fat intake compared with parent–child dyads in the control condition. White et al. (2004) found family climate to be a significant mediator of adolescent weight management and adherence to the study protocol. These findings support social learning theory, suggesting that parents can model healthy eating, exercise habits, and adherence to the program, which can provoke similar behaviors in adolescents. Parents' willingness to change their own eating behavior likely affects their children's weight loss. White et al. (2004) concluded that the Internet may be an effective mechanism for the promotion of health-related behavior. The authors suggested that the most efficacious use of the Internet in weight-loss treatment may be in school- or community-based overweight prevention programs.

Commercial Weight Loss Programs

As the use of the Internet has proliferated, so too have online commercial weight-loss programs. An increasing number of existing weight-loss programs such as Weight Watchers and Jenny Craig, have developed online components to their programs. Table 7.2 provides examples of several online commercial weight-loss programs, selected by highest rankings (determined by "hit" rates, i.e., frequency of use) on google.com. Even more Web-based programs have arisen in response to the increasing demand for online health information. (See shapeup.org, a nonprofit weight-management organization, for a more complete list of programs.)

Very few commercial weight-loss programs have been subject to empirical review. In one of these rare studies, Womble et al. (2004) compared the effectiveness of a commercial Web-based program (eDiets.com) with a weight-loss manual (LEARN, described subsequently). The eDiets.com program consisted of prescribed meal plans that reduced overall caloric intake, customized grocery lists, and tailored physical activity goals according to self-reported endurance and strength. Social support was provided through professionally moderated online meetings, bulletin board support groups, and a "find a buddy" program that allowed participants to form e-mail relationships with each other. The eDiets.com program also included an animated fitness instructor, access to a 24-hour help desk, e-mail reminders about goals, and biweekly newsletters. The manual-based program, the *LEARN Program for Weight Management 2000 and Maintenance Survival Guide* (Brownell, 2000) involved reduced caloric intake, increased physical activity, stimulus control, and cognitive restructuring. Participants in the manual condition were also encouraged to self-monitor food intake for 16 weeks, which was consistent with the self-monitoring in the eDiets.com condition.

Womble et al. (2004) found that women in the manual group lost significantly more weight than those in the eDiets.com condition (16 weeks, $d = 0.79$; 52 weeks, $d = 0.65$). Results also demonstrated a relationship between the frequency of program use and weight loss, such that users who logged onto the eDiets.com program more often lost more weight than participants who logged on less often. Womble et al. (2004) hypothesized that the differences between program success rates was partly a result of the amount of structure provided by each program. The authors found eDiets.com to be less regimented than the LEARN manual. The results suggest that it may be useful to require participants to submit daily food records and to provide individualized feedback in order to increase a program's structure.

Maintenance of Change and Relapse Prevention

Maintaining weight loss is difficult. Wadden and Bell (1990) found that a year after participating in behavioral weight-loss therapy, patients usually have regained 37% of the weight they lost in treatment. Once individuals cease participating in a structured treatment program, they typically regress to their former eating and exercise habits. In order to make lasting lifestyle changes, weight-loss patients should engage in regular follow-up sessions, complete sporadic self-monitoring inventories, and receive feedback about their progress. Perri et al. (1993) found a combination of four strategies to be most effective in maintaining weight loss: (1) continued professional guidance involving therapist contact posttreatment, (2) skills training to help cope with high-risk situations, (3) structured exercise, and (4) social support. Participants with all four factors maintained 74% of weight loss versus 6% for the control group. Internet-delivered programs have the capability of offering the aforementioned weight-maintenance components. Table 7.1 additionally summarizes several randomized controlled trials for online weight-maintenance programs.

Harvey-Berino et al. (2002) compared an in-person behavioral weight-loss maintenance treatment with a similar program delivered over the Internet. Participants received the same initial treatment, attending 15 one-hour therapist-moderated group meetings. The initial weight-loss program involved reducing overall caloric intake, lifestyle changes (including nutritious eating and exercise), and principles of behavior modification, such as stimulus control, problem solving, social skills training, and relapse prevention. Following treatment, participants were randomized to maintenance conditions involving either continued in-person sessions and phone support or Internet-delivered video sessions and e-mail support. Participants receiving in-person treatment were instructed to complete self-monitoring diaries, attend group meetings, stay within a preset calorie goal, meet or exceed exercise goals, and initiate contact with other group members. Therapist-led group discussions focused on solving difficult eating and exercise situations. During weeks in which the groups did not meet, participants received phone support from the group therapist. Participants in the Internet condition entered self-monitoring data on the website, viewed online videos of the group therapist, and received e-mail support. An online bulletin board served as a discussion forum for participants in the Internet condition, and participants were encouraged to establish e-mail contact with other group members. Participants in both conditions had the opportunity to win money for adherence to the study protocol.

Harvey-Berino et al. (2002) found that participants assigned to the in-person group reported higher satisfaction with their group assignment and attended meetings more regularly. However, attrition rates and the overall number of peer support contacts were not significantly different between the groups. In the first 6 months of weight-maintenance treatment, the Internet group gained significantly more weight than did the group receiving in-person treatment ($d = 0.56$). This pattern was consistent with the postassessment, which indicated that the Internet group sustained a significantly smaller weight loss than did the group receiving in-person support

(d = 0.77). Interestingly, all peer support contacts by both groups were made through e-mail, suggesting some degree of preference for online social support. These results indicate that online interventions may not be as effective as in-person treatment.

In an additional study, Harvey-Berino, Pintauro, Buzzell, and Casey Gold (2004) investigated a 12-month weight-maintenance program involving three conditions: frequent in-person support, minimal in-person support, and Internet-delivered support. All participants initially participated in a 6-month behavioral weight-loss treatment conducted over interactive television (ITV). During ITV sessions, participants could see the therapist at all times and could hear and be heard by all other participants speaking into their own microphones. Participants were also always visible when they were speaking, as the audio system alerted the video camera.

Participants in the frequent in-person support group condition met biweekly for 1 year. Participants turned in their self-monitoring diaries, were weighed, and participated in the therapist-led group discussion. During the weeks in which the group did not meet, participants received phone support from the therapist and submitted self-monitoring data by postcard. Participants in the minimal in-person support condition met monthly over ITV for the first 6 months of the 12-month weight-maintenance condition. Participants in this condition were not contacted between monthly meetings and received no contact from the therapist during weeks 7–12. Participants in the Internet-delivered support condition attended an initial meeting to review logistics of logging on and using the program website. Participants in the Internet condition were expected to attend biweekly Internet chat sessions facilitated by a group therapist and to enter self-monitoring data online. Social support consisted of therapist and peer e-mail contact, online bulletin board access, and a chat room. The authors found no significant differences in weight loss among the groups at 18-month follow-up (d = 0.36). The authors concluded that an Internet-based intervention may be an effective mechanism for promoting long-term weight maintenance.

The treatment studies described in this section indicate that online weight-control programs are a promising alternative to standard care. These interventions appear to be equally as effective as, if not more than, effective standard care, and can be delivered at a lower cost to consumers, and require less time for providers. The future directions and implications of Internet-based interventions are numerous and are described briefly in the following section.

CONCLUSIONS AND FUTURE DIRECTIONS

Internet technology has enabled exciting advances and innovation in the way prevention and treatment interventions are delivered. Health care providers can incorporate online technology into existing treatment programs, such as utilizing scheduled automated e-mails to remind patients to access a website to elicit information about current weight, food consumption, and physical activity. Web-based programs can be used to give consumers and providers instant feedback, such as the instruction to schedule an appointment with their providers or to complete a self-monitoring assessment daily. Online groups can be used as adjuncts to individual "booster" sessions with therapists in the maintenance phase of treatment. "Graduate" groups can be moderated by "recovered" patients to decrease the time required from providers. As Harvey-Berino, Pintauro, and Casey Gold (2000) state, the Internet may hold promise as a method for maintaining contact with patients to facilitate long-term behavior change. Furthermore, Internet-based interventions will allow prevention and treatment to be delivered to a greater percentage of the population.

The rapidly progressing field of computer and Internet technology requires that online interventions remain dynamic and change to meet the expectations and norms of current users. In order for prevention and treatment programs to be effectively utilized, these interventions must create online environments that are normative to savvy users and that employ the latest technology. Commercial obesity treatment programs have begun to utilize the potential of the Internet to provide information and interventions combined with groups and, more recently, to create online "communities" of individuals with similar experience and goals. In our work we have begun to address the problem of adherence in adolescence by reconceptualizing how adolescents use media. Adolescents use a variety of media outlets for pleasure and communication—they may text-message one set of friends, provide extensive personal details on a public "personal space" website, share their deepest thoughts on personal blogs, post and share pictures of friends, trade songs—all in a rapidly changing and dynamic fashion.

The challenge, we believe, is to capitalize on the ability of this technology to connect with students and patients in brief periods rather than the prolonged periods that are used in conventional programs. The next generation of programs needs to find ways to develop communities of at-risk individuals devoid of commercial and financial interests but, rather, focused completely on the problem at hand. For instance, as part of her e-life, an adolescent at risk of overweight might belong to a "health community" existing on a common website and participate in a program that provides standard information and, additionally, innovative features, including the ability to send instant messages and even pictures of healthy meals to other participants.

Technological advances such as Internet2 and Next Generation Internet will ensure the rapid transfer of new network services and applications to the broader Internet community and enable revolutionary Internet applications. Information and images will be accessed more quickly due to increased bandwidth, interconnection and communication between computer devices (e.g., wireless connections to telephones), and increased microprocessor speed. Faster connection speed will allow richer images and more complex graphical material to be conveyed via animation, audio, and video rather than the present heavy reliance on text and still images in today's online interventions. Multidimensional forums will also allow users to adopt three-dimensional avatars (i.e., visual icons to represent oneself online) to interact with other users and facilitate navigation through programs. Virtual reality programs can be adapted for computer administration, allowing users to practice skills and solve problems in simulated situations. This new technology will improve the quality of interpersonal connections made online, which may consequently improve adherence to treatment protocols. Advances in computer and Internet technology have opened a new frontier for the delivery of prevention and treatment of a range of medical and psychological disorders. The existing research suggests that Internet technology can effectively address the growing problem of obesity and body dissatisfaction in the United States and perhaps across the globe.

REFERENCES

Abascal, L., Brown, J., Winzelberg, A. J., Dev, P., & Taylor, C. B. (2004). Combining universal and targeted prevention for school-based eating disorder programs. *International Journal of Eating Disorders, 35*, 1–9.

Austin, S. B., Field, A. E., Wiecha, J., Peterson, K. E., & Gortmaker, S. L. (2005). The impact of a school-based obesity prevention trial on disordered weight-control behaviors in early adolescent girls. *Archives of Pediatric Adolescent Medicine, 159*, 225–230.

Berland, G. H., Elliott, M. N., Morales, L. S., Algazy, J. I., Kravitz, R. L., Broder, M. S., et al. (2001). Health information on the Internet: Accessibility, quality, and readability in English and Spanish. *Journal of the American Medical Association, 285*, 2612–2621.

Brownell, K. D. (2000). *The LEARN program for weight management 2000 and maintenance survival guide.* Dallas, TX: American Health.

Bruning Brown, J., Winzelberg, A. J., Abascal, L. B., & Taylor, C. B. (2004). An evaluation of an Internet-delivered eating disorder prevention program for adolescents and their parents. *Journal of Adolescent Health, 35*, 290–296.

Burnett, K. F., Taylor, C. B., & Agras, W. S. (1985). Ambulatory computer-assisted therapy for obesity: A new frontier for behavior therapy. *Journal of Consulting and Clinical Psychology, 53*, 698–703.

Burnett, K. F., Taylor, C. B., & Agras, W. S. (1992). Ambulatory computer-assisted therapy for obesity: An empirical model for examining behavioral correlates of treatment outcome. *Computers in Human Behavior, 8*, 239–248.

Cash, T. F. (1991). *Body-image therapy: A program for self-directed change.* New York: Guilford Press.

Celio, A. A. (2005). *Early intervention of eating- and weight-related problems via the Internet in overweight adolescents: A randomized controlled trial.* Unpublished doctoral dissertation, University of California, San Diego, and San Diego State University.

Celio, A. A., Winzelberg, A. J., Wilfley, D. E., Eppstein-Harald, D., Springer, E. A., Dev, P., et al. (2000). Reducing risk factors for eating disorders: Comparison of an Internet- and a classroom-delivered psychoeducation program. *Journal of Consulting and Clinical Psychology, 68,* 650–657.

Centers for Disease Control and Prevention. *Health objectives for the nation: Prevalence of overweight among adolescents: United States 1988–1991.* Retrieved November 11, 1994, from http://www.cdc.gov/mmwr/preview/mmwrhtml/00033492.htm

Cooper, P. J., Taylor, M. J., Cooper, Z., & Fairburn, C. G. (1987). The development and validation of the Body Shape Questionnaire. *International Journal of Eating Disorders, 6,* 485–494.

Fontaine, K. R., & Allison, D. B. (2002). Obesity and the Internet. In K. Brownell & C. Fairburn (Eds.), *Eating disorders and obesity: A comprehensive handbook* (2nd ed., pp. 609–612). New York: Guilford Press.

Fotheringham, M. J., Wonnacott, R. L., & Owen, N. (2000). Computer use and physical inactivity in young adults: Public health perils and potentials of new information technologies. *Annals of Behavioral Medicine, 22,* 269–275.

Fox, S., & Rainie, L. (2002). *Vital decisions: How Internet consumers decide what information to trust when they or their loved ones are sick.* Retrieved October 1, 2005, from the Pew Internet and American Life Project website. www.pewinternet. org/report_display.asp?r=59

Gleason, N. A. (1995). A new approach to disordered eating using an electronic bulletin board to confront social pressure on body image. *Journal of American College Health, 44,* 78–80.

Glenny, A. M., O'Meara, S., Melville, A., Sheldon, T. A., & Wilson, C. (1997). The treatment and prevention of obesity: A systematic review of the literature. *International Journal of Obesity and Related Metabolic Disorders, 21,* 715–737.

Gollings, E. K., & Paxton, S. J. (2006). Comparison of Internet and face-to-face delivery of a group body image and disordered eating intervention for women: A pilot study. *Eating Disorders: Journal of Treatment and Prevention, 14,* 1–15.

Harvey, E., Glenny, A. M., Kirk, S., & Summerbell, C. (2002). An updated systematic review of interventions to improve health professionals' management of obesity . *Obesity Reviews, 3,* 45–55.

Harvey-Berino, J., Pintauro, S. J., Buzzell, P., & Casey Gold, E. (2004). Effect of Internet support on the long-term maintenance of weight loss. *Obesity Research, 12,* 320–329.

Harvey-Berino, J., Pintauro, S. J., Buzzell, P., DiGiulio, M., Casey Gold, E., Moldovan, C., et al. (2002). Does using the Internet facilitate the maintenance of weight loss? *International Journal of Obesity, 26,* 1254–1260.

Harvey-Berino, J., Pintauro, S. J., & Casey Gold, E. (2000). The feasibility of using Internet support for the maintenance of weight loss. *Behavior Modification, 26,* 103–116.

Jacobi, C., Morris, L. Beckers, C. Bronisch-Holtze, J., Winter, J., Winzelberg, A. J., et al. (2006). Maintenance of internet-based prevention: A randomized controlled trial. *International Journal of Eating Disorders, 40,* 114–119.

Jacobi, C., Morris, L., Bronisch-Holtze, J., Winter, J., Winzelberg, A., & Taylor, C. B. (2006). Reduction of risk factors for disordered eating behavior: Adaptation and initial results of an internet-supported prevention program.. *Zeitschrift für Gesundheitspsychologie, 13*(2), 92–101.

Jeffery, R. W., Drewnowski, A., Epstein, L. H., Stunkard, A. J., Wilson, G. T., Wing, R. R., et al. (2000). Long-term maintenance of weight loss: Current status. *Health Psychology, 19,* 5–16.

Jeffery, R. W., Wing, R. R., Thorsen, C., Burton, L. R., Raether, C., Harvey, J., et al. (1993). Strengthening behavioral interventions for weight loss: A randomized trial for food provision and monetary incentives. *Journal of Consulting and Clinical Psychology,* *61,* 1038–1045.

Kiernan, M., King, A. C., Kraemer, H. C., Stefanick, M. L., & Killen, J. D. (1998). Characteristics of successful and unsuccessful dieters: An application of signal detection methodology. *Annals of Behavioral Medicine, 20,* 1–6.

Killen, J. D., Taylor, C. B., Hayward, C. H., Haydel, F., Wilson, D. M., Hammer, L., et al. (1996). Weight concerns influence the development of eating disorders: A four-year prospective study. *Journal of Consulting and Clinical Psychology, 64,* 936–940.

Killen, J. D., Taylor, C. B., Hayward, C. H., Wilson, D. M., Haydel, F., Hammer, L. D., et al. (1994). Pursuit of thinness and onset of eating disorder symptoms in a community sample of adolescent girls: A three-year prospective analysis. *International Journal of Eating Disorders, 16,* 227–238.

Kirk, S. (1999). Treatment of obesity: Theory into practice. *Proceedings of the Nutrition Society, 58,* 53–58.

Kopelman, P. G. (2000). Obesity as a medical problem. *Nature, 404,* 635–643.

Low, K. G., Charanasomboon, S., Lesser, J., Reinhalter, K., Martin, R., Winzelberg, A., et al. (2006). Effectiveness of a computer-based interactive eating disorders prevention program at long term follow-up. *Eating Disorders, 14,* 17–30.

Luce, K. H., Osborne, M. I., Winzelberg, A. J., & Taylor, C. B. (2004). Application of an algorithm-driven protocol to simultaneously provide universal and targeted prevention programs. *International Journal of Eating Disorders, 37,* 1–7.

McKnight Investigators. (2003). Risk factors for the onset of eating disorders in adolescent girls: Results of the McKnight longitudinal risk factor study. *American Journal of Psychiatry, 160,* 248–254.

Ogden, C. L., Flegal, K. M., Carroll, M. D., & Johnson, C. L. (2002). Prevalence and trends in overweight among U.S. children and adolescents, 1999–2000. *Journal of the American Medical Association, 288,* 1728–1732.

Osborne, M., Luce, K. H., House, T., & Taylor, C. B. (2005). *Evaluation of an Internet-delivered school-based universal and targeted health curriculum.* Manuscript submitted for publication.

Perri, M. G., Nezu, A. M., Patti, E. T., & McCann, K. L. (1989). Effect of length of treatment on weight loss. *Journal of Consulting and Clinical Psychology, 57,* 450–452.

Perri, M. G., Nezu, A. M., & Viegener, B. J. (1992). *Improving the long-term management of obesity: Theory, research and clinical guidelines* (pp. 110–145). New York: Wiley.

Perri, M. G., Sears, S. F., Jr., & Clark, J. E. (1993). Strategies for improving maintenance of weight loss: Toward a continuous care model of obesity management. *Diabetes Care, 16,* 200–209.

Sansone, R. A. (2001). Patient-to-patient e-mail: Support for clinical practices. *Eating Disorders: Journal of Treatment and Prevention, 9,* 373–375.

Spiegel, A. M., & Alving, B. M. (2005). Executive summary of the Strategic Plan for National Institutes of Health Obesity Research. *American Journal of Clinical Nutrition, 82,* 211S–214S.

Springer, E. A., Winzelberg, A. J., Perkins, R., & Taylor, C. B. (1999). Effects of a body image curriculum for college students on improved body image. *International Journal of Eating Disorders, 26,* 13–20.

Tate, D. F., Jackvony, E. H., & Wing, R. R. (2003). Effects of Internet behavioral counseling on weight loss in adults at risk for type 2 diabetes. *Journal of the American Medical Association, 289,* 1833–1836.

Tate, D. F., Wing, R. R., & Winett, R. A. (2001). Using Internet technology to deliver a behavioral weight-loss program. *Journal of the American Medical Association, 285,* 1172–1177.

Taylor, C. B., Agras, W. S., Losch, M., & Plante, T. G. (1991). Improving the effectiveness of computer-assisted weight loss. *Behavior Therapy, 22,* 229–236.

Taylor, C. B., Bryson, S., Luce, K. H., Cunning, D., Celio Doyle, A., & Abascal, L. B. (2006). Prevention of eating disorders in at-risk college-age women. *Archives of General Psychiatry, 63*, 831–888.

U.S. Department of Commerce. (2002). *A nation online: How Americans are expanding their use of the Internet.* Washington, DC: U.S. Government Printing Office.

Wadden, T. A., & Bell, S. T. (1990). Obesity. In A. S. Bellack, M. Hersen, & A. E. Kazdin (Eds.), *International handbook of behavior modification and therapy* (2nd ed., pp. 449–473). New York: Plenum Press.

Wadden, T. A., & Butryn, M. L. (2003). Behavioral treatment of obesity. *Endocrinology and Metabolism Clinics of North America, 32*, 981–1003.

White, M. A., Martin, P. D., Newton, R. L., Walden, H. M., York-Crowe, E. E., Gordon, S. T., et al. (2004). Mediators of weight loss in a family-based intervention presented over the Internet. *Obesity Research, 12*, 1050–1059.

Wing, R. R., Venditti, E. V., Jakicic, J. M., Polley, B. A., & Lang, W. (1998). Lifestyle intervention in overweight individuals with a family history of diabetes. *Diabetes Care, 21*, 250–258.

Winzelberg, A. J., Eppstein, D., Eldredge, K., Wilfley, D., Dasmahapatra, R., Dev, P., et al. (2000). Effectiveness of an Internet-based program for reducing risk factors for eating disorders. *Journal of Consulting and Clinical Psychology, 68*, 346–350.

Womble, L. G., Wadden, T. A., McGuckin, B. G., Sargent, S. L., Rothman, R. A., & Krauthamer-Ewing, E. S. (2004). A randomized controlled trial of a commercial Internet weight-loss program. *Obesity Research, 12*, 1011–1018.

Yager, J. (2001). Implementing the revised American Psychiatric Association practice guidelines for the treatment of patients with eating disorders. *Psychiatry Clinics of North America, 24*, 185–199.

8

Computer-Based Intervention for Bulimia Nervosa and Binge Eating

ULRIKE SCHMIDT *and* MIRIAM GROVER

Many young people with common mental health problems are unlikely to seek professional help for their problems and hold self-help strategies in higher esteem than treatments delivered by health professionals. Those in the age group of 16–24 are least likely to seek professional help for a mental health disorder (Oliver, Pearson, Coe, & Gunnell, 2005). In a large community-based study in which people were asked about their views on the effectiveness of interventions for common mental disorders (Jorm et al., 2004), different types of self-help intervention were thought to be effective by 41–84% of people, whereas only 27% of people thought that therapist-aided cognitive-behavioral therapy (CBT) would be effective. In another survey, one in four potential users of self-help treatment said that they would rather use the Internet for help, advice, and counseling than see a doctor (Graham, Franses, Kenwright, & Marks, 2001). The reasons quoted for this were ease and rapidity of access, lack of stigma and embarrassment associated with self-help, and not wanting a mental health record. The vast majority of potential users (91%) wanted to access self-help therapy via a computer.

Thus it seems that many health care consumers want to take a more active approach in terms of dealing with any mental health problems rather than accepting the role of the passive recipient of care, and computerized treatments may bridge this gap by placing the consumer in the position of being the "agent of change."

Stand-alone therapeutic computer programs for common mental disorders have existed since the 1970s. Three stages of the development of computerized therapy can be distinguished (Cavanagh & Shapiro, 2004). These stages parallel the development and predominant use of particular therapies. Thus the first generation of therapy computers, most notably Eliza, developed by Joseph Weizenbaum in 1966, provided a client-centered simulation of therapist–patient dialogue. The second wave of therapy computers provided behavioral training, exposure therapy, psychoeducation, and simple cognitive strategies. We have now reached the third stage in this development, in which interactive multimedia programs, typically based on cognitive-behavioral models, have been developed for a number of common mental health problems (for a review, see Proudfoot, 2004). Research into computerized CBT (C-CBT) for anxiety and depression is the most advanced, and the existing evidence has been summarized in a number of systematic and narrative reviews (National Institute of Clinical Excellence [NICE], 2002; Kaltenthaler et al., 2002; Proudfoot, 2004). C-CBT is more effective than treatment as usual, is as effective and acceptable as therapist-aided CBT or bibliotherapy, and requires less therapist time than conventional CBT. A meta-analysis of five studies of C-CBT for depression (Cavanagh & Shapiro, 2004) found that C-CBT was better than a waiting-list condition. A second finding was that C-CBT did somewhat less well than therapist-provided CBT, but the numbers included in this comparison were very low.

Taken together, these findings suggest that computerized interventions might have potential in the treatment of bulimia nervosa (BN) or binge-eating disorder (BED). The majority of sufferers with BN fall precisely into the age group in which seeking help from professionals is low.

In what follows we discuss the packages available and the research based on them and also look at patient and therapist variables that may influence acceptance and outcomes of treatment.

COMPUTER-BASED SELF-HELP INTERVENTIONS FOR BULIMIA NERVOSA

The *Overcoming Bulimia* Program

Overcoming Bulimia is a cognitive-behavioral multimedia self-help package for BN and related disorders (Williams, Aubin, Cottrell, & Harkin, 1997). The program consists of eight modules. Module 1 describes BN and its physical, emotional, and social consequences and introduces readers to the cognitive model of the maintenance of BN and how this might apply to them. Module 2 introduces the topic of why people develop eating disorders and how food, shape, and weight are perceived in our society. Additionally, self-monitoring of eating, thoughts, and feelings is introduced. There is also a section on increasing motivation to change. Module 3 covers the question of how to change; for example, how to fight cravings for food and how to break the vicious circle of BN. Additionally, patients are taught how to eat healthily. Module 4 addresses the role of thoughts in bingeing, including unhelpful thinking styles and how to change extreme and unhelpful thinking. Module 5 tackles the area of assertiveness and how to increase daytime activity. Module 6 looks at problem solving, that is, the role of thinking and coping in the face of practical difficulties. Module 7 is called "Living Life to the Full" and attends to the topics of how to face up to one's fears, how to build confidence and enjoy life more, how to start doing things one has stopped doing, and how to use an activity diary to increase feelings of pleasure and achievement in life. Module 8 addresses the topic of planning for the future and reviews what has been learned. Patients have to work through the modules in order and can proceed to the next module only once the previous module has been completed. Each module requires about 45 minutes at the computer. Patient workbooks and "putting into practice what you have learned" (homework) tasks accompany each session. Self-assessment tools in the program provide patients with feedback on their progress. This package has been evaluated in two pilot studies in a large catchment area–based specialist eating-disorder service. Patients with BN and eating disorder not otherwise specified (EDNOS) who were consecutively referred to the clinic by their general practitioners, were included. In the first of these pilot studies, a cohort of 60 patients were offered the package without therapist support (Bara-Carril et al., 2004). Patients accessed the treatment program in the clinic and were introduced to it and booked in for computer appointments by a research worker. Patients were encouraged to complete the program over a period of 4 to 8 weeks by working through one to two computer modules per week. Forty-seven of those 60 who were offered the intervention accepted it. Follow-up showed significant reductions in bingeing and compensatory behaviors, most clearly in self-induced vomiting.

The second pilot study conducted within the Eating Disorders Service of the South London and Maudsley NHS Trust aimed to examine whether the addition of therapist support to the CD-ROM intervention would improve treatment acceptance, adherence, and outcome. It compared outcomes from the first cohort with those from a second cohort who were offered three brief focused support sessions with a therapist (Murray et al., 2007). The two cohorts were compared on treatment acceptance, adherence and outcome. Patients in both groups improved significantly. There were no significant differences between the two groups in terms of treatment acceptance, adherence, or outcome, except that the group with therapist guidance more often achieved a reduction of excessive exercise at follow-up.

Overcoming Bulimia is currently undergoing trials to compare it with a waiting-list group of adults with BN. Furthermore, this intervention has now been adapted for use on the Internet and is being piloted in adolescents with BN in a randomized controlled trial in students with BN in the United Kingdom.

The SALUT Project

An Internet-based cognitive-behavioral self-help guide for the treatment of bulimia (*www.2salut-ed.org/demo/*) was developed within a European Multicenter Study ("Self-Help Guide for Bulimia," 2004). The program consists of seven sequential steps that include: motivation, self-observation, and modification of behavior; dietary plan and strategies for warding off or avoiding binges; observation and modification of automatic thoughts; problem solving; self-affirmation; conclusion; and relapse prevention. Each step is divided into lessons, exercises, and examples. Patients work through the self-help guide at their own speed. However, a minimum amount of time that patients should spend on each step has been predefined so as to make sure that participants do not go through the whole program within a few days.

Studies evaluating the efficacy and acceptability of the self-help guide were conducted in Switzerland, Sweden, Germany, and Spain (Carrard et al., 2006; Rouget, Carrard, & Archinard, 2005; Fernández-Aranda, 2005). The studies followed a common protocol and targeted adult women between 18 and 30 with BN (purging or nonpurging BN and EDNOS). During the 4-month self-help treatment phase, patients were supported by a "coach." They had three face-to-face evaluations and one e-mail contact per week during the program and optional e-mail support during the 2-month follow-up period. Results from the full study are not available yet.

A pilot study conducted in Switzerland using this self-help guide consisted of a cohort of 45 patients with BN or EDNOS (Carrard et al., 2006; Rouget et al., 2005). Sixty-four percent completed outcome questionnaires at 4 months, and 51% completed them at 6 months. Dropout during treatment was 36%. "Completers" and "dropouts" differed on frequency of bingeing and vomiting, with "completers" having less severe symptoms. After 4 months of treatment, 17.2% of participants were abstinent from bingeing and vomiting. The proportion of abstinent participants was maintained at follow-up.

Participants were highly satisfied with the idea of using Internet-based self-help, the ease of use of the program, its usefulness, and the e-mail support. Participants thought that the self-help treatment was about equally effective as therapist treatment. Some but not all satisfaction measures were correlated with positive outcomes.

Treatment compliance was measured in two ways: (1) Compliance with self-monitoring assessed as the difference between the number of days actually completed in the dietary notebook and the number of potential days to be completed; and (2) the treatment step reached in the treatment at the last follow-up evaluation. The former did not correlate with improvement, whereas the latter did.

In Spain, a controlled (but not randomized) trial of 93 DSM-IV patients with BN was conducted using the self-help guide (Fernández-Aranda, 2005). Thirty-one patients received the Internet-based therapy. There were two control groups: 31 patients who received brief psychoeducational group therapy (PET) and 31 patients who remained on a waiting list. At the end of treatment, 32.3% of patients in the Internet-treatment group had a full remission of bulimic symptoms compared with 37.6% of patients in the PET group and only 3% in WL. There were no significant differences between the two treatment conditions on dropout rates (35.5% Internet-based treatment vs. 16.1% in the PET group).

COMPUTER-BASED SELF-HELP
INTERVENTIONS FOR BINGE-EATING DISORDER

An as yet unpublished randomized controlled trial compared traditional group CBT with a CD-ROM–based CBT program and with a waiting-list control group for the treatment of overweight adults with BED (Shapiro, Bulik, Reba, & Dymek-Valentine, 2005). Sixty-six participants were randomized to one of the treatment conditions. Participants in the group-therapy condition received 10 weekly sessions of CBT for BED. Individuals in the CD-ROM condition received the CD and a suggested 10-week schedule for completion and were instructed to contact the research assistant as needed for technical questions or concerns about their clinical condition. The wait-list-control condition lasted 10 weeks. Following this period participants were given the option of either group therapy or self-help with CD-ROM. Preliminary results at the end of the treatment phase indicated that the group-CBT condition had a significantly higher dropout rate than CD-ROM or wait-list-control conditions. At the end of the treatment phase in comparison with the wait-list control, both the CD-ROM and group-treatment conditions showed trends toward decreased weight, increased daily fruit and vegetable consumption, and decreased fast-food consumption. Finally, 76% of those who completed the wait-list condition chose to receive the CD-ROM over group therapy.

PATIENT FACTORS AFFECTING
ACCEPTANCE OF COMPUTERIZED SELF-HELP

One study has examined in detail the characteristics and subjective appraisals of patients who choose to accept or decline to use the *Overcoming*

Bulimia CD-ROM self-help package (Murray et al., 2003). In this study of 81 patients, sociodemographic background, severity of symptoms, duration of illness, and comorbidity did not differ between those patients who agreed to use the CD-ROM package and those who declined. There was also no significant difference between the groups in patients' attitudes toward self-help, perceptions of usefulness of self-help for others, or previous use of self-help treatments. The only significant factor identified was that the patients who agreed to use the CD-ROM package significantly more commonly endorsed the view that this treatment would be useful for them (Murray et al., 2003). This study also had a qualitative component that suggested that patients who began the treatment were more "willing to give it a try" (p. 250) and understood that self-help was a first step in treatment. In contrast, those who did not begin the program saw the CD-ROM "as a replacement of a human therapist" (p. 251) and as a kind of cheap or "ersatz" therapy.

THERAPISTS' KNOWLEDGE, BELIEFS ABOUT, AND ATTITUDES TOWARD COMPUTERIZED SELF-HELP

One study to date has examined therapists' attitudes toward the use of computerized self-help treatments for BN (Hitchman, 2004). A focus group with professionals working for a specialist eating-disorders service within the National Health Service (NHS) informed the development of a 27-item questionnaire probing into knowledge of, attitudes toward, and potential usage of computerized self-help treatments for patients with eating disorders. A survey of 83 accredited eating-disorder therapists and practitioners working both within the U.K. NHS and in private practice in London was conducted. Perhaps unsurprisingly, therapists who identified themselves as using a predominantly cognitive-behavioral therapeutic orientation held significantly more positive attitudes toward computerized self-help than therapists from other orientations, such as psychodynamic, systemic, and humanistic therapists. Overall, one-third (32.5%) of respondents were not familiar with any computerized self-help treatments for psychological disorders, and almost half (48.2%) had not worked with patients who had used this method of treatment. Despite this seemingly low level of familiarity with computerized treatment, virtually all of the respondents felt that self-help had at least some role to play in the treatment of patients with eating disorders. Most thought that in terms of its efficacy, computerized self-help would be somewhere in the middle, between written formats of self-help (which were seen as less effective) and face-to-face therapies (which were seen as more effective). Respondents thought that the more interactive and structured nature of the CD-ROM intervention aided patients in working through the interaction systematically rather than "dipping in," which can often be the case with manualized self-help treatments. Most thought that computerized self-help would be more beneficial to patients with BN than to those with anorexia nervosa (AN) and more beneficial to those patients with BN who had a shorter duration of illness and mild to moderate bulimic symptom levels. Therapists also identified a number of concerns regarding the use of computerized treatment for BN—for example, that the lack of a therapeutic relationship, emotional response, and feedback from the computer might result in a less attractive and beneficial experience for the patient. Other concerns included beliefs that the use of computerized therapies could reinforce and exacerbate the interpersonal and emotional processing difficulties common with this disorder.

The study included an assessment of therapist attitudes to self-help before and after a 1-day training course in the use of a computerized self-help program. After the training there was a significant improvement in therapists' knowledge of computerized self-help packages and a shift in the direction of more positive therapist attitudes toward this mode of treatment delivery (Hitchman, 2004).

DISCUSSION

These are exciting times in terms of the development of technology-based treatments for eating disorders. Advances in technologies coupled with a greater understanding of what works in terms of treatments for BN and BED have led to a point at which enthusiasts argue that computer-based self-help treatments now so closely resemble current evidence-based treatments that the only reason that they are dubbed "self-help" is that a health professional is not physically present (Richards, 2004). However, in trying to get the best out of these packages, a number of factors need to be considered.

Patient Selection

Computerized treatments are unlikely to appeal to all potential users, and some may feel "put off" by the concept of computerized treatment, seeing it as cold and impersonal. Others, however, see it as a desirable means of engaging in the process of change and often as helpful preparation for individual therapy (Murray et al., 2003). We still know very little about who will begin, persist with, and benefit most from computerized or Web-based treatments for BN and BED. This is perhaps unsurprising, given that our knowledge of these factors is limited for *any* type of treatment of BN and BED, not just for computerized self-help. What is clear so far is that those people who have a positive view of self-help approaches in general are more likely to accept computerized treatment than those who are less positive about the usefulness of self-help treatments for themselves. What underlies these beliefs is not clear. It is conceivable that beliefs about the efficacy of self-help are linked in a complicated fashion to other illness beliefs and self-beliefs a person may hold. However, we also need to learn much more about how symptom severity, different types of comorbidity, and the availability of social support affect acceptance and efficacy of computerized treatments in different eating disorders.

Delivery of Treatment

Much thought must be put into establishing optimum methods of access to and delivery of computerized treatments. Computer treatments can be used as a stand-alone treatment, and in the future many will perhaps be commercially available, just as many self-help books are. Alternatively, they can be used as part of a stepped-care model of treatment within clinical services with different levels of clinician support (Mains & Scogin, 2003).

Packages such as *Overcoming Bulimia* have been successfully used within eating-disorder clinics, where access to support by specialist professionals is readily available should the person using the package feel "stuck," experience difficulty using the package, or have a crisis. Additionally, the sense of inclusion within a clinical service has been reported by people using the package to promote adherence to the package. This method of delivery, however, is often less flexible for those people for whom treatment must be incorporated into a busy lifestyle that does not accommodate clinic hours. For those individuals, private use at home or in a more accessible venue (such as in a primary care facility, public access area, or public library), either through possession of the package or access via the Internet, may feel more acceptable. In the one currently available study of Internet-based self-help treatments for BN and BED, a high number of study participants did in fact predominantly use the package in the evenings and on weekends (Fernández-Aranda et al., 2005). This kind of increased flexibility for the patient is mirrored by increased flexibility for supporting clinicians, who can give e-mail support at a time and place convenient for them. Very little is known about the frequency, type, and nature of support needed to optimize outcomes.

For some people, however, the appeal of computerized treatments may be precisely their potential independence from clinical services and the avoidance of stigma that can be associated with seeking psychological treatment through conventional health care channels. Using treatment in this way does require the person using the package to be highly self-directed to keep up with the sessions without prompting from service staff, if the treatment is sought entirely independently of services. This method of delivery, without any connection to formal or voluntary health care services, may be more problematic should the person using the package experience problems in terms of lack of progress or acute crises.

One must also consider the C-CBT user's need for technical support when using such a treatment package. If this is used as a stand-alone treatment outside of clinical services, one must consider how package users will gain technical support should they experience difficulties using the package. One must also consider how package updates might be disseminated to users; perhaps this would be done via an Internet website, as is currently the case with software packages for the computer.

Clinicians' Views

In the only survey so far of eating disorder therapists' views about computerized treatments, therapists from different therapeutic orientations differed in their attitudes toward computerized self-help-based treatments, with those practicing CBT being most open to the idea, whereas those with training in other treatment modalities (family, psychodynamic) usually were more skeptical and had more concerns (Hitchman, 2004). Similar concerns have also been identified by therapists in relation to computer-assisted therapies for other disorders (Newman, 2004).

This difference between CBT practitioners and those of different therapeutic orientations in respect to computerized treatments is not surprising. Within CBT, although a positive working alliance is considered important, the central focus is on teaching patients new skills and how to practice in the "real world" as "homework" between sessions in order to make meaningful and lasting changes to their disorders. The CBT stance of "what you put in is what you get out" is very much in keeping with what happens in self-help approaches. In contrast, therapists trained in treatments in which the "curative relationship" holds the central role as the method of change (Newman, Erickson, Przeworski, & Dzus, 2003) may find that a package designed for skills development based on an adult learning model of therapy does not sit easily with their idea of what is helpful to their patients.

Thus, in any clinical setting in which computerized treatments are to be used, training of therapists in the package and how to deliver it is vital for the successful implementation of the package.

CONCLUSIONS AND FUTURE DIRECTIONS

These are early days in relation to the development of computerized treatments for BN and BED, and there is much exciting opportunity for increasing our currently rather limited knowledge of how these treatments work and what works for whom. Clinical trials are currently under way within a number of centers, including our own to address some of these questions.

REFERENCES

Bara-Carril, N., Williams, J., Pombo-Carril, M. G., Reid, Y., Murray, K., Aubin, S., et al. (2004). A preliminary investigation into the feasibility and efficacy of a CD-ROM-based cognitive-behavioral self-help intervention for bulimia nervosa. *International Journal of Eating Disorders, 35,* 538–548.

Carrard, I., Rouget, P., Fernández-Aranda, F., Volkart, A-C., Damoiseau, M., & Lam, T. (2006). Evaluation and deployment of evidence-based patient self-management support program for bulimia nervosa. *International Journal of Medical Informatics, 75,* 101–109.

Cavanagh, K., & Shapiro, D. (2004). Computer treatment for common mental health problems. *Journal of Clinical Psychology, 60,* 239–251.

Fernández-Aranda, F. (2005, April). *Internet-based self-help: Guide for treatment of bulimia.* Paper presented at the conference of the Academy of Eating Disorders, Montreal, Quebec, Canada.

Graham, C., Franses, A., Kenwright, M., & Marks, I. (2000). Psychotherapy by computer: A postal survey of responders to a teletext article. *Psychiatric Bulletin, 24,* 331–332.

Hitchman, E. (2004). *An investigation into the attitudes of healthcare professionals towards the use of computerised self-help for patients with eating disorders.* Unpublished manuscript.

Jorm, A. G., Griffiths, K. M., Christensen, H., Korten A. E., Parslow, R. A., & Rodgers, B. (2004). Actions taken to cope with depression at different levels of severity: A community survey. *Psychological Medicine, 34,* 293–299.

Kaltenthaler, E., Shackley, P., Stevens, K., Beverley, C., Parry, G., & Chilcott, J. (2002). A systematic review and economic evaluation of computerised cognitive behaviour therapy for depression and anxiety. *Health Technology Assessments, 6,* 1–89.

Mains, J. A., & Scogin, F. R. (2003). The effectiveness of self-administered treatments: A practice-friendly review of the research. *Journal of Clinical Psychology, 59,* 237–246.

Murray, K., Pombo-Carril, M. G., Bava-Carril, N., Grover, M., Reid, Y., Largh, CF., et al. (2000). Factors determining uptake of a CD-ROM-based CBT self-help treatment for bulimia: Patient characteristics and subjective appraisals of self-help treatment. *European Eating Disorders Review, 11,* 243–260.

Murray, K., Schmidt, U., Pombo-Carril, M. G., Grover, M., Alenya, J., Treasure, J., et al. (2007). Does therapist guidance improve uptake, adherence and outcome from a CD-ROM-based cognitive-behavioural intervention for the treatment of bulimia nervosa? *Computers in Human Behaviour, 23,* 850–859.

National Institute of Clinical Excellence. (2002). *Guidance on the use of computerised cognitive behavioural therapy for anxiety and depression.* Retrieved from *www.nice.org.uk.*

Newman, M. G. (2004). Technology in psychotherapy: An introduction. *Journal of Clinical Psychology, 60,* 141–145.

Newman, M. G., Erickson, T., Przeworski, A., & Dzus, E. (2003). Self-help and minimal contact therapies for anxiety disorders: Is human contact necessary for therapeutic efficacy? *Journal of Clinical Psychology, 59,* 251–274.

Oliver, M. I., Pearson, N., Coe, N., & Gunnell, D. (2005). Help-seeking behaviour in men and women with common mental health problems: Cross-sectional study. *British Journal of Psychiatry, 186,* 297–301.

Proudfoot., J. G. (2004). Computer-based treatment for anxiety and depression: Is it feasible? Is it effective? *Neuroscience and Biobehavioral Reviews, 28,* 353–363.

Richards, D. (2004) Self-help: Empowering service users or aiding cash strapped mental health services? *Journal of Mental Health, 13*(2), 117–123.

Rouget, P., Carrard, I., & Archinard, M. (2005). Self-treatment for bulimia on the Internet: First results in Switzerland. *Revue Medicale Suisse, 2,* 359–361.

Self-help guide for bulimia. (2004). Retrieved October 29, 2005, from *www.cordis.lu/itt/ itt-en/04-4/prog01.htm*

Shapiro, J. R., Bulik, C. M., Reba, L., & Dymek-Valentine, M. (2005, April). *CD-ROM and Web-based CBT treatment for BED and obesity.* Paper presented at the Academy of Eating Disorders International Conference, Montreal, Quebec, Canada.

Williams, C. J., Aubin, S. D., Cottrell, D., & Harkin, P. J. R. (1998). *Overcoming bulimia: A self-help package* [CD-ROM]. Available from *www.calipso.co.uk/mainframe.htm*

PART IV

GROUP SELF-HELP

Perhaps the most commonly sought forms of self-help for weight management are those that use group therapy as the primary treatment modality. Commercial and organized self-help programs provide an environment of structured group support. Treatment techniques are recommended by the program and discussed by its members, and meetings give participants the opportunity to talk about their problems with each other and with a professional or volunteer group leader.

The efficacy of commercial and noncommercial group self-help programs is reviewed in Chapter 9. Chapters 10 and 11 review ways to improve the efficacy of group treatment over the long term. Chapter 10 presents the research evidence on improving the management of obesity by extending the length of treatment in guided group support. Chapter 11 discusses the utility of continuing care in the long-term treatment of obesity and the implications of this approach for group self-help.

9

Commercial and Organized Self-Help Programs for Weight Management

ADAM GILDEN TSAI *and* THOMAS A. WADDEN

The United States is experiencing an epidemic of obesity, and health care providers from a variety of disciplines must play a role in its prevention and treatment. A joint task force of the National Heart, Lung, and Blood Institute (NHLBI) and the North American Association for the Study of Obesity (NAASO) has issued guidelines for the assessment and treatment of obesity (NHLBI & NAASO, 2000). Assessment includes calculation of the patient's body mass index (BMI), measurement of the waist circumference, and determination of cardiovascular risk factors. The risk of diabetes and other comorbidities increases with increasing BMI and waist circumference (NHLBI, 1998). Weight losses as little as 5–7% of initial weight, combined with increased physical activity, may be sufficient to ameliorate or prevent many of the medical complications of obesity (NHLBI, 1998; Diabetes Prevention Program Research Group, 2002; World Health Organization, 2000; Institute of Medicine, 1995; Blackburn, 1995; Tuomilehto et al., 2001; Frank, 1993).

The joint task force proposed a treatment algorithm that recommends more intensive interventions for patients with higher BMIs and in which lifestyle modification (i.e., dietary counseling, increased physical activity, and behavior therapy) is the cornerstone of treatment for all obese patients (NHLBI & NAASO, 2000). The U.S. Preventive Services Task Force (2003) has concluded that only intensive interventions (i.e., more than one visit per month for the first 3 months) are effective for weight loss. Physicians and other health care providers, however, are often not prepared to provide intensive counseling to assist patients with lifestyle modification (Frank, 1993; Stafford, Farhat, Misra, & Schoenfeld, 2000). In addition, reimbursement for weight management has usually been suboptimal (Downey, 2002). As a result, numerous commercial and proprietary weight-management programs have arisen (Cleland et al., 2001).

The chapters in this volume describe self-help interventions for weight control and the management of eating disorders. As noted by Latner (2001), limited payment for professional treatment and the growing clinical need may render self-help programs the only feasible model for long-term weight management. In this chapter, we review the largest commercial and self-help programs in the United States (as defined by numbers of participants). Our review considers only organized programs, which are interventions that require regular counseling visits, either in person or online. These programs vary in the degree to which they provide active support. For example, some interventions offer weekly group treatment, whereas others provide individual treatment several times a week. The amount and type of treatment provided by program differs widely.

We reviewed programs by drawing from two prior publications (Womble, Wang, & Wadden, 2002; Tsai & Wadden, 2005) and by using criteria proposed by an expert panel convened by the Federal Trade Commission (Cleland et al., 2001). The panel recommended that commercial weight-loss providers disclose information about four aspects of their interventions: (1) central program components; (2) staff qualifications; (3) costs; and (4) risks of treatment (see Table 9.1). (Several panel members also called for disclosure of outcome data, but some members from industry suggested that they did not have adequate resources or expertise to provide such data.) We used a previously developed system (Stern et al., 1995) to classify programs as nonmedical, medically supervised, or self-help, to which we added Internet-based.

PLAN OF THE REVIEW

A description of the intervention is provided for each program, including the type and frequency of counseling, provider qualifications, and costs. For purposes of comparison, we estimated the cost of participating in each program for 12 weeks. We then reviewed the studies that have been published of each program. In our search for clinical trials, we focused first on randomized trials, followed by multicenter and/or prospective observational studies. Lowest priority was given to retrospective observational

TABLE 9.1. Voluntary Guidelines for Disclosure by Commercial
Weight-Loss Programs

Criteria	Description
Program content	• Major components of weight-loss program (educational format, specifics of diet, physical activity programs, behavioral counseling)
Staff qualifications	• Program staff training, certification, and experience
Costs	• One-time costs (entry or termination fees) • Recurring costs (weekly fees, meals) • Optional costs (long-term maintenance program) • Refundable costs (based on weight loss)
Program risks	• Specific program risks (risk from medications, supplements, physical activity provided in the program) • Risk of rapid weight loss (cholelithiasis)

Note. Data from Partnership for Healthy Weight Management (www.consumer.gov/weightloss). Adapted from Womble, Wang, and Wadden (2002). Copyright 2002 by The Guilford Press. Adapted by permission.

studies, in which data are reported for only a subset of participants, such as program completers or individuals with long-term follow-up data. Such studies provide the weakest evidence. Descriptions are provided of several programs that have not been formally evaluated, simply because they treat such large numbers of individuals. As mentioned, the review includes only programs that require in-person or online visits. Thus diet books and foods are not considered here (see Chapter 2, this volume, for a review).

NONMEDICAL COMMERCIAL PROGRAMS

Nonmedical programs are defined by their use of nonphysician personnel to facilitate clients' weight loss. As shown in Table 9.2, staff members at such programs may include former clients, peer counselors, or laypersons trained by the parent company. Occasionally, degree-trained professionals (i.e., dietitians, exercise specialists, nurses, etc.) may provide counseling, often as a backup to lay providers. These programs do not provide medical supervision. Thus persons with obesity-related diagnoses need to be monitored by their own primary care providers while participating in such programs. Nonmedical commercial programs aim to induce a weight loss of 1–2 pounds a week (0.4–0.9 kg/week), which is considered safe (NHLBI & NAASO, 2000; NHLBI, 1998). The three largest nonmedical commercial programs in the United States currently are Weight Watchers, Jenny Craig, and LA Weight Loss.

TABLE 9.2. Central Program Components of Selected Commercial and Self-Help Weight-Loss Programs

Program	Staff qualifications	Diet	Physical activity	Behavior modification	Support
Weight Watchers	Successful lifetime member	LCD; exchange diet; clients prepare own meals	"Get Moving" booklet distributed	Behavioral weight-control methods	Group sessions, weekly meetings
Jenny Craig	Company-trained counselor	LCD; Jenny Craig meals required	Audiotapes for walking	Manual on weight-loss strategies provided	Individual sessions, weekly contact
LA Weight Loss	Company-trained counselor	LCD; clients prepare own meals	Optional walking videotape	Included in counseling sessions	Individual sessions, three times weekly
HMR	Licensed physician and other health care providers	LCD/VLCD using meal replacement products; three-phase program	Walking and calorie charts provided in lifestyle classes	Included in lifestyle classes; accountability and skill acquisition emphasized	Group sessions, weekly classes; some telephone support
OPTIFAST	Licensed physician and other health care providers	LCD using meal-replacement products; three-phase program	Physical activity modules taught in lifestyle classes	Included in lifestyle classes; stress management and social support emphasized	Group sessions, weekly classes; some telephone support
Medifast/TSFL	Company-trained counselor (TSFL only)	LCD/VLCD using meal-replacement products; three-phase program	Included in TSFL	Included in TSFL	Included in TSFL
eDiets.com	Company-trained counselor and company dietitians	LCD using "virtual dietitian" program; clients prepare own meals	Physical activity seminar[a] as part of eDiets.com U	Included in eDiets.com U;[a] stress management emphasized	Individual and group Internet support
TOPS	Group leader elected by local chapter	LCD exchange plan recommended	Members make plan with their health care providers	Included in TOPS curriculum	Group format; weekly sessions
OA	Volunteer chapter leaders	No specific recommendation	Members make plan with their health care providers	12-step program	Group format; weekly sessions; sponsors

Note. LCD, low-calorie diet; VLCD, very-low-calorie diet; TSFL, Take Shape for Life; TOPS, Take Off Pounds Sensibly; OA, Overeaters Anonymous; HMR, Health Management Resources.

[a] eDiets.com University.

182

Weight Watchers

Program Components

Weight Watchers provides 1-hour weekly meetings, which include dietary counseling and group support (see Table 9.2). The dietary plan is similar to the exchange diet developed by the American Diabetic Association. The plan assigns point values to foods. Participants can estimate portion sizes using commonly found objects and do not need to count calories. The meal plan is a moderately restricted (hypocaloric) diet, and participants may expect to lose up to 2 pounds (0.9 kg) per week (Weight Watchers, 2003). The weekly meetings also provide social support, instruction in traditional behavioral weight-control techniques, and educational materials that encourage clients to increase their physical activity. Participants are encouraged to select a final goal weight that falls in a "normal" BMI range (20–25 kg/m^2). Persons who reach their goal weight and maintain it for 6 weeks become "lifetime members." This entitles them to attend meetings free of charge as long as they maintain their weight loss within 2 pounds of goal (see Table 9.2; Weight Watchers, 2003).

Costs

Weight Watchers costs approximately $167 for 12 weeks. This includes a $35 membership fee and a $12 weekly pay-as-you-go fee (Table 9.3).

Outcomes

Weight Watchers has sponsored three controlled evaluations of its program (Heshka et al., 2003; Rippe et al., 1998; Djuric et al., 2002) and a fourth (publicly funded) study has recently been published (Dansinger, Gleason, Griffith, Selker, & Schaefer, 2005). In the largest of these studies, 426 participants at six sites were randomly assigned either to weekly Weight Watchers visits or to a self-help intervention that included two 20-minute dietitian visits. Individuals in the Weight Watchers group lost 5.3% of initial weight at year 1 and 3.2% at year 2, whereas those in self-help lost 1.5% and 0%, respectively ($p < 0.001$ at both times). Attrition was 27% and was similar in the two arms (Heshka et al., 2003).

In a second, single-site study (Djuric et al., 2002), 48 women with a history of breast cancer were randomized to: (1) usual care; (2) Weight Watchers (i.e., weekly group counseling); (3) individual counseling provided by a dietitian; or (4) the two latter interventions combined. At a 1-year follow-up assessment, individuals in usual care had gained 0.9 kg, whereas those in the other groups had lost 2.6, 8.0, and 9.4 kg, respectively. Total attrition after 1 year was 19%. (The authors did not state whether this number differed by group.) Persons in groups 3 and 4 lost significantly

TABLE 9.3. Estimated Program Costs for Commercial, Proprietary, and Self-Help Weight Loss Programs

Program	Costs Membership fee/initial cost	Periodic fees	Meal plan	Other	Estimated cost for 3-month program[a]
Weight Watchers	$35 for first week (membership fee)	$12/week, pay-as-you-go fee	Not required	None	$167
Jenny Craig	$199 for 1 year, $399 for 3 years	None	$70–$105/week ($10–$15/day)	$10 for second of two weight-loss manuals	$1,249
LA Weight Loss	$79	Upfront costs of $7/week x no. of weeks calculated to reach goal weight	None	$10 for optional walking videotape	Not calculated[b]
HMR	$150–$300 for medical evaluation	$35/week for medical visits and lab tests; $35/week for behavior modification	$68–86/week for VLCD plan	Maintenance visits at extra cost	$1,800–$2,000
OPTIFAST	$150–$300 for medical evaluation	$35/week for physician visits, $10/week for behavior modification	$97/week for "full fast" meal replacement	Laboratory tests, EKGs, and maintenance visits at extra cost	$1,800–$2,000
Medifast/ TSFL	None	Not required	$70 or $56/week (full or partial meal replacement)	Physician visits at extra cost	$840[c]
eDiets.com	None	$65/3 months	None	Individual counseling with experts at extra cost	$65
TOPS	$20/year	$0.50–$1.00/week	None	None	$26
OA	None	Donations	None	None	$0

Note. HMR, Health Management Resources; VLCD, very-low-calorie diet; TSFL, Take Shape for Life; TOPS, Take Off Pounds Sensibly; OA, Overeaters Anonymous. Costs were estimated from discussions with company representatives and calls to programs in the Philadelphia area. Costs are estimated in 2003 U.S. dollars and should be considered approximate and subject to change (with special offers, incentives, and other considerations). Costs also may vary within the same program from site to site and with geographic region.
[a]The estimated cost includes charges for the first visit (e.g., membership fee or initial evaluation) and 12 subsequent visits. "Other" costs are not included in the estimated cost for the 3 months.
[b]Costs for LA Weight Loss were not estimated because of insufficient information. Applicants are given a weight-loss goal at their initial evaluation and are requested (at this visit) to pay for the number of weeks (of consultation) required to reach their goal (at a cost of $7 a week). Persons who withdraw early are reimbursed for unused visits minus a fee of $149.
[c]Costs are estimated for full meal-replacement plan.

more weight than those in group 1 (both ps < 0.05), and there were no other differences between groups (Djuric et al., 2002). Thus, in this small study, Weight Watchers was not more beneficial than usual care or when added to individual counseling. In a third study, 80 women at one site were randomly assigned to Weight Watchers or to usual care. At 12 weeks, participants lost 7.5% and 1.6%, respectively, of initial weight (p < 0.001), with attrition of 25 and 65%, respectively. No long-term data were reported (Rippe et al., 1998). Finally, in a recent study, 160 persons were randomly assigned to Weight Watchers, the Atkins Diet, the Ornish Diet, or the Zone Diet (Dansinger et al., 2005). Weight losses at 1 year (as a percentage of initial weight) were 3.1%, 2.1%, 3.2%, and 3.2%, respectively, with no significant differences between groups. Attrition was 35%, 47%, 50%, and 35%, respectively (p = .08 for the comparison of Atkins and Ornish with Weight Watchers and Zone), with no significant differences between groups among participants who submitted food records. It is unclear why participants in the Weight Watchers arm in this study lost less weight at 1 year than persons in the study by Heshka et al. (2003). (Participants in the Heshka et al. study attended actual Weight Watchers meetings and thus could have received more intensive coaching and social support; see also Chapter 1, this volume.)

There are two published case series reports of Weight Watchers (Christakis & Miller-Kovach, 1996; Lowe, Miller-Kovach, & Phelan, 2001). In the first of these, 1,200 Weight Watchers lifetime members were interviewed by telephone. In subgroups based on time since participation, 97%, 80%, 53%, and 37% of individuals were within 5 pounds of goal weight at 1, 2, 3–4, and 5–12 years after the program, respectively (Christakis & Miller-Kovach, 1996). In the second report, 1,002 Weight Watchers lifetime members were sampled, and a separate sample of 258 persons was evaluated in person to develop a correction factor for underreporting of weight. These 1,002 lifetime members had lost 15.4% of initial weight to reach their goal. When corrected for underreporting, subgroups based on time since participation maintained losses of 10.5%, 7.1%, 6.2%, 3.4%, and 3.6% of initial weight at 1, 2, 3, 4, and 5 years after the program, respectively (Lowe et al., 2001). Neither of these two studies accounted for individuals who refused to participate in the telephone surveys.

Jenny Craig

Program Components

The main components of the Jenny Craig program are: (1) individual dietary counseling and (2) prepackaged meals (see Table 9.2; Jenny Craig,

2003). Counselors meet weekly with clients, either in person or by phone, to help them plan their menus (Jenny Craig, 2003). Participants also may call in for additional support 24 hours a day, 7 days a week. The purchase of Jenny Craig meals is strongly encouraged. The meals provide a balanced, hypocaloric diet (1,200–2,300 kcal/day), which is expected to induce a weight loss of approximately 1–2 pounds (0.5–0.9 kg) per week (Jenny Craig, 2003). Clients are encouraged to select a goal BMI of between 20 and 25 kg/m^2. At the time of inquiry, Jenny Craig offered a "gold" membership for 1 year or a "platinum" membership that usually lasts for 3 years or more and includes monthly maintenance counseling sessions after the first year.

Costs

Jenny Craig costs approximately $1,249 for 12 weeks, which includes the $199 sign-up fee for the 1-year standard plan and $10–15/day for food (Table 9.3). The platinum plan would cost approximately $1,549, including the sign-up fee.

Outcomes

There are two published reports of the Jenny Craig program. In the first, a national sample of participants ($n = 60,164$) was tracked from enrollment until discontinuation for up to 1 year (Finley, 2006). On average, clients used the program for 11 weeks, losing an average of 5.0 kilograms (5.6% of initial weight). Retention rates were 73%, 42%, 22%, and 7% at 4, 13, 26, and 52 weeks, respectively. Weight losses were greater with increasing duration in the program (1.1 %, 8.3%, 12.6%, and 15.6%, respectively).

The second report from Jenny Craig was a retrospective case series of 517 individuals who completed the program and who reached (or nearly reached) their goal weight. Of these 517 persons, 256 participated in a I-year follow-up evaluation (conducted by telephone). Women and men in the study lost 19% and 20% of initial weight during active treatment and at 1-year follow-up were maintaining weight losses of 16.3% and 15.4%, respectively (Wolfe, 1996). Jenny Craig is currently conducting a randomized trial of its program, the initial results of which are expected sometime in 2007.

LA Weight Loss

Program Components

LA Weight Loss uses in-person counseling to emphasize dietary education and behavior modification. Visits take place three times per week (Table

9.2). The intervention is conducted in three phases: (1) a weight-loss phase (which varies according to the individual's current and ideal body weight), during which clients aim to lose 2 pounds (0.9 kg) per week while consuming a moderately restricted hypocaloric diet; (2) a stabilization program that lasts approximately 6 weeks; and (3) a long-term maintenance phase (LA Weight Loss, 2003). The length of counseling sessions reportedly varies according to client need. Participants consume a hypocaloric diet of conventional foods; no prepackaged meals are required (LA Weight Loss, 2003). However, clients are encouraged to use measuring devices and scales to estimate portion size and calories. Individuals select a goal weight, but it does not have to fall in the BMI range of 20–25 kg/m^2 (Table 9.2).

Costs

It is difficult to estimate the costs of the LA Weight Loss program. Participants are asked to pay, in advance, $7 per week, multiplied by the number of weeks needed to reach goal weight (Table 9.3). There is also a sign-up fee of $79. For example, an individual who needs to lose 25 pounds to reach goal weight would require 12 weeks at a total cost of $569 ($79 sign-up fee plus 12 weeks active weight loss x $7 plus 58 weeks of stabilization and maintenance x $7).

Outcomes

Our search revealed no published articles on the efficacy of LA Weight Loss.

Summary of Nonmedical Commercial Programs

Weight Watchers is the only nonmedical program whose efficacy has been evaluated in randomized trials. Participants who adhere to the program can expect to lose approximately 5% of initial weight, the goal recommended by several scientific panels (NHLBI, 1998; World Health Organization, 2000; Institute of Medicine, 1995). Individuals in the Weight Watchers studies by Heshka et al. (2003) and Dansinger et al. (2005) regained weight during the latter half of the trials. This is typical for persons treated with lifestyle modification (Tate, Jackvony, & Wing, 2003; Wadden, Berkowitz, Sarwer, Prus-Wisniewski, & Steinberg, 2001). However, in the Heshka study, participants who attended the most group sessions during the 2 years of the study maintained the largest weight losses. This demonstrates the importance of encouraging patients to attend treatment regularly.

Jenny Craig and LA Weight Loss, though widely available, are not as well supported by evidence. Controlled studies of these two programs are needed. (The randomized trial of Jenny Craig will be a useful comparison.) However, the national study sponsored by Jenny Craig is a good example of a naturalistic analysis, in which all participants enrolling in the program are tracked until their time of discontinuation. These data provide a more realistic estimate of weight loss in commerical programs (in the report by Finley et al., 5.6% of initial weight during an average of 11 weeks of participation). The results from Jenny Craig are consistent with an older study (not described in detail here because average weight loss could not be calculated), in which 50% and 70% of participants stopped attending Weight Watchers after 6 and 12 weeks, respectively (Volkmar, Stunkard, Woolston, & Bailey, 1981).

Regarding cost, Weight Watchers is moderately priced at $12 a week, although it is probably still too expensive for some populations with high rates of obesity (persons of low socioeconomic status, including those from some ethnic minority groups). The cost of prepackaged meals renders Jenny Craig an expensive program, although, if the cost of conventional table foods is considered, the costs of Weight Watchers and Jenny Craig are more similar. The costs of LA Weight Loss are difficult to determine, as described previously.

Participants in Weight Watchers and LA Weight Loss are counseled to follow a meal plan of their own choice (composed of conventional foods). Jenny Craig provides most or all meals during the weight-loss phase; participants may have difficulty transitioning from this diet to a diet of conventional foods. All three programs provide counseling for physical activity and behavior modification, although the ultimate benefit of this support for LA Weight Loss cannot be determined in the absence of data.

MEDICALLY SUPERVISED PROPRIETARY PROGRAMS

Medically supervised programs include physician care. Thus they are suitable for individuals with obesity-related health complications. In the past, these programs used very-low-calorie diets (VLCDs), which contain fewer than 800 kcal per day and include large amounts of protein (70–100 g/d) to preserve lean body mass (National Task Force on the Prevention and Treatment of Obesity, 1993). (Medically supervised programs have generally shifted to low-calorie, partial-meal-replacement diets that provide 800–1,500 kcal/day, although some companies continue to offer VLCD plans.) VLCDs usually induce losses of 3 pounds or more per week (1.4 kg/week) during the first few months. VLCDs carry a greater risk of side effects than low-calorie regimens, but the diets are considered safe for selected patients under medical supervision (National Task Force on the Prevention and

Treatment of Obesity, 1993). The largest medically supervised proprietary programs are Health Management Resources (HMR), OPTIFAST, and Medifast.

We found a large number of published reports on HMR and OPTIFAST and/or their meal-replacement plans. We review here only studies in which both the diet and the behavioral intervention were provided *as they were offered to the general public* at that time. These are contrasted with studies in which a company's meal-replacement products were combined with an investigator's own behavioral protocol. We note that the studies reviewed here were published a decade or more ago and thus may not accurately reflect the current efficacy of medically supervised diet plans.

Health Management Resources

Program Components

HMR currently offers three weight-loss plans, all of which include meal replacements. The first is a VLCD that includes a range of medical supervision, depending on patients' initial weight and comorbidities (Table 9.2). Participants consume 500–750 kcal per day during the rapid-weight-loss phase and may expect to lose 3 to 6 pounds per week (1.4–2.7 kg). The second plan ("Healthy Solutions"), a low-calorie diet (1,200 kcal/day) designed to induce more gradual weight loss, combines the use of meal replacements with conventional foods. The third HMR offering is a telephone-based program. This plan also is a low-calorie diet, designed to induce more moderate weight loss. Patients can expect to lose 1–2 pounds (0.5–0.9 kg) per week with the moderate plans.

Participants in the two in-person programs attend weekly 90-minute lifestyle modification classes. The curriculum emphasizes accountability (e.g., record keeping). Physical activity is encouraged, especially walking, and participants receive information on the number of calories expended by different amounts and types of activity. The lifestyle modification classes last 18–20 weeks. If participants do not attain their goal weight, they may continue to attend extra classes (and continue using meal replacements) until they do so. The VLCD program takes place in three phases: (1) rapid weight loss (approximately 13 weeks); (2) transition to conventional foods (approximately 6–8 weeks); and (3) maintenance (variable duration). VLCD clients reportedly attend treatment for an average of 18–20 weeks, whereas individuals in the moderately restricted plan generally participate for 13 weeks (Health Management Resources, 2003). The telephone-based program lasts for 6 weeks. HMR encourages all clients to take part in monthly weight maintenance visits after they reach goal weight.

Costs

HMR costs approximately $1,800–2,000 for 12 weeks of treatment. This includes fees for the initial history and physical examination, the cost of meal replacements, and periodic fees for physician visits, lab tests, and classes. Follow-up costs (after the end of the transition phase) are not included in this estimate (Table 9.3).

Outcomes

There are numerous published reports of the HMR program; all of these evaluated the very-low-calorie diet plan (Anderson, Hamilton, Crown-Weber, Riddlemoser, & Gustafson, 1991; Anderson, Brinkman, & Hamilton, 1992; Anderson, Brinkman-Kaplan, Hamilton, et al., 1994; Anderson, Brinkman-Kaplan, Lee, & Wood, 1994; Anderson, Vichitbandra, Qian, & Kryscio, 1999; Bryner et al., 1999; Collins & Anderson, 1995; Daly, 2000; Donnelly, Jacobsen, & Whatley, 1994; Donnelly, Jacobsen, Jakicic, & Whatley, 1994; Hartman, Stroud, Sweet, & Saxton, 1993). Of these studies, five tested the HMR program as it was offered to the public (Anderson et al., 1991, 1992, 1999; Anderson, Brinkman-Kaplan, Hamilton, et al., 1994; Hartman et al., 1993). In the first of these, which was a randomized trial, 40 obese patients with type 2 diabetes were assigned to one of two 800-kcal diets. The first diet provided only HMR liquid meal replacements, whereas the second included meal replacements with one meal per day of conventional foods. Both groups participated in the HMR protocol of intensive lifestyle modification. Weight losses after 12 weeks in the two groups were 15.3% and 14.1%, respectively, of initial weight, with attrition of 0% and 2.5%, respectively. Of the original sample, 36 persons (92%) participated in a 1-year follow-up, at which time they had maintained an 8.4% loss. Results by group were not given separately (Anderson, Hamilton, et al., 1994).

The other four reports of HMR were single-site observational studies. In the longest of these trials, 154 of 426 consecutive enrollees were asked to participate in a follow-up study (Anderson et al., 1999). These 154 individuals had *completed the 12-week core program and lost at least 10 kg during treatment.* Of these 154 invited to participate, 112 provided at least one follow-up weight 2 or more years after the end of treatment (with 70% of weights assessed on site and 30% by self-report). These 112 individuals, clearly a select subset of the original 426 enrollees, lost 27.5% of initial weight during 5 months of treatment. Seventy-six individuals completed a 3-year follow-up, at which time they were maintaining a 6.9% loss. At 5 and 7 years, 15 and 32 patients were maintaining 5.5% and 4.9% losses, respectively. (Some individuals were recaptured between 5 and 7 years; Anderson et al., 1999). A second observational study evaluated 100 consecutive enrollees (71 women, 29 men). Of these, 69 completed at least 17 weeks of treatment (Anderson et al., 1991). Women lost 20.0% and men 16% of initial weight. Three-year weight losses (assessed by telephone) among 58 participants were 7.6% and 6.2%, respectively. In a third study, 80 consecutive enrollees were assessed. Of these, 69 completed the program and lost a mean of 27.3% of initial weight (Anderson et al., 1992). These persons were provided an intensive weight-loss-maintenance program, with every other week meetings after active treatment was completed. Of the 80 patients who enrolled, 46 participated in a 2-year follow-up (either on site or by telephone) and maintained a loss of 13.1%. Finally, a fourth study assessed 138 consecutive enrollees, of whom 102 participated in a 2–3 year telephone follow-up. (The percentage of enrollees completing treatment was not given.) Among the 102 with follow-up data, 73 women and 29 men lost a mean of 24.8% and 28.9% of initial weight, respectively, during the first 22 weeks of treatment. At follow-up, they maintained losses of 9.7% and 12.9%, respectively (Hartman et al., 1993).

All of the data in these five studies, including those for the randomized trial, represent a best-case scenario because of significant attrition during treatment and incomplete follow-up of patients. In addition, the company's meal plans have changed. Studies of the moderate weight loss plans are needed.

OPTIFAST

Program Components

The primary components of the OPTIFAST program are similar to those of HMR (i.e., meal replacements, physician monitoring, and a curriculum of group lifestyle modification; Table 9.2). The meal replacements include shakes, snack bars, and soups. The major difference between the two programs is that OPTIFAST clients are no longer offered a VLCD meal plan. Rather, they are prescribed a low-calorie liquid diet of 800–960 kcal/per day during the period of rapid weight loss. (The majority of published OPTIFAST studies used VLCD meal plans with 420 kcal/day; thus our evaluation of the program may not reflect the effectiveness of the company's current offerings.) The supervising physician conducts the initial history and physical exam and reviews electrocardiograms and periodic laboratory tests. A nurse or physician monitors obesity-related health complications (Table 9.2; OPTIFAST, 2003; see also Chapter 2).

As with HMR, the treatment program has three phases. During the 12- to 16-week full-meal-replacement phase, patients consume only OPTIFAST. This is followed by a 4 to 6 week transition phase in which conventional table foods are gradually reintroduced (OPTIFAST, 2003). Patients attend weekly lifestyle modification classes (of approximately 60 minutes) during the first two phases. The classes are taught by behaviorists, dietitians, or exercise specialists who are, in turn, retained by the supervising physician. In the third phase, patients are encouraged to attend monthly visits to prevent weight regain and may do so indefinitely (at extra cost; OPTIFAST, 2003).

Costs

OPTIFAST costs approximately $1,800–2,000 for 12 weeks of treatment. This includes fees for an initial history and physical examination, as well as the costs of meal replacements and of the lifestyle modification classes and follow-up physician visits. This estimate does not include lab tests, electrocardiograms (EKGs), or follow-up visits after the first two phases of treatment (Table 9.3).

Outcomes

There have been multiple studies of the OPTIFAST program (Barrows & Snook, 1987; Beliard, Kirschenbaum, & Fitzgibbon, 1992; Doherty et al., 1991; Flynn & Walsh, 1993; Genuth, Castro, & Vertes, 1974; Grodstein et al., 1996; Kanders, Blackburn, Lavin, & Norton, 1989; Kirschner, Schneider, Ertel, & Gorman, 1988; Vertes, Genuth, & Hazelton, 1977; Wadden, Foster, Letizia, & Stunkard, 1992; Wadden & Frey, 1997). Five of these reports, all observational studies, tested the program as it was offered to the public (Flynn & Walsh, 1993; Grodstein et al., 1996; Kanders et al., 1989; Wadden et al., 1992; Wadden & Frey, 1997). The highest quality of these was a prospective multicenter analysis that enrolled 517 consecutive persons. Two hundred eighty-five participants (55%) finished the 26-week program (Wadden et al., 1992). Women who completed treatment lost 21% and men lost 25% of initial weight. (Women and men who dropped out lost 13.6% and 15.5%, respectively.) In a 1-year follow-up, with weights measured on site, 118 treatment completers participated out of 160 who were invited. These 118 individuals maintained losses of 13% (women) and 15.4% (men; Wadden et al., 1992). A second multicenter evaluation surveyed 929 participants who completed at least 3 weeks of treatment (Kanders et al., 1989). Over 16 weeks, women and men lost 19 and 20.0% of initial weight, respectively. The percentage of patients who completed the program was not reported. A 1-year follow-up of 704 women and men (i.e., 76% of the sample that completed 3 weeks' treatment), conducted by telephone, revealed losses of 14.3 and 14.8%, respectively. (These 704 persons participated in a weight-maintenance program after the completion of active treatment.)

   In addition to the studies described here, three studies of OPTIFAST included follow-up evaluations at or after 2 years, with weights assessed by telephone or mail (Flynn & Walsh, 1993; Grodstein et al., 1996; Wadden

& Frey, 1997). One study evaluated 306 consecutive enrollees at a single OPTIFAST program. Two-year follow-up data were obtained on a subset of 255 of these individuals (Flynn & Walsh, 1993). The 255 individuals studied lost 19.6% of initial weight during 24 weeks of treatment; 112 of the 255 (44%) completed treatment. After 2 years, the 255 patients reported a mean loss of 5.6% (Flynn & Walsh, 1993). A second study, this one a multicenter study, obtained follow-up data on 621 of 1,283 patients who completed a 26-week program (Wadden & Frye, 1997). Among the 621 participants, weight losses at the end of active treatment were 22.6% for women and 25.5% for men. At the 2-year follow-up, mean losses declined to 9.1 and 13.1%, respectively. A total of 337 participants participated in a 5-year assessment, at which time women and men maintained losses of 5.1 and 7.3%, respectively. A third study, also multicenter, mailed a questionnaire to 325 individuals who completed an 18-week or 26-week OPTIFAST program (Grodstein et al., 1996). A total of 192 persons responded to the questionnaire. These individuals had lost 21% of initial weight during treatment but maintained a loss of only 2.9% at 3-year follow-up (Grodstein et al., 1996).

Medifast

Program Components

Medifast offers a meal plan that provides 450 or more kcal per day (Table 9.2; Medifast, 2003). Unlike HMR and OPTIFAST, Medifast is sold directly to the public. At the time of inquiry, clients were instructed to use the meal replacements either as a sole source of nutrition (i.e., the "complete plan") or as a supplement to one meal a day of lean meat and low-carbohydrate vegetables (i.e., the "modified plan"; Medifast, 2003). Participants were told to expect a loss of 3 to 7 pounds (1.4 to 3.2 kg) a week with the complete plan and 2 to 4 pounds (0.9 to 1.8 kg) a week with the modified plan (Medifast, 2003). Thus the "complete plan" is clearly a VLCD, whereas the "modified plan" falls close to the 800 kcal/per day cutoff between a VLCD and a low-calorie diet. (The rate of weight loss with the modified plan almost certainly requires medical monitoring, however.) All Medifast clients can obtain free telephone consultation from company representatives and, when necessary, with the company's registered nurses. Medifast recommends that the meal replacement program last approximately 16 weeks, with a period of 3 to 6 weeks for resuming consumption of conventional foods (Table 9.2).

Medifast states that its VLCD plans require medical monitoring to reduce the risk of side effects (Medifast, 2003), and the company retains a network of physician referrals to provide medical monitoring. However, documentation of physician care is not required for clients to order the product. Instead, participants are reportedly screened by telephone to determine whether they are receiving appropriate medical supervision. This screening may be performed by a company-trained employee or by a nurse, depending on the individual's comorbidities and meal plan. Thus Medifast is not consistently provided to consumers in accordance with guidance for the use of VLCDs suggested by several expert panels, including the National Task Force on the Prevention and Treatment of Obesity (2003). Serious complications, including death, have been reported in obese individuals who consumed VLCDs in the absence of medical supervision (Wadden, Stunkard, Brownell, & Van Itallie, 1983). Additionally, for participants who do actually undergo medical monitoring through their physicians, provision of a concurrent lifestyle modification program (required by HMR and OPTIFAST) is at the discretion of the supervising provider. Participants in Take Shape for Life, a subsidiary of Medifast at the time of inquiry, *do* receive support from a health advisor trained by the company (Take Shape for Life, 2003).

Costs

The cost of Medifast is approximately $840 for 12 weeks. This includes only the cost of meal replacements (Table 9.3).

Outcomes

We were unable to identify any evaluations of the Medifast program. The company's website reports abstracts of two studies, but neither of these has been published.

Summary of Medically Monitored Programs

Results of studies sponsored by HMR and OPTIFAST suggest that persons who complete a comprehensive low-calorie or very-low-calorie diet program may lose approximately 15–25% of initial weight during the first 4–6 months of treatment. Successful program completers can expect to maintain an average loss of 8–9% of initial weight at 1 year after treatment, 7% at 3 years, and 5% at 4 years (Anderson et al., 1991; Anderson, Brinkman-Kaplan, Lee, & Wood, 1994; Anderson, Brinkman-Kaplan, Hamilton, et al., 1994; Flynn & Walsh, 1993; Wadden et al., 1992). However, these values certainly represent a best-case estimate. They do not account for individuals who dropped out of treatment or declined follow-up assessments (Beliard et al., 1992). Finally, several studies used self-reported weights. This method is likely to have overestimated program efficacy.

An ideal study of either the HMR or the OPTIFAST program would randomize participants to a (very) low-calorie meal replacement program or to a balanced 1,200–1,500 kcal/per day diet of conventional foods (i.e., a diet that does not require intensive medical monitoring). Given the high costs of medically supervised programs, such a study would also include an economic analysis. Because of the large initial weight losses and substantial reductions maintained by some patients several years after treatment, some investigators have argued in favor of VLCDs (Anderson, Konz, Frederich, & Wood, 2001; Astrup & Rossner, 2000). However, after reviewing the results of randomized trials that compared VLCDs and low-calorie diets (LCDs), the NHLBI expert panel did not recommend the use of VLCDs (NHLBI, 1998). Our own meta-analysis that compared VLCDs and LCDs confirmed the conclusions of the NHLBI expert panel (Tsai & Wadden, 2006). Finally, the studies reviewed here are now 10 to 15 years old. Both HMR and OPTIFAST have shifted their focus to LCDs. Studies of these newer diet plans are needed.

HMR and OPTIFAST are both expensive (i.e., $1,800–$2,000 for 3 months of treatment). As mentioned previously, this high cost limits access among patient populations with high rates of obesity, including low-SES populations and some minority groups. Medifast is significantly less expensive than HMR or OPTIFAST, but this is only because the company fails to require medical supervision or behavior modification. We reiterate that mandatory medical supervision is critical to the safe use of VLCDs.

INTERNET-BASED COMMERCIAL WEIGHT-LOSS PROGRAMS

Internet-based programs represent the newest form of weight management. Such programs include advice and/or participant contact with counselors, provided by e-mail or accessed via company websites. In this review, we discuss eDiets.com, the only commercial Internet program that has, to our knowledge, been evaluated in a published clinical trial. Many other commercial Internet-based programs are available to the public, including nutrisystem.com, WebMD, DietWatch, CaloriesCount, Weight Watchers online, a-personaldietitian.com, MDdiets, and others (see also Chapter 7, this volume). Clinicians who want more information about Internet weight-loss programs may consult Shape Up America!, a nonprofit weight-management organization that provides a list of online programs (www.shapeup.org).

eDiets.com

Program Components

eDiets.com recommends a hypocaloric diet, designed to induce a loss of up to 2 pounds (0.9 kg) per week, in conjunction with online counseling (Table 9.2; eDiets.com, 2003). Participants choose from 13 different diets, based on their nutritional preferences. The company provides clients with shopping lists and recipes for the diet selected. Participants purchase and prepare all of their own meals. eDiets.com provides additional services with the membership package, including weekly online chats and personalized e-mail counseling from company experts, many of whom are registered dietitians or psychologists.

Costs

eDiets.com charges $65 for 13 weeks' participation in the program (Table 9.3).

Outcomes

eDiets.com had not sponsored any evaluations of its program at the time of this writing. However, Womble and colleagues (Womble et al., 2004) randomized 46 individuals to either eDiets.com (as available on the Internet from February 2001 to September 2002) or to treatment with a behavioral weight-loss manual (i.e., *The LEARN Program for Weight Management 2000*) (Brownell, 2000). Each person was provided with five 20-minute visits with a psychologist to review his or her progress, as well as 11 brief assessment visits at which weight was measured. Participants in eDiets.com lost 0.7 kg (0.9%) and 0.8 kg (1.1%) at weeks 16 and 52, respectively, compared with 3.0 kg (3.6%) and 3.3 kg (4.0%) for patients in the weight-loss-manual group. Using a last-observation-carried-forward analysis, differences in weight loss were statistically significant ($p < .05$) at both time points. Attrition was 34% at both week 16 and week 52 and did not differ significantly between groups.

Summary of Internet-Based Programs

Currently, minimal evidence exists to recommend *commercial* Internet interventions for weight loss. Results of the study by Womble et al. (2004) are likely to be a best-case scenario concerning the efficacy of eDiets.com (as provided in 2001–2002). The reason is that participants were provided frequent on-site assessment visits and multiple meetings with a psychologist, neither of which is offered to eDiets.com subscribers. Thus larger controlled evaluations are needed to assess the efficacy of eDiets.com and other Internet-based commercial weight-loss programs.

The results of two randomized trials from Internet programs *based at an academic medical center* suggest that participants should keep daily records of their food intake and physical activity, as they do when attending a behavioral weight-loss clinic (Tate, Wing, & Winett, 2001; Tate et al.,

2003). Participants who kept such records and who received regular e-mail feedback on their performance lost over twice as much weight (i.e., approximately 4.5 kg vs. 2 kg) as did participants who received information alone (on proper eating and activity habits; Tate et al., 2003). In addition, a follow-up study demonstrated that after a 6-month behavioral weight-loss program, Internet support was not inferior to frequent in-person support during 18 months of weight maintenance (Harvey-Berino, Pintauro, Buzzell, & Gold, 2004). It is not known whether any of the results just described can be reproduced in commercial programs.

ORGANIZED SELF-HELP PROGRAMS

Organized self-help programs have two important differences when compared with commercial programs. First, they are not for profit, and thus they charge no or minimal fees. Second, they are led by locally selected volunteers. The theory of self-help is that persons who have experienced the same condition (i.e., obesity or overeating) may be more effective counselors. Thus self-help group leaders are individuals who have struggled with weight or eating disorders in the past.

Take Off Pounds Sensibly

Program Components

The Take Off Pounds Sensibly (TOPS) program consists of group meetings that provide social support and a curriculum on diet, physical activity, and behavior change (Table 9.2; Take Off Pounds Sensibly, 2005). The recommended diet is a 1,200, 1,500, or 1,800 kcal/per day meal plan (TOPS, 2005) based on an exchange plan (similar to both the American Diabetes Association diet and the Weight Watchers points system). Members who wish to have additional direction are referred to their individual health care provider. Participants are not asked to set a weight-loss goal.

Costs

TOPS charges a membership fee of $20 per year. In addition, local chapters charge 50 cents or 1 dollar per week to support their costs. Thus, 12 weeks of participation would cost $26–$32 (Table 9.3).

Outcomes

The TOPS website states that its members lost 1,271,466 pounds in 2003, equivalent to over 6 pounds (2.7 kg) per member (TOPS, 2005). These numbers were taken from weekly weigh-ins. There are no recent studies of the TOPS program. Levitz and Stunkard (1974), in an older study, assigned 16 chapters of TOPS to one of four conditions: (1) behavior modification conducted by a professional therapist; (2) behavior modification provided by a TOPS leader; (3) nutrition education conducted by a TOPS leader; or (4) the TOPS program as it was provided in 1974. After 1 year, attrition rates in the four groups were 38%, 41%, 55%, and 67%, respectively. Only those in the first group maintained a significant weight loss (3.2% of initial weight) at the follow-up assessment (Levitz & Stunkard, 1974). The results of this study apparently led to the incorporation of behavior modification in the TOPS program (Womble et al., 2002).

Overeaters Anonymous

Program Components

The theory underlying Overeaters Anonymous (OA) is that obesity is the result of compulsive eating, which in turn is the consequence of anger, sadness, loneliness, and other negative emotions (Overeaters Anonymous, 2003). For many participants, overeating is seen as an addiction to food. Thus the goal of OA is to guide members to physical, emotional, and spiritual recovery (OA, 2003). The program's philosophy and 12-step approach are modeled after those of the older Alcoholics Anonymous. Program content features supportive group meetings and a one-to-one "sponsor" relationship with an established member of the group (Table 9.2). New members are encouraged to call their sponsors daily to discuss weight-management efforts (Anonymous, 1989). Also, participants are asked to explore the underlying social or emotional problems that are leading them to overeat and to then work on these problems (Anonymous, 1989). OA does not recommend any particular diet or exercise plans. Rather, each participant develops his or her own plan. Finally, members are encouraged to attend group meetings indefinitely to maintain their recovery. Apparently, each OA chapter is slightly different; thus patients may need to sample more than one to find the best fit.

Costs

OA relies entirely on member donations to support its program. There are no mandatory fees (Table 9.3).

Outcomes

Our search revealed no studies of the efficacy of OA for weight loss.

Summary of Organized Self-Help Programs

There is minimal scientific evidence to support organized self-help programs. It is unlikely that rigorous studies will be conduced, given the limited financial resources of programs such as TOPS and OA. However, it would seem unreasonable to discourage a patient from using one these of programs, given the minimal financial or physical risks involved. (The OA program, however, should not serve as a substitute for treatment by a trained mental health professional for persons with eating disorders.) Based on the experience of one of us (TAW) in reviewing patients' dieting histories, we believe that only a small minority of patients will lose 5% or more of initial weight by attending TOPS or OA. The TOPS program is similar to Weight Watchers in that it recommends an exchange diet and includes weekly weigh-ins. Conversely, OA may be appropriate for patients who seek intensive emotional support for weight management. Both programs place responsibility for long-term lifestyle modification with the member. Interested clinicians can help their patients by familiarizing themselves with TOPS or OA chapters in their areas.

CONCLUSIONS

Among the nonmedical commercial programs, only Weight Watchers has been demonstrated to be effective in a randomized trial. In their largest study (Heshka et al., 2003), 2-year weight losses were modest (i.e., 3.2% of initial weight) and of questionable clinical significance. However, patients who regularly attend the program may lose approximately 5% of initial weight, which in conjunction with increased physical activity may be sufficient to prevent or improve obesity-related health complications. Regarding medically supervised programs, patients who complete a comprehensive weight-loss program (that includes a lifestyle modification curriculum and medical monitoring) may lose 15–25% of initial weight. However, the probability of weight regain is high, and attrition is close to 50% in such programs. There is little evidence to support commercial Internet or organized self-help programs, although the latter category is a reasonable option given its low cost. Weight Watchers is moderately priced but is probably too costly for many patients in need of treatment. The high cost of medically supervised programs is a deterrent to their use, as discussed earlier.

Supporting Patients' Weight-Loss Efforts

Clinicians may refer to the practical guide developed by the NHLBI/NAASO panel to help them determine which patients have the greatest need for weight loss (NHLBI & NAASO, 2000). For patients participating in organized programs, the provider can facilitate weight management by regularly reviewing changes in diet and activity, weight, and obesity-related diagnoses (Anderson et al., 1999). The clinician should praise patients' success, both for weight loss and for the prevention of weight gain, and should be empathetic toward patients who continue to gain weight. In this fashion, clinicians who treat obese patients can help control the epidemic of obesity.

The intensive degree of counseling needed by some individuals to lose and maintain weight is burdensome, both for the provider and for the clinicians, and, as mentioned earlier, may not be feasible in the current health care system. Thus self-help methods are increasingly important for weight management. Interventions that can help patients build long-term weight management skills (in contrast to those interventions that induce weight loss but that are not as successful with maintenance) will be the most valuable. Some providers, after reading this review, may decide that there is not enough research to recommend commercial or self-help programs to obese individuals. The evidence clearly is modest. Such an assessment, however, would not relieve the clinician of his or her responsibility to assist patients with weight control. Neither practitioners nor their patients can afford to overlook the epidemic of obesity with its profound clinical and economic consequences.

REFERENCES

Anderson, J., Brinkman-Kaplan, V., Lee, H., & Wood, C. (1994) Relationship of weight loss to cardiovascular risk factors in morbidly obese individuals. *Journal of the American College of Nutrition, 13*, 256–261.

Anderson, J., Hamilton, C., Crown-Weber, E., Riddlemoser, M., & Gustafson, N. (1991). Safety and effectiveness of a multidisciplinary very-low-calorie-diet program for selected obese individuals. *Journal of American Diet Association, 91*, 1582–1584.

Anderson, J., Vichitbandra, S., Qian, W., & Kryscio, R. (1999) Long-term weight maintenance after an intensive weight-loss program. *Journal of the American College of Nutrition, 18*, 620–627.

Anderson, J. W., Brinkman, V. L., & Hamilton, C. C. (1992). Weight loss and 2-year follow-up for 80 morbidly obese patients treated with intensive very-low-calorie diet and an education program. *American Journal of Clinical Nutrition, 56*, 244S–246S.

Anderson, J. W., Brinkman-Kaplan, V., Hamilton, C. C., Logan, J. E., Collins, R. W., & Gustafson, N. J. (1994). Food-containing hypocaloric diets are as effective as liquid-supplement diets for obese individuals with NIDDM. *Diabetes Care, 17*, 602–604.

Anderson, J. W., Konz, E. C., Frederich, R. C., & Wood, C. L. (2001). Long-term weight-loss maintenance: A meta-analysis of U.S. studies. *American Journal of Clinical Nutrition, 74*, 579–584.

Anonymous. (1989). *Take it off and keep it off: Based on the successful methods of Overeaters Anonymous.* Chicago, IL: Contemporary Books.

Astrup, A., & Rossner, S. (2000). Lessons from obesity management programmes: Greater initial weight loss improves long-term maintenance. *Obesity Reviews, 1*, 17–19.

Barrows, K., & Snook, J. (1987). Effect of a high-protein, very-low-calorie diet on resting metabolism, thyroid hormones, and energy expenditure of obese middle-aged women. *American Journal of Clinical Nutrition, 45,* 391–398.

Beliard, D., Kirschenbaum, D. S., & Fitzgibbon, M. L. (1992). Evaluation of an intensive weight control program using a priori criteria to determine outcome. *International Journal of Obesity, 16,* 505–517.

Blackburn, G. (1995). Effect of degree of weight loss on health benefits. *Obesity Research, 3,* 211S–216S.

Brownell, K. D. (2000). *The LEARN program for weight management 2000.* Dallas, TX: American Health.

Bryner, R., Ullrich, I., Sauers, J., Donley, D., Hornsby, G., Kolar, M., et al. (1999). Effects of resistance vs. aerobic training combined with an 800-calorie liquid diet on lean body mass and resting metabolic rate. *Journal of the American College of Nutrition, 18,* 115–121.

Christakis, G., & Miller-Kovach, K. (1996). Maintenance of weight goal among Weight Watchers lifetime members. *Nutrition Today, 31,* 29–31.

Cleland, R., Graybill, D., Hubbard, V., Khan, L. K., Stern, J. S., Wadden, T. A., et al. (2001). Commercial weight loss products and programs: What consumers stand to gain and lose. *Critical Reviews in Food Science and Nutrition, 41,* 45–70.

Collins, R., & Anderson, J. (1995). Medication cost savings associated with weight loss for obese non-insulin-dependent diabetic men and women. *Preventive Medicine, 24,* 369–375.

Daly, A. (2000). Successful long-term maintenance of substantial weight loss: One program's experience. *Journal of the American Dietetic Association, 100,* 1456.

Dansinger, M. L., Gleason, J. A., Griffith, J. L., Selker, H. P., & Schaefer, E. J. (2005). Comparison of the Atkins, Ornish, Weight Watchers, and Zone diets for weight loss and heart disease risk reduction: A randomized trial. *Journal of the American Medical Association, 293,* 43–53.

Diabetes Prevention Program Research Group. (2002). Reduction in the incidence of type 2 diabetes with lifestyle intervention or metformin. *New England Journal of Medicine, 346,* 393–403.

Djuric, Z., DiLaura, N. M., Jenkins, I., Darga, L., Jen, C. K., Mood, D., et al. (2002). Combining weight-loss counseling with the Weight Watchers plan for obese breast cancer survivors. *Obesity Research, 10,* 657–665.

Doherty, J., Wadden, T. A., Zuk, L., Letizia, K., Foster, G., & Day, S. (1991). Long-term evaluation of cardiac function in obese patients treated with a very-low-calorie diet: A controlled clinical study of patients without underlying cardiac disease. *American Journal of Clinical Nutrition, 53,* 854–858.

Donnelly, J., Jacobsen, D., Jakicic, J., & Whatley, J. (1994). Very-low-calorie diet with concurrent versus delayed and sequential exercise. *International Journal of Obesity, 18,* 469–475.

Donnelly, J., Jacobsen, D., & Whatley, J. (1994). Influence of degree of obesity on loss of fat-free mass during very-low-energy diets. *American Journal of Clinical Nutrition, 60,* 874–878.

Downey, M. (2002). Insurance coverage for obesity treatments. In D. H. Bessesen & R. Kushner (Eds.), *Evaluation and management of obesity* (pp. 112–119). Philadelphia: Hanley & Belfus.

eDiets. com. (2003). *Company overview.* Retrieved October 3, 2003, from www.ediets. com/ company

Finley C. E., Barlow C. E., Greenway F. L., Rock C. L., Rolls B. J., & Blair S. N. (2006). Retention rates and weight loss in a commercial weight loss program. *International Journal of Obesity,* advance online publication, 6 June; doi:10.1038/sj.ijo.0803395

Flynn, T., & Walsh, M. (1993). Thirty-month evaluation of a popular very-low-calorie-diet program. *Archives of Family Medicine, 2,* 1042–1048.

Frank, A. (1993). Futility and avoidance: Medical professionals in the treatment of obesity. *Journal of the American Medical Association, 269,* 2132–2133.

Genuth, S. M., Castro, J. H., & Vertes, V. (1974). Weight reduction in obesity by outpatient semistarvation. *Journal of the American Medical Association, 230,* 987–991.

Grodstein, F., Levine, R., Troy, L., Spencer, T., Colditz, G., & Stampfer, M. (1996). Three-year follow-up of participants in a commercial weight loss program: Can you keep it off? *Archives of Internal Medicine, 156,* 1302–1306.

Hartman, W., Stroud, M., Sweet, D., & Saxton, J. (1993). Long-term maintenance of weight loss following supplemented fasting. *International Journal of Eating Disorders, 14,* 87–93.

Harvey-Berino, J., Pintauro, S., Buzzell, P., & Gold, E. C. (2004). Effect of Internet support on the long-term maintenance of weight loss. *Obesity Research, 12,* 320–329.

Health Management Resources. (2003). *About us.* Retrieved October 2, 2003, from *www.yourbetterhealth.com*

Heshka, S., Anderson, J. W., Atkinson, R. L., Greenway, F. L., Hill, J. O., Phinney, S. D., et al. (2003). Weight loss with self-help compared with a structured commercial program: A randomized trial. *Journal of the American Medical Association, 289,* 1792–1798.

Institute of Medicine. (1995). *Weighing the options: Criteria for evaluating weight management programs.* Washington, DC: Government Printing Office.

Jenny Craig. (2003). *Jenny Craig weight loss programs.* Retrieved October 2, 2003, from *www.jennycraig.com/programs*

Kanders, B., Blackburn, G., Lavin, P., & Norton, D. (1989). Weight loss outcome and health benefits associated with the OPTIFAST program in the treatment of obesity. *International Journal of Obesity, 13,* 131S–134S.

Kirschner, M., Schneider, G., Ertel, N., & Gorman, J. (1988). An eight-year experience with a very-low-calorie formula diet for control of major obesity. *International Journal of Obesity, 12,* 69–80.

LA Weight Loss. (2003). *A record of success.* Retrieved October 2, 2003, from *www.laweightloss.com*

Latner, J. D. (2001). Self-help in the long-term treatment of obesity. *Obesity Reviews, 2,* 87–97.

Levitz, L., & Stunkard, A. J. (1974). A therapeutic solution for obesity: behavior modification and patient self-help. *American Journal of Psychiatry, 131,* 423–427.

Lowe, M., Miller-Kovach, K., & Phelan, S. (2001). Weight-loss maintenance in overweight individuals one to five years following successful completion of a commercial weight loss program. *International Journal of Obesity, 25,* 325–331.

Medifast. (2003). *About us.* Retrieved October 2, 2003, from *www.medifast.net*

National Heart, Lung, and Blood Institute. (1998). Clinical guidelines on the identification, evaluation, and treatment of overweight and obesity in adults: The evidence report. *Obesity Research, 6,* 51S–209S.

National Heart, Lung, and Blood Institute and North American Society for the Study of Obesity. (2000). *Practical guide to the identification, evaluation, and treatment of overweight and obesity in adults.* Retrieved September 30, 2003, from *www.nhlbi.nih.gov/guidelines/obesity/practgde.htm*

National Task Force on the Prevention and Treatment of Obesity. (1993). Very-low-calorie diets. *Journal of the American Medical Association, 270,* 967–974.

OPTIFAST. (2003). *Why choose OPTIFAST?* Retrieved October 3, 2003, from *www.optifast.com/why_choose_optifast.jsp*

Overeaters Anonymous. (2003). *About OA.* Retrieved October 2, 2003, from *www.oa.org*

Rippe, J. M., Price, J. M., Hess, S. A., Kline, G., DeMers, K. A., Damitz, S., et al. (1998). Improved psychological well-being, quality of life, and health practices in moderately overweight women participating in a 12–week structured weight loss program. *Obesity Research, 6,* 208–218.

Stafford, R. S., Farhat, J. H., Misra, B., & Schoenfeld, D. A. (2000). National patterns of physician activities related to obesity management. *Archives of Family Medicine, 9,* 631–638.

Stern, J. S., Hirsch, J., Blair, S. N., Foreyt, J. P., Frank, A., Kumanyika, S. K., et al. (1995). Weighing the options: Criteria for evaluating weight-management programs. *Obesity Research, 3,* 591–604.

Take Off Pounds Sensibly. (2005). *About TOPS/information.* Retrieved April 1, 2005, from *www.tops.org*

Take Shape for Life. (2003). *Our company.* Retrieved October 3, 2003, from *www.makemethinner.com*

Tate, D. F., Jackvony, E. H., & Wing, R. R. (2003). Effects of Internet behavioral counseling on weight loss in adults at risk for type 2 diabetes: A randomized trial. *Journal of the American Medical Association, 289,* 1833–1836.

Tate, D. F., Wing, R. R., & Winett, R. A. (2001). Using Internet technology to deliver a behavioral weight loss program. *Journal of the American Medical Association, 285,* 1172–1177.

Tsai, A. G., & Wadden, T. A. (2005). Systematic review: an evaluation of major commercial weight loss programs in the United States. *Annals of Internal Medicine, 142,* 56–66.

Tsai, A. G., & Wadden, T. A. (2006). The evolution of very-low-calorie diets: An update and meta-analysis. *Obesity, 14,* 1283–1293.

Tuomilehto, J., Lindstrom, J., Eriksson, J. G., Valley, T. T., Hamalainen, H., Parikka-Ilanne, P., et al. (2001). Prevention of type 2 diabetes mellitus by changes in lifestyle among subjects with impaired glucose tolerance. *New England Journal of Medicine, 344,* 1343–1350.

U. S. Preventive Services Task Force. (2003). Screening for obesity in adults: Recommendations and rationale. *Annals of Internal Medicine, 139,* 930–939.

Vertes, V., Genuth, S. M., & Hazelton, I. M. (1977). Supplemented fasting as a large-scale outpatient program. *Journal of the American Medical Association, 238,* 2151–2153.

Volkmar, F. R., Stunkard, A. J., Woolston, J., & Bailey, R. A. (1981). High attrition rates in commercial weight reduction programs. *Archives of Internal Medicine, 141,* 426–428.

Wadden, T. A., Berkowitz, R. I., Sarwer, D. B., Prus-Wisniewski, R., & Steinberg, C. (2001). Benefits of lifestyle modification in the pharmacologic treatment of obesity: A randomized trial. *Archives of Internal Medicine, 161,* 218–227.

Wadden, T. A., Foster, G. D., Letizia, K. A., & Stunkard, A. J. (1992). A multicenter evaluation of a proprietary weight reduction program for the treatment of marked obesity. *Archives of Internal Medicine, 152,* 961–966.

Wadden, T. A., & Frey, D. L. (1997). A multicenter evaluation of a proprietary weight loss program for the treatment of marked obesity: A five-year follow-up. *International Journal of Eating Disorders, 22,* 203–212.

Wadden, T. A., Stunkard, A. J., Brownell, K. D., & Van Itallie, T. B. (1983). The Cambridge diet: More mayhem? *Journal of the American Medical Association, 250,* 2833–2834.

Weight Watchers. (2003). *About us, plan and products, flex points, FAQs.* Retrieved October 1, 2003, from *www.weightwatchers.com*

Wolfe, B. L. (1992). Long-term maintenance following attainment of goal weight: A preliminary investigation. *Addictive Behaviors, 17,* 469–477.

Womble, L., Wang, S., & Wadden, T. A. (2002). Commercial and self-help weight loss programs. In T. A. Wadden & A. Stunkard (Eds.), *Handbook of obesity treatment* (pp. 395–415). New York: Guilford Press.

Womble, L. G., Wadden, T. A., McGuckin, B. G., Sargent, S. L., Rothman, R. A., Krauthamer-Ewing, E. S. (2004). A randomized controlled trial of a commercial Internet weight loss program. *Obesity Research, 12*, 1011–1018.

World Health Organization. (2000). Obesity: Preventing and managing the global epidemic. *World Health Organization Technical Report Series, 894*, 1–253.

10

Guided Group Support and the Long-Term Management of Obesity

VANESSA A. MILSOM, MICHAEL G. PERRI,
and W. JACK REJESKI

Helping obese individuals to maintain treatment-induced weight losses is a difficult endeavor. Indeed, the majority of people who lose a significant amount of weight regain most of their lost weight within 5 years (Institute of Medicine [IOM], 1995; Field, Wing, Manson, Spiegelman, & Willett, 2001). This sobering statistic has led many to conclude that obesity should be viewed as a chronic condition requiring continuous care (Klein et al., 2004; Latner et al., 2000; Perri, Nezu, & Viegener, 1992), and some have proposed that guided group support may be an effective modality to assist in the long-term management of obesity (Perri et al., 1988; Wing & Jeffery, 1999).

In this chapter, we examine the use of group interventions in the long-term treatment of obesity. After a brief look at factors that contribute to posttreatment weight gain, we review the impact of guided group support as an approach to helping obese individuals maintain posttreatment weight losses. We compare the results of treatment interventions *with* and *without* guided support during follow-up, and we discuss the structure and function of groups in the long-term management of behavior change. We conclude the chapter with a discussion of clinical implications and directions for future research.

LIFESTYLE INTERVENTIONS
FOR THE MANAGEMENT OF OBESITY

Rooted in learning and social-cognitive theories, "lifestyle" or "behavioral" interventions for weight management induce weight loss through moderate changes in eating and physical activity patterns. Most often this is accomplished in a structured group therapy format *without* the use of very-low-calorie diets (i.e., < 800 kcal/day) or pharmacotherapy. Cognitive-behavioral strategies, such as goal setting, self-monitoring, stimulus control, and cognitive restructuring, are used to help group members adopt and maintain changes in their eating and physical activity patterns (Brownell, 2000; Wing, 2002).

Reviews of randomized trials (IOM, 1995; Jeffery et al., 2000; National Heart, Lung, and Blood Institute [NHLBI], 1998; Perri & Fuller, 1995; Perri, 1998; Wadden, Sarwer, & Berkowitz, 1999; Wadden & Butryn, 2003; Wing, 2002) show that behavioral treatments delivered in 16–26 weekly group sessions typically produce initial body-weight reductions of 8–10%, with approximately half of the lost weight regained at 1-year follow-ups. For obese individuals, body-weight losses of 5% or more are associated with meaningful improvements in risk factors for heart disease (Klein, 2001; Klein et al., 2004; NHLBI, 1998; Pi-Sunyer, 1996) and the prevention of type 2 diabetes (Diabetes Prevention Program Research Group, 2002). However, these benefits are unlikely to remain if the lost weight is regained (Klein, 2001; Wing, Venditti, Jakicic, Polley, & Lang, 1998). Thus the "maintenance problem" represents a critical challenge in the management of obesity. Although numerous strategies have been employed to prevent the regaining of lost weight, the use of guided group support following initial treatment (i.e., group sessions led by a treatment provider during the follow-up period) has received the greatest amount of research attention and thus is the focus of this chapter.

CONTRIBUTORS
TO POSTTREATMENT WEIGHT GAIN

Before we examine the impact of group interventions on the maintenance of lost weight, it is important to consider briefly some of the physiological, environmental, and psychological factors that contribute to the regaining of lost weight. Following an extended period of reduced caloric intake, physiological changes occur that include a reduction in resting metabolic rate (Leibel, Rosenbaum, & Hirsch, 1995) and an increase in ghrelin, a gut peptide associated with the sensation of hunger (Cummings et al., 2002). These changes make the dieter vulnerable to a regaining of lost weight. Moreover, after an interval of restricted intake, dieters experience a heightened sensitivity to palatable foods (Rodin, Schank, & Streigel-Moore, 1989). As a result, when surrounded by an environment rich in tasty high-calorie foods, they may be particularly susceptible to a loss of dietary control (Hill, Wyatt, Reed, & Peters, 2003).

Faced with these potent environmental and biological challenges, it is not surprising that many overweight individuals experience difficulty maintaining their posttreatment weight losses. Moreover, weight loss, which represents the most rewarding aspect of treatment for obese individuals, usually ends with cessation of intervention. As a result, many individuals perceive a high behavioral "cost" associated with continued dietary control at the same time that they are experiencing diminished "benefits" in terms of little or no additional weight loss. Consequently, discouragement is common. Small posttreatment weight gains often lead to attributions of personal ineffectiveness that can trigger negative emotions, a sense of hopelessness, and an abandonment of the weight-control effort (Foreyt et al., 1995; Goodrick, Raynaud, Pace, & Foreyt, 1992; Jeffery, French, & Schmid, 1990).

LONG-TERM EFFECTS OF GUIDED GROUP SUPPORT

Following the completion of group-based treatment for weight loss, additional group contacts conducted under the guidance of a treatment provider may improve the maintenance of lost weight (Perri et al., 1987; Perri et al., 1988). To assess this proposition, we examined the results of group-based lifestyle intervention studies reported in the past decade. We conducted a computerized literature search via the PubMed database for articles published between January 1, 1995, and June 30, 2005, using the terms "behavioral treatment of obesity," "behavioral weight control," "lifestyle modification," and "obesity treatment." We selected only randomized trials of group-based lifestyle interventions conducted with overweight or obese adults on an outpatient basis, in which (1) weight change was the primary outcome, (2) the initial intervention period lasted at least 16 weeks, and (3) participants were followed for 1 year (or more). At a minimum, each study had one "standard" group-based lifestyle intervention condition, and most had various other conditions that allowed testing the benefits of additional components (e.g., meal replacements, specific exercise regimens, financial incentives, etc.).

Eleven randomized studies met the criteria noted (Anderson et al., 1999; Carels, Darby, Douglass, Cacciapaglia, & Rydin, 2005; Jakicic, Winters, Lang, & Wing, 1999; Jeffery, Wing, Thorson, & Burton, 1998; Jeffery, Wing, Sherwood, & Tate, 2003; Leermakers, Perri, Shigaki, & Fuller, 1999; Perri et al., 2001; Ramirez & Rosen, 2001; Wadden, Vogt, Foster, & Anderson, 1998; Wing et al., 1996; and Wing et al., 1998). These 11 studies included a total of 31 lifestyle weight-management conditions; 20 of the treatment conditions included guided group support during follow-up and 11 did not.

Across the 31 intervention groups, the mean pretreatment weights of participants ranged from 83.6 to 104.8 kg (overall M = 92.2 kg, unadjusted for intervention n). The length of initial treatment varied from 16 to 28 weeks, and the mean initial weight changes ranged from 5.6 to 18.6 kg. The largest mean loss, of 18.6 kg (Wadden et al., 1998), was observed in a trial that involved a portion-controlled diet of 925 kcal per day for the initial 16 weeks of treatment. Omitting this "outlier," we observed initial weight losses ranging from 5.6 kg to 12.0 kg, with an overall mean of 8.7 kg (unadjusted for n). When viewed as percentage of body weight lost, the mean reduction across interventions was 9.4%, with a range of 6.1–13.1%. These findings mirror the results from earlier research reviews (Jeffery et al., 2000; Perri, 1998; Perri & Corsica, 2002; Perri & Fuller, 1995; Wadden et al., 1999; Wing, 2002), indicating that group-based lifestyle interventions commonly produce substantial short-term reductions in body weight.

Next, we examined the impact of providing participants with extended care during the period following initial treatment. We did this by summarizing the findings for interventions *with* and *without* guided group support during the year following initial treatment. Table 10.1 summarizes weight-loss outcomes for lifestyle interventions *with* guided group support, and Table 10.2 presents the findings for interventions *without* additional support. We used three evaluative criteria to make comparative judgments of long-term success: (1) the net change in body weight (kg) from baseline to follow-up; (2) the percentage of posttreatment weight loss maintained; and (3) whether or not a "successful" weight-loss outcome was achieved as defined by the IOM's (1995) criterion (i.e., > 5% reduction from baseline weight observed at follow-up of 1 year or more after initial treatment).

At 1-year follow-ups, lifestyle treatments *with* guided group support showed a mean net weight loss of 7.3 kg (unadjusted for intervention n) compared with a mean net loss of 5.3 kg for interventions *without* group contacts during follow-up. Participants who received extended contact also maintained a greater percentage of their initial weight loss when compared with those *without* extended contact (73 vs. 57%, respectively). Finally, a higher percentage of interventions *with* guided group support, compared with those *without* such contact, had mean weight changes that met the IOM (1995) criteria for successful outcome (85 vs. 55%, respectively). Taken collectively, these findings suggest that extending treatment through the use of guided group support improves long-term outcome in the management of obesity.

During the year following initial treatment, the interventions *with* guided group support held an average of 14.6 group sessions. Our review

TABLE 10.1. Lifestyle Interventions with Extended Care Provided via Guided Group Support during Follow-up

Study	n^a	Pretreatment (kg)	Initial treatment type	Initial treatment length (week)	Initial weight loss (kg)	No. Of sessions during follow-up	Net loss at 1-year follow-up	% initial loss maintained	IOM criteria for success met
Jakicic et al. (1999)	37	89.2	BT + LB exerc	24	8.2	18	5.8	70.7	Yes
	36	90.3	BT + SB exerc	24	7.5	18	3.7	49.3	No
	42	87.5	BT + SB exerc + exerc equip	24	9.3	18	7.4	79.6	Yes
Jeffery et al. (1998)	40	85.6	BT	24	8.3	12	7.6	91.6	Yes
	41	87.1	BT + supv exerc	24	6.0	12	3.8	63.3	No
	42	84.7	BT + trainer	24	5.6	12	2.9	51.8	No
	37	87.7	BT + incentive	24	6.7	12	4.5	67.2	Yes
	36	85.7	BT + trainer + incentive	24	7.9	12	5.1	64.6	Yes
Jeffery et al. (2003)	74	91.6^b	BT + moderate PA	24	8.1	18	6.1	75.3	Yes
	84	91.6^b	BT + high PA	24	9.0	18	8.5	94.4	Yes
Leermakers et al. (1999)	38	94.0^b	BT	26	9.6	13	5.2	54.2	Yes
	29	94.0^b	BT	26	8.7	13	7.9	90.8	Yes

(continued)

209

TABLE 10.1. (*continued*)

Study	n[a]	Pretreatment (kg)	Initial treatment type	Initial treatment length (week)	Initial weight loss (kg)	No. Of sessions during follow-up	Net loss at 1-year follow-up	% initial loss maintained	IOM criteria for success met
Perri et al. (2001)	28	97.0	BT	20	9.1	26	5.9	64.8	Yes
	34	98.0	BT	20	8.4	26	10.8	128.6	Yes
Wadden et al. (1998)	21	95.8[b]	BT	28	17.7	10	11.3[c]	86.4	Yes
	21	95.8[b]	BT + aerobic exerc	28	15.8	10	11.0[c]	85.4	Yes
	18	95.8[b]	BT + strength training	28	17.8	10	13.7[c]	97.2	Yes
	17	95.8[b]	BT + aerobic exerc + strength training	28	18.6	10	12.6[c]	89.2	Yes
Wing et al. (1998)	37	99.6	BT + diet	24	9.1	12	5.5	60.4	Yes
	40	98.7	BT + exerc	24	10.3	12	7.4	71.8	Yes
Summary	N = 752	M = 92.3 kg		M = 24.6 weeks	M = 10.1 kg	M = 14.6	M = 7.3 kg	M = 72.7%	% Yes = 85.0

Note. IOM, Institute of Medicine; BT, behavior therapy; LB, long-bout (40 minutes, 1 time/day); SB, short-bout (10 minuters, 4 times/day); exerc, exercise; equip, equipment; supv, supervised; PA, physical activity.

[a]Number of participants who began treatment.

[b]Baseline weights were not provided by condition; thus, the baseline weight for the entire sample is given.

TABLE 10.2. Lifestyle Interventions without Extended Care Provided via Guided Group Support during Follow-Up

Study	n^a	Pretreatment (kg)	Initial treatment type	Initial treatment length (week)	Initial weight loss (kg)	Net loss at 1-year follow-up	% initial loss maintained	IOM criteria for success met
Anderson et al. (1999)	20	83.6	BT + aerobic exercise	16	8.3	6.7	80.7	Yes
	20	90.5	BT + lifestyle activity	16	7.9	7.8	99.0	Yes
Carels et al. (2005)	20	104.8	BT	20	8.2	3.7	37.8	No
	20	101.2	BT + glycemic education	20	7.1	2.6	36.6	No
Perri et al. (2001)	18	94.7	BT	20	9.5	4.1	43.4	No
Ramirez & Rosen (2001)	27	91.0	BT	16	9.3	3.4	36.6	No
	38	101.1	BT + body image therapy	16	8.8	5.7	64.4	Yes
Wing et al. (1996)	40	86.4	BT	26	8.0	3.3	41.3	No
	41	87.4	BT+ meal plan	26	12.0	6.9	57.5	Yes
	41	87.5	BT + meal plan + buy food	26	11.7	7.5	64.1	Yes
	41	84.5	BT + meal plan + free food	26	11.4	6.6	57.9	Yes
Summary	$N = 326$	$M = 92.1$ kg		$M = 20.7$ weeks	$M = 9.3$ kg	$M = 5.3$ kg	$M = 57.0\%$	% Yes = 54.5

Note. IOM, Institute of Medicine; BT, behavior therapy.
[a]Number of participants who began treatment.

cannot answer the question of whether the benefits of guided group support are derived specifically from ongoing contacts with the treatment group or from contact with the treatment provider. To our knowledge there are no randomized trials that address the effects of individual versus group contact for the *maintenance* of lost weight.

However, the comparative effects of individual versus group therapy in the *initial* treatment of obesity have been studied. In an early trial, Kingsley and Wilson (1977) found comparable losses in individual and group therapy after 8 weeks of treatment and enhanced long-term effects for group treatment at a 12-month follow-up. In a more recent study, Renjilian and colleagues (2001) found that over the course of 6 months of treatment, group therapy produced greater weight loss than individual therapy (Ms = 11.0 vs. 9.1 kg, respectively; $p < .02$, $\eta2 = .14$). The superiority of group over individual treatment was observed even among participants who had initially indicated that they preferred to be treated individually rather than in a group. So although we do not have a direct comparison of the effectiveness of individual versus group therapy in maintaining weight loss, it appears reasonable to assume that extended care via group contacts would be at least as effective as individual contacts. Moreover, the lower costs associated with group treatment argue for its use as a first-line strategy in the management of obesity.

The studies described in our review all employed health professionals with advanced training in psychology, nutrition, or exercise science as group leaders. Consequently, we are not able to assess the impact of interventions led by lay health counselors (LHCs), who commonly have been used to deliver weight-management programs in health promotion trials, particularly those targeting members of minority communities (Winkleby, Feldman, & Murray, 1997). Some promising results have been achieved using LHCs to promote dietary changes aimed at increasing fruit and vegetable consumption (Buller et al., 1999; Larkey et al., 1999), and two church-based studies have used LHCs to deliver weight-management programs to African American participants (Kennedy et al., 2005; Quinn & McNabb, 2001). In the latter studies, the participants achieved mean weight losses of 3 to 4 kg, which represented body weight reductions of less than 5%. It is not possible to discern whether these modest weight losses were attributable to the use of LHCs or to the composition of the study samples; African American participants commonly experience smaller weight changes than are commonly observed in European American participants (Kumanyika, 2002).

Commercial and self-help programs often use successful former participants as leaders of weight-management groups (Latner, 2001; Rosenblatt, 1988). However, relatively little information is available about their effectiveness. To our knowledge, only one randomized trial has examined the use of peers to lead weight-management groups. In an early study, Perri and colleagues (Perri et al., 1987) evaluated the effectiveness of a peer-based *posttreatment* program designed to enhance the maintenance of lost weight. Following a 5-month initial weight-loss intervention, participants were randomly assigned to maintenance programs led either by peers or by therapists or to a control group that received no additional contact. At a 7-month follow-up, participants in the therapist-led groups showed significantly greater weight-loss progress compared with those assigned to the peer and control conditions. However, an 18-month follow-up revealed equivalent relapses across conditions, with mean net losses of 6.3 and 6.4 kg for the therapist- and peer-led groups, respectively, and 3.1 kg for the control group.

The use of LHCs or peers to deliver weight-management service offers many attractive features, including the potential to serve as a cost-efficient approach to widespread dissemination of weight-management services. Nonetheless, more research is needed regarding the effectiveness of programs led by LHCs or peers, as well as the training required to prepare nonprofessional counselors to deal with the range of problems that commonly arise in the group management of obesity.

THE STRUCTURE AND FUNCTION OF GROUP TREATMENT IN WEIGHT LOSS

In the previous section, we identified and described the effects of extended-care interventions centered on the use of guided group support. In examining the specific content of the various group conditions, rarely was it possible to describe precisely what occurred within these groups and how it was related to improved outcome. Often, no clear operational description was provided for "group treatment," and it appeared that interventionists conducted "group treatment" with widely divergent models guiding their behavior. In some instances, the group sessions were used to review and reinforce the training that occurred during the initial phase of treatment. In other cases, new intervention techniques, such as relapse prevention training or problem-solving therapy, were introduced. Therefore, without a clear delineation of what occurred during the group support sessions, it is difficult to determine what factors may be responsible for benefits of extended care.

If we were to query obesity researchers about the "effective ingredients" in guided group contacts, it is likely that they would attribute the benefits to the combination of therapist advice and group support. Greater attention is generally given to the content of the advice and guidance provided by the group leader than to the role played by the group itself. Nonetheless, group processes may play an instrumental role in the success of individual members. Often, the group provides individuals with opportunities to learn by observing others who are coping with similar challenges. This may help to normalize the experience of dealing with problems that arise during the maintenance phase, and it may instill the hope that successful coping can be achieved.

Group Cohesion

In his classic text *The Theory and Practice of Group Psychotherapy*, Irvin Yalom (1985) concluded that *group cohesion* is fundamental to what makes group therapy a powerful agent of change. In fact, Yalom made a distinction between two independent forms of social cohesion: one that represents the *social integration* of the group as a unit and a second that describes the individual's level of *social attraction* to the group. Indeed, the importance of this distinction has been echoed in the group dynamics literature (Cartwright, 1953) and in research on team sports (Carron, Hausenblas, & Mack, 1996).

Within the context of guided group support, it is desirable to employ strategies that enhance both the integration of the group as a unit and the attraction that specific individuals may have to the group. For example, one strategy that we have used to increase the social integration of the group is to have participants create a formal name or identity for their group and then to display it on a large banner that remains in the area where their group sessions are held (Rejeski et al., 2003). Alternatively, social attraction to the group for specific participants can be augmented by promoting activities that increase their interest in fellow participants and by incorporating strategies into treatment that encourage self-disclosure and emotional expression.

Small-group research in both industry and sports has emphasized the value of *task cohesion*, both at the level of the group and of the individual (Carron, Widmeyer, & Brawley, 2005). Group-integrated task cohesion is perhaps most obvious when sports teams, which at times may appear disjointed with respect to social group cohesion, demonstrate an exceptional level of group integration in completing tasks that are central to team success. Although the application of this concept to weight loss may seem less obvious, we believe that the introduction of group procedures that require task cohesion can be valuable during the maintenance phase of treatment (e.g., having the group work as a team to prepare a lesson plan on coping with "slips").

One element common in weight-management groups is the *attraction* that individuals have for the group experience as a function of task-related cohesion. Participants can feel attracted to the group because the group is an integral part of their individual weight-loss experience. We often hear group members make comments such as: "If not for the people that I have come to know in this group and the sense of responsibility that I have to them, it is unlikely that I would have had the success that I have experienced—their role in my weight loss has been huge." Nonetheless, there have been few attempts to develop and evaluate strategies in weight-management programs that might influence this motive. Potential tactics might include: (1) creating weight-loss partners within the group who are rotated periodically during the extended care period, (2) having group members contact each other between sessions, either by phone or by Internet, to discuss progress in their weight-control efforts, and (3) structuring food preparation exercises in which participants bring highly desirable but unhealthy dishes to a session followed by group problem solving of ways to modify the dishes to make them healthier.

Social Support

When obesity researchers discuss the merits of group treatment, the most common explanations concern social support and, more specifically, the emotional support and friendships that develop within the group. Participants often comment on the value of social support as it relates to emotional needs and friendship, but we also hear comments such as the following: "there are people in the group who need me"; "there are days that I can barely drag myself to group, but I come because I know that I will feel better when I leave"; "it is reassuring to know that other people have setbacks"; and "it is good to be with a group of people who have a similar problem." These and other experiences that relate in one way or another to social support are what drive the two central components of group cohesion, specifically the *social integration* of the group and the *social attraction* that the group has for specific individuals.

Wing and Jeffery (1999) attempted to capitalize on the potential advantages of social attraction and group cohesion in a weight-management study with a 6-month follow-up. These researchers examined the effects of recruiting participants with friends and increasing social support for weight loss and maintenance. The participants who were recruited either alone or with a team of three friends or family members were randomly assigned to either standard behavioral treatment or standard treatment plus social support strategies. The social support intervention included *intragroup* activities to develop task cohesion (e.g., planning of a group party), as well as *intergroup* competitions during follow-up, using group contingencies to encourage maintenance of lost weight (e.g., monetary awards to teams in which all members maintained their lost weight). Wing and Jeffery (1999) found that recruiting participants with friends *and* treating them with a social support intervention decreased the number of dropouts and increased the percentage of individuals who maintained 100% of their initial weight reductions during the 6-month follow-up period. These findings and those of earlier studies (Perri et al.,

1988) highlight the potential of social influence manipulations in the management of obesity.

Mechanisms of Actions

How do group factors affect a group member's efforts at weight management? The social- and task-related functions of the group may have direct effects on a participant's eating and physical activity patterns. In addition, it is likely that these group processes influence the individual through social-cognitive mechanisms. For example, evidence in the exercise literature indicates that social support has a positive influence on the exercise behavior of older adults. This effect appears to be due to the influence of social support on *self-efficacy*, namely, the individual's perceived ability to adhere to an exercise regimen and to cope with barriers to exercise performance (Duncan & McAuley, 1993).

We recently conducted a group-mediated strength-training study with older adults (Rejeski, Katula, Rejeski, Rowley, & Sipe, 2005) and found that change in desire for strength was a strong predictor of change in strength-related self-efficacy beliefs. In other words, increasing the desire for an outcome represents one potential source of enhancing self-efficacy. Thus, in the context of group weight-loss treatment, increases in group cohesion may elevate the desire of group members to be more physically active, to control caloric intake, and hence to lose weight. In fact, the impact of group processes on increasing the desire to engage in weight-control behaviors may have direct effects on eating and physical activity, as well as indirect effects through increases in self-efficacy.

FUTURE DIRECTIONS

Guided group support is far from the perfect solution to the maintenance problem. Indeed, although our review highlights some of the benefits of extended group contacts, it also underscores the need for further attention to the limitations of extended care programs centered on group support. During the year following initial treatment, participants in interventions *with* group support regained on average more than one-quarter of their post-treatment losses. Although this amount was less than the amount regained by those *without* continued support, it illustrates that more work needs to be done.

Greater attention must be given to the problematic attendance and attrition associated with long-term care. For example, in the Perri et al. (2001) study, we observed attendance rates of 90% during initial treatment but only 58% during the follow-up intervention. Moreover, compared with the initial treatment period, the attrition rate was twice as high in the follow-up program (15% vs. 32%, respectively). Wadden, Butryn, and Byrne (2004) have recently noted that participants sometimes describe extended care sessions as "monotonous" and even "demoralizing." Often they perceive that there is an absence of "new" information and an overemphasis on group members who are struggling with lapses and regaining of weight. Moreover, this typically occurs at a point at which participants have been involved in treatment for a year or more and very few, if any, are continuing to lose weight. As participation in group sessions becomes less rewarding, some individuals may decrease or discontinue their involvement in follow-up care (Wing, Blair, Marcus, Epstein, & Harvey, 1994).

To counter the lag in morale that sometimes accompanies long-term treatment, it may be important to infuse novelty and enjoyment into group sessions. One strategy is to employ short-term campaigns that focus on *group cohesion* and the achievement of group goals. We have used this approach in promoting physical activity among older adults (Rejeski et al., 2003) and among rural residents in a weight-management program (Perri et al., 2005). For example, one of our weight-control groups recently undertook a "Walk America" campaign. Using a large map of the U.S., the group identified a target destination. At each session during the campaign, the group tallied the miles walked by individual members since their previous meeting. The group then plotted on the map their progress in walking across America to their virtual destination. Having each member make a contribution toward a common goal may make the group experience more enjoyable and more productive.

The use of campaigns involving group tasks is also an integral part of the maintenance phase of treatment in the Look AHEAD (Action for Health in Diabetes) Trial, a current large-scale multisite investigation examining the effect of weight loss on cardiovascular events in obese adults with type 2 diabetes (Ryan et al., 2003). However, we are not aware of any published studies that have examined the specific value of task-related group integration on promoting the maintenance of behavior change in lifestyle interventions.

Varying the frequency and timing of support sessions may also improve participant motivation and success. In most studies, group support meetings have been provided on an interval schedule, usually once or twice per month. It may be helpful to consider alternative schedules that involve "planned breaks" and "minicourses" offered at select times of the year to maximize motivation and sustain interest. For example, "refresher" campaigns that begin in January would seem a good fit to capitalize on the natural cycle of heightened motivation for weight loss that accompanies the beginning of a new year. Alternatively, a minicourse offered in November could be used to help participants develop strategies to prevent the weight gains that commonly occur during the holiday season. Indeed, some research has demonstrated the benefits of having participants develop plans for intensive self-monitoring during the holiday season (Boutelle, Kirschen-baum, Baker, & Mitchell, 1999).

In future research, there is a need to focus on both the processes and outcomes associated with group support. For example, a better under-standing is needed of the specific mechanisms of group treatment that influ-ence long-term outcome. Toward this end, it is important that investigators include process measures that evaluate group factors such as task cohesion, social attraction, and social support (Gottlieb, 1988). Further investigation is needed to determine what aspects of group treatment enhance or hinder its effectiveness. Such information would aid clinicians in their efforts to improve treatment delivery.

Finally, it may be useful to employ an overarching conceptual frame-work to guide the design and evaluation of group-based maintenance strat-egies. The "social provisions" model of Cutrona (1987) may be quite useful in this regard. Cutrona and colleagues (Cutrona, Russell, & Gardner, 2005) have identified different provisions inherent in social relationships. They in-clude the following domains: *attachment* (i.e., having a strong emotional bond with at least one other person), *social integration* (i.e., feeling that you are a part of a group that shares your attitudes and beliefs), *reassur-ance of worth* (i.e., believing that others admire your talents and abilities), *reliable alliance* (i.e., knowing that there are others you can depend on for help), *guidance* (i.e., believing there is a trustworthy person you could turn to for advice), and the opportunity for *nurturance* (i.e., believing that there are others who depend on you for help). These six domains constitute potential targets for group-based interventions. The development of thera-peutic approaches to enhance these social provisions may improve the ef-fectiveness of group interventions. Moreover, such an approach would clearly be consistent with a continuous-care model of obesity management.

CONCLUSIONS

The findings from our selective review of lifestyle interventions conducted in the past decade suggest that the group-based extended care programs im-prove the long-term effects of behavioral treatment. When we compared the results at 1-year follow-ups for interventions *with* and *without* guided group support, we found what appears to be a clear benefit for the use of guided group support. Indeed, the superiority of interventions *with* versus *without* guided support seems evident in all three evaluative criteria: net change in body weight from baseline to follow-up (7.3 vs. 5.3 kg, respec-tively); percentage of initial weight loss maintained during the year follow-ing treatment (73% vs. 57%); and evidence of a 5% or greater body weight reduction 1 year after the completion of initial treatment (85 vs. 55%).

Groups can serve multiple purposes in weight-loss treatment, and a number of factors have been suggested as mechanisms responsible for group treatment's effectiveness, including social support, group cohesion, and task cohesion. Both support- and task-related functions warrant further consideration, with strategies directed both to the group as a unit and to the manner in which individuals relate to the group. Indeed, we believe that it is timely and prudent to consider, in a systematic manner, how groups may be put to greater use to facilitate the long-term maintenance of weight loss.

ACKNOWLEDGMENT

This chapter was completed, in part, with the support of Grant R01 HL 73326 to Michael G. Perri and R01 HL076441 to W. Jack Rejeski from the National Institutes of Health.

REFERENCES

Anderson, R. E., Wadden, T. A., Bartlett, S. J., Zemel, B., Verde, T. J., & Franckowiak, S. C. (1999). Effects of lifestyle activity vs. structured aerobic exercise in obese women. *Journal of the American Medical Association, 281,* 335–340.

Boutelle, K. N., Kirschenbaum, D. S., Baker, R. C., & Mitchell, M. E. (1999). How can obese weight controllers minimize weight gain during the high risk holiday season? By self-monitoring very consistently. *Health Psychology, 18,* 364–368.

Brownell, K. D. (2000). *The LEARN program for weight management 2000.* Dallas, TX: American Health.

Buller, D. B., Morrill, C., Taren, D., Aickin, M., Sennott-Miller, L., Buller, M. K., et al. (1999). Randomized trial testing the effect of peer education at increasing fruit and vegetable intake. *Journal of the National Cancer Institute, 91,* 1491–1500.

Carels, R. A., Darby, L. A., Douglass, O. M., Cacciapaglia, H. M., & Rydin, S. (2005). Education of the glycemic index of foods fails to improve treatment outcomes in a behavioral weight loss program. *Eating Behaviors, 6,* 145–150.

Carron, A. V., Hausenblas, H. A., & Mack, D. (1996). Social influence and exercise: A meta-analysis. *Journal of Sport and Exercise Psychology, 18,* 1–16.

Carron, A. V., Widmeyer, W., & Brawley, L. R. (2005). The development of an instrument to assess cohesion in sport teams: The group environment questionnaire. *Journal of Sport Psychology, 4,* 123–138.

Cartwright, D. C. (1953). *Group dynamics: Research and theory.* New York, NY: Harper & Row.

Cummings, D. E., Weigle, D. S., Frayo, R. S., Breen, P. A., Ma, M. K., Delinger, E. P., et al. (2002). Plasma ghrelin levels after diet-induced weight loss or gastric bypass surgery. *New England Journal of Medicine, 346,* 1623–1630.

Cutrona, C. E. (1987). The provisions of social relationships and adaptation to stress. In W. H. Jones (Ed.), *Advances in personal relationships* (pp. 37–67). Greenwich, CT: JAI Press.

Cutrona, C. E., Russell, D. W., & Gardner, K. A. (2005). The relationship enhancement model of social support. In T. A. Revenson, K. Kayser, & G. Bodenmann (Eds.), *Cou-*

ples coping with stress: Emerging perspectives on dyadic coping (pp. 73–95). Washington DC: American Psychological Association.

Diabetes Prevention Program Research Group. (2002). Reduction in the incidence of type 2 diabetes with lifestyle intervention or metformin. *New England Journal of Medicine, 346*, 393–403.

Duncan, T. E., & McAuley, E. (1993). Social support and efficacy cognitions in exercise adherence: A latent growth curve analysis. *Journal of Behavioral Medicine, 16*, 199–218.

Field, A. E., Wing, R. R., Manson, J. E., Spiegelman, D. L., & Willett, W. C. (2001). Relationship of a large weight loss to long-term weight change among young and middle-aged U.S. women. *International Journal of Obesity, 25*, 1113–1128.

Foreyt, J. P., Brunner, R. L., Goodrick, G. K., Cutter, G., Brownell, K. D., & St. Jeor, S. T. (1995). Psychological correlates of weight fluctuation. *International Journal of Eating Disorders, 17*, 263–275.

Goodrick, G. K., Raynaud, A. S., Pace, P. W., & Foreyt, J. P. (1992). Outcome attribution in a very low calorie diet program. *International Journal of Eating Disorders, 12*, 117–120.

Gottlieb, B. (1988). Marshaling social support: The state of the art in research and practice. In B. Gottlieb (Ed.), *Marshaling social support* (pp. 11–51). Newbury Park, CA: Sage.

Hill, J. O., Wyatt, H. R., Reed, G. W., & Peters, J. C. (2003). Obesity and the environment: Where do we go from here? *Science, 299*, 853–855.

Institute of Medicine. (1995). *Weighing the options: Criteria for evaluating weight-management programs.* Washington, DC: National Academies Press.

Jakicic, J. M., Winters, C., Lang, W., & Wing, R. R. (1999). Effects of intermittent exercise and use of home exercise equipment on adherence, weight loss, and fitness in overweight women: A randomized trial. *Journal of the American Medical Association, 282*, 1554–1560.

Jeffery, R. W., Drewnowski, A., Epstein, L. H., Stunkard, A. J., Wilson, G. T., Wing, R. R., et al. (2000). Long-term maintenance of weight loss: Current status. *Health Psychology, 19*, 5–16.

Jeffery, R. W., French, S. A., & Schmid, T. L. (1990). Attributions for dietary failures: Problems reported by participants in the Hypertension Prevention Trial. *Health Psychology, 9*, 315–329.

Jeffery, R. W., Wing, R. R., Sherwood, N. E., & Tate, D. F. (2003). Physical activity and weight loss: Does prescribing higher physical activity goals improve outcome? *American Journal of Clinical Nutrition, 78*, 669–670.

Jeffery, R. W., Wing, R. R., Thorson, C., & Burton, L. R. (1998). Use of personal trainers and financial incentives to increase exercise in a behavioral weight-loss program. *Journal of Consulting and Clinical Psychology, 66*, 777–783.

Kennedy, B. M., Paeratakul, S., Champagne, C. M., Ryan, D. H., Hersha, D. W., McGee, B., et al. (2005). Lower Mississippi Delta nutrition intervention research initiative. *Ethnicity and Disease, 15*, 373–378.

Kingsley, R. G., & Wilson, G. T. (1977). Behavior therapy for obesity: A comparative investigation of long-term efficacy. *Journal of Consulting and Clinical Psychology, 45*, 288–298.

Klein, S. (2001). Outcome success in obesity. *Obesity Research, 9*, 354S–358S.

Klein, S., Burke, L. E., Bray, G. A., Blair, S., Allison, D. B., Pi-Sunyer, F. X., et al. (2004). Clinical implications of obesity with specific focus on cardiovascular disease. *Circulation, 110*, 2952–2967.

Kumanyika, S. K. (2002). Obesity treatment in minorities. In T. A. Wadden & A. J. Stunkard (Eds.), *Handbook of obesity treatment* (pp. 416–446). New York: Guilford Press.

Larkey, L. K., Alatorre, C., Buller, D. B., Morrill, C., Klein, B. M., Taren, D., et al. (1999).

Communication strategies for dietary change in a worksite peer educator intervention. *Health Education Research, 14,* 777–790.

Latner, J. D. (2001). Self-help in the long-term treatment of obesity. *Obesity Reviews, 2,* 87–97.

Latner, J. D., Stunkard, A. J., Wilson, G. T., Jackson, M. L., Zelitch, D. S., & Labouvie, E. (2000). Effective long-term treatment of obesity: A continuing care model. *International Journal of Obesity, 24,* 893–898.

Leermakers, E. A., Perri, M. G., Shigaki, C. L., & Fuller, P. R. (1999). Effects of exercise-focused versus weight-focused maintenance programs on the management of obesity. *Addictive Behaviors, 24,* 219–227.

Leibel, R. L., Rosenbaum, M., & Hirsch, J. (1995). Changes in energy expenditure resulting from altered body weight. *New England Journal of Medicine, 332,* 673–674.

National Heart, Lung, and Blood Institute. (1998). Clinical guidelines on the identification, evaluation, and treatment of overweight and obesity in adults: The evidence report. *Obesity Research, 6,* 51S–209S.

Perri, M. G. (1998). The maintenance of treatment effects in the long-term management of obesity. *Clinical Psychology: Science and Practice, 5,* 526–543.

Perri, M. G., & Corsica, J. A. (2002). Improving the maintenance of weight lost in behavioral treatment of obesity. In T. A. Wadden & A. J. Stunkard (Eds.), *Handbook of obesity treatment* (pp. 357–382). New York: Guilford Press.

Perri, M. G., Fox, L. D., Durning, P. E., Limacher, M. C., Martin, A. D., Bobroff, L. B., et al. (2005). Treatment of obesity in underserved rural setting (TOURS): Preliminary findings. *Annals of Behavioral Medicine, 29,* S130.

Perri, M. G., & Fuller, P. R. (1995). Success and failure in the treatment of obesity: Where do we go from here? *Medicine, Exercise, Nutrition and Health, 4,* 255–272.

Perri, M. G., McAdoo, W. G., McAllister, D. A., Lauer, J. B., Jordan, R. C., Yancey, D. Z., et al. (1987). Effects of peer support and therapist contact on long-term weight loss. *Journal of Consulting and Clinical Psychology, 55,* 615–617.

Perri, M. G., McAllister, D. A., Gange, J. J., Jordan, R. C., McAdoo, W. G., & Nezu, A. M. (1988). Effects of four maintenance programs on the long-term management of obesity. *Journal of Consulting and Clinical Psychology, 56,* 529–534.

Perri, M. G., Nezu, A. M., McKelvey, W. F., Shermer, R. L., Renjilian, D. A., & Viegener, B. J. (2001). Relapse prevention training and problem-solving therapy in the long-term management of obesity. *Journal of Consulting and Clinical Psychology, 69,* 722–726.

Perri, M. G., Nezu, A. M., & Viegener, B. J. (1992). *Improving the long-term management of obesity: Theory, research, and clinical guidelines.* New York: Wiley.

Pi-Sunyer, F. X. (1996). A review of long-term studies evaluating the efficacy of weight loss in ameliorating disorders associated with obesity. *Clinical Therapeutics, 18,* 1006–1035.

Quinn, M. T., & McNabb, W. L. (2001). Training lay health educators to conduct a church-based weight-loss program for African American women. *Diabetes Educator, 27,* 231–238.

Ramirez, E. M., & Rosen, J. C. (2001). A comparison of weight control and weight control plus body image therapy for obese men and women. *Journal of Consulting and Clinical Psychology, 69,* 440–446.

Rejeski, W. J., Brawley, L. R., Ambrosius, W. T., Brubaker, P. H., Focht, B. C., Foy, C. G., et al. (2003). Older adults with chronic disease: The benefits of group mediated counseling in the promotion of physically active lifestyles. *Health Psychology, 22,* 414–423.

Rejeski, W. J., Katula, J., Rejeski, A. F., Rowley, J., & Sipe, M. (2005). Strength training in older adults: Does desire determine confidence? *Journal of Gerontology: Psychological Sciences, 60,* 335–337.

Renjilian, D. A., Perri, M. G., Nezu, A. M., McKelvey, W. F., Shermer R. L., & Anton, S. D. (2001). Individual versus group therapy for obesity: Effects of matching participants to their treatment preferences. *Journal of Consulting and Clinical Psychology, 69,* 717–721.

Rodin, J., Schank, D., & Striegel-Moore, R. (1989). Psychological features of obesity. *Medical Clinics of North America, 73,* 47–66.

Rosenblatt, E. (1988). Weight-loss programs: Pluses and minuses of commercial and self-help groups. *Postgraduate Medicine, 6,* 137–148.

Ryan, D. H., Espeland, M. A., Foster, G. D., Haffner, S. M., Hubbard, V. S., Johnson, K. C., et al. (2003). Look AHEAD (Action for Health in Diabetes): Design and methods for a clinical trial of weight loss for the prevention of cardiovascular disease in type 2 diabetes. *Controlled Clinical Trials, 24,* 610–628.

Wadden, T. A., & Butryn, M. L. (2003). Behavioral treatment of obesity. *Endocrinology and Metabolism Clinics of North America, 32,* 981–1003.

Wadden, T. A., Butryn, M. L., & Byrne, K. J. (2004). Efficacy of lifestyle modification for long-term weight control. *Obesity Research, 12,* 151S–162S.

Wadden, T. A., Sarwer, D. B., & Berkowitz, R. I. (1999). Behavioral treatment of the overweight patient. *Clinical Endocrinology and Metabolism, 13,* 93–107.

Wadden, T. A., Vogt, R. A., Foster, G. D., & Anderson, D. A. (1998). Exercise and the maintenance of weight loss: 1-year follow-up of a controlled clinical trial. *Journal of Consulting and Clinical Psychology, 66,* 429–433.

Wing, R. R. (2002). Behavioral weight control. In T. A. Wadden & A. J. Stunkard (Eds.), *Handbook of obesity treatment* (pp. 301–316). New York: Guilford Press.

Wing, R. R., Blair, E., Marcus, M., Epstein, L. H., & Harvey, J. (1994). Year-long weight loss treatment for obese patients with type II diabetes: Does including an intermittent very-low-calorie diet improve outcome? *American Journal of Medicine, 97,* 354–362.

Wing, R. R., & Jeffery, R. W. (1999). Benefits of recruiting participants with friends and increasing social support for weight loss and maintenance. *Journal of Consulting and Clinical Psychology, 67,* 132–138.

Wing, R. R., Jeffery, R. W., Burton, L. R., Thorson, C., Sperber Nissinoff, K., & Baxter, J. E. (1996). Food provision vs. structured meal plans in the behavioral treatment of obesity. *International Journal of Obesity, 20,* 56–62.

Wing, R. R., Venditti, E., Jakicic, J. M., Polley, B. A., & Lang, W. (1998). Lifestyle intervention in overweight individuals with a family history of diabetes. *Diabetes Care, 21,* 350–355.

Winkleby, M. A., Feldman, H. A., & Murray, D. (1997). Joint analysis of three U.S. community intervention trials for reduction of cardiovascular disease risk. *Journal of Clinical Epidemiology, 50,* 645–658.

Yalom, I. D. (1985). *The theory and practice of group psychotherapy* (3rd ed.). New York: Basic Books.

11

Continuing Care and Self-Help in the Treatment of Obesity

JANET D. LATNER *and* G. TERENCE WILSON

Behavioral weight-loss (BWL) treatment, focusing on lifestyle change, remains the most widely used approach to weight control (Wadden, Butryn, & Byrne, 2004). The nature of this treatment is described in Chapters 12 and 14 of this volume. The therapeutic efficacy of BWL has been shown to be consistent across different investigators and clinical research settings. The short-term effects are uniformly positive. A typical treatment of 24 weeks reliably results in an average weight loss of about 10% of body weight. Binge eating is reduced, if not eliminated; body image is improved, self-esteem enhanced, and depressed mood decreased. Blood pressure and cholesterol level tend to drop. Long-term effects, however, are another matter.

Relapse—weight regain following treatment—has proved to be a remarkably robust phenomenon (Jeffery et al., 2000). In a recent summary of the efficacy of BWL, Wadden et al. (2004) concluded that patients regain approximately "30% to 35% of their lost weight in the year after treatment. Weight regain slows after the first year, but by 5 years, 50% or more of patients are likely to have returned to their baseline weight" (p. 153S). For example, in the Diabetes Prevention Program (DPP; Diabetes Prevention Program Research Group, 2002), arguably one of the most sophisticated lifestyle interventions for obesity to date, participants gradually regained about one-third of the weight they had lost in treatment over the following 4 years. Moreover, this weight regain occurred despite an intensive (and expensive) maintenance treatment program designed to preserve weight loss.

TOWARD AN EXPLANATION OF WEIGHT
REGAIN FOLLOWING TREATMENT

Several factors help explain the seemingly inevitable relapse following BWL. Probable biological contributors identified by Wadden et al. (2004) include reductions in resting energy and leptin and increases in the gut peptide ghrelin. Here we focus on the effects of what Brownell and Horgen (2003) have called the "toxic environment."

The Toxic Environment

As has been extensively documented elsewhere (e.g., Brownell & Horgen, 2003), in the United States today we have easy access to excess when it comes to eating. The ready availability of enticing, calorically dense, varied, cheap, and aggressively marketed foods represents an unprecedented environmental challenge to healthy weight regulation. Portions have increased dramatically over the past two decades, as has obesity. People need to eat several times a day—hence they have multiple exposures to different primary reinforcers (varieties of food) that are particularly problematic for individuals who are genetically predisposed to favoring these reinforcers.

An evolutionary perspective suggests that people overeat because the presence, expectation, and even the thought of high positive-incentive value foods promotes hunger. The problem is that humans naturally suited to an environment of paucity now live in environments with the greatest possible variety and abundance of palatable foods (Pinel, Assanand, & Lehman, 2000). Given these conditions, a behavioral analysis suggests that relapse is predictable rather than unexpected. The self-regulatory strategies that BWL comprises are likely to be overwhelmed by environmental forces, especially in vulnerable individuals.

The "toxic environment" is not limited to the physical abundance and availability of food. Cultural influences undermine self-control. People have a quick-fix mentality—looking for the magic pill or diet—that works against the patience and perseverance required for lasting lifestyle change. People have unrealistic expectations of how much weight can be lost, so that even successful outcomes of current BWL might result in disappointment, a sense of failure, and lowered self-efficacy that undermines self-control (Cooper, Fairburn, & Hawker, 2003; Rothman, 2000). The contemporary United States, as someone once said, can be called a country that is too fat trying to be too thin too quickly.

Costs of Weight Maintenance in the Toxic Environment

It is useful to analyze the poor maintenance of weight lost in terms of the response costs and benefits (Jeffery, Kelly, Rothman, Sherwood, & Boutelle, 2004). The costs of maintaining treatment-induced weight loss involve continual vigilance (including active self-regulation of eating) in the face of unremitting temptations and pressure to eat. We know a lot about the short-term benefits, as noted earlier. But in an innovative and provocative descriptive analysis, Jeffery et al. (2004) found that patient-perceived benefits decline over the first six months of treatment. A measure asking patients "to evaluate benefits of weight loss relative to the effort was favorable in the first three months and then dropped to near zero in the last three months" (p. 104). In view of these findings, it is hardly surprising that participants would not continue to invest time and effort in often challenging self-regulatory activities. Physiological factors, such as compensatory metabolic responses (e.g., reductions in energy expenditure and leptin, increases in ghrelin), may make it even more difficult to maintain lost weight (Wadden et al., 2004).

Other health behavior changes, such as smoking cessation, demand high initial cost and stress that diminish over time, with rewards that become increasingly apparent with time. Long-term weight loss, however, requires that the initial efforts, such as restriction, deprivation, exercise, planning, and monitoring food intake, be consistently applied (Jeffery, French, & Rothman, 1999). The efforts are often accompanied by large initial rewards; during active weight loss individuals may observe with pride (and receive favorable comments from others on) their steady weight reductions, changes in clothing size, improved facial appearance, physical stamina, and so forth. They may also perceive subtler changes in the responses of others, such as greater acceptance, less stigmatization, or more romantic or sexual attention. These changes may at first be reinforcing and satisfying enough to maintain motivation. However, individuals adapt to these improvements, which may remain in place but stop increasing, once maximal weight loss (the amount of which is often unsatisfactory) is achieved. Longer term benefits of weight maintenance include the amelioration of the severity of diseases such as non-insulin-dependent diabetes mellitus, osteoarthritis, and hypertension (Pi-Sunyer, 1996). In the DPP study described previously, although patients regained a third of their weight, they experienced a clinically significant reduction in their risk for developing diabetes (Diabetes Prevention Program Research Group, 2002). However, these health benefits are often not obvious to patients, and the cost and difficulty of maintaining weight loss remains high.

Whereas initial weight-loss efforts are motivated by a desire to reach a favorable goal state (being thin and all that it entails; Rothman, 2000), maintenance efforts may be motivated by a desire to avoid an unfavorable goal state (going back to one's heaviest weight). Even when individuals are aware that maintenance requires special effort and possess the skills to make this effort (which may rarely be the case; Cooper et al., 2003), behaviors motivated by an approach-oriented process (e.g., initiation of weight loss) are thought to be far more likely to occur than avoidance-oriented behaviors (e.g., maintenance of weight loss; Rothman, 2000).

Cooper and Fairburn (2002) postulated that patients typically fail to maintain weight losses for two reasons. First, they have unrealistic expectations about weight loss. Patients overestimate not only the amount of weight they will lose but also the life changes that weight loss will bring about. Cooper and Fairburn (2002) suggested that treatment should help patients separately identify and address these "primary goals" as distinct from their "weight goals." (This cognitive-behavioral treatment has been described in greater detail by Cooper et al., 2003, but outcome data on this professionally led, individual treatment are not yet available.) Second, patients fail to learn active maintenance skills or to learn even the fact that maintaining weight loss requires skills that can be distinct from those initially used to lose weight. These two obstacles interact with and exacerbate each other. Because patients undervalue their initial weight losses, which they consider too small and too inconsequential in improving their quality of life, they may feel that it is hardly worth the effort to acquire and practice the behaviors needed to maintain these losses. Finch and colleagues (2005) found that patients with overly positive expectations early in treatment were less successful at maintaining their weight losses at 18 months after an 8-week behavioral treatment. On the other hand, the individuals who do maintain weight losses may be those who are more aware of the long-term benefits. People who successfully maintain long-term weight losses report improvements in energy, mobility, mood, health, and self-confidence (Klem, Wing, McGuire, Seagle, & Hill, 1997). Successful men and women both report better physical condition, and women also report less loneliness and greater life satisfaction (Sarlio-Lahteenkorva, Rissanen, & Kaprio, 2000).

CONTINUING CARE AND OVERCOMING THE OBSTACLES TO MAINTENANCE

The problems in maintaining weight loss have resulted in BWL programs that offer continuing maintenance or booster sessions after treatment (see Chapter 10, this volume, for a review). However, it is clear that participants in these studies fail to take advantage of this offer and are unwilling to attend regular clinic-based maintenance sessions. For example, attendance at meetings dropped from 89% in the first 26 weeks of treatment to 77% in the second 26 weeks of treatment (Wadden, Foster, & Letizia, 1994). Why?

Wadden et al. (2004) speculate that participants drop out because they are frustrated with the lack of sufficient weight loss or find the maintenance sessions too monotonous and demoralizing.

In contrast to these findings, data from a small number of long-term treatment studies have suggested that behavioral and nutritional treatments can produce long-term weight loss. Several professionally administered treatment programs, all outside the United States, have been examined. Bjorvell and Rossner (1985) treated 68 patients with initial very-low-calorie diet (VLCD) and behavior modification in an intensive, 6-week hospital-based program in Sweden. They continued treatment for a period of 4 years with weekly meetings, weigh-ins, advice from dietitians, and the opportunity to reenroll in the more intensive treatment if relapse began. Patients maintained substantial weight losses at 4 years (12.6 kg) and 10 years (10.5 kg; Bjorvell & Rossner, 1990) after treatment initiation. Attrition rates were surprisingly low compared with those usually seen in the United States (Jeffery et al., 2000), with 56 patients still participating after 4 years.

A German study found weight losses of 8.4% of initial weight (9.5 kg) and health improvements among patients given energy-controlled meal and snack replacements over a 3-month treatment and over a 48-month maintenance period. Interestingly, much smaller losses (3.2%; 4.1 kg) were achieved by patients given only dietary advice for the first 3 months and meal replacements for the final 48 months (Flechtner-Mors, Ditschuneit, Johnson, Suchard, & Adler, 2000).

Another Swedish study offered 2 years of treatment of dietary and behavioral counseling, with or without VLCD, to 113 patients (Lance, Peltonen, Agren, & Torgerson, 2003). The 87 patients who completed these first 2 years of treatment were offered another 2 years of further monthly counseling with a nurse or dietitian. Of the 70 who chose to participate in this second 2 years of continuing treatment, 55 completed it. Randomization to VLCD or no VLCD made no difference to outcomes, but completers of the 4-year continuing-care program lost more weight than noncompleters (7.0 vs. 5.4 kg). This group difference remained at a subsequent 8-year follow-up, when completers maintained a 3.3-kg weight loss and noncompleters had gained 3.2 kg. Of course, the completers in this study were a self-selected group, but the fact that nearly half (49%) of the originally randomized participants completed 4 years of treatment is encouraging.

These randomized trials included comparison groups and had high internal validity, but they tell us less about the effects of continuing care in its natural settings (external validity). In Italy, a naturalistic study examined 15 medical centers that used a variety of treatment procedures (dieting, cognitive-behavior therapy, medication) but provided continuing care by beginning with an intensive initial treatment (3–6 months) followed by contact every 2–4 months. Dalle Grave and colleagues (2005) found that 36 months after treatment began, the 15.7% of patients still in treatment had maintained greater weight losses than those who had dropped out (5.2% vs. 3.0% of initial weight). However, selected subgroups of dropouts who stopped treatment because they were satisfied with their results or had confidence that they could lose weight on their own achieved even greater weight losses than treatment completers (9.6% and 6.5%, respectively). This suggests that not everyone may need continuing care, particularly individuals with the self-efficacy and self-determination to lose weight independently (e.g., Williams, Grow, Freedman, Ryan, & Deci, 1996; see also Chapter 1, this volume).

The Trevose Behavior Modification Program (TBMP) in the United States, a lay-directed self-help program that provides continuing care, has achieved results that are similar to those of professionally administered continuing care. Weekly meetings in groups of 10 teach traditional behavior modification principles and provide social support. The program is highly disciplined, with strict rules mandating regular attendance, self-monitoring of food intake, and specific personalized weight-loss goals. Members who fail to meet these requirements are dismissed from the program, and individuals are permitted to join the group only once. Members who remained in the program (47% at 2 years and 22% at 5 years) had lost 19% (18 kg) of their initial weight at 2 years and 17% (16 kg) at 5 years (Latner et al., 2000). The proportion of people remaining in TBMP over the long term was similar to or higher than that found in large medication studies: At one year, 70% remained in TBMP, compared with 67% who remained in treatment with orlistat at 1 year (and lost 8.8 kg; Davidson et al., 1999) and 51% who remained in treatment at 1 year with the new obesity medication rimonabant (and lost 6.3 kg; Pi-Sunyer, Aronne, Heshmati, Devin, & Rosenstock, 2006).

The treatment approach used by TBMP appears to be portable, as it has been replicated with similar results in several different settings (Latner, Wilson, Stunkard, & Jackson, 2002). The treatment may produce weight loss even in those participants with frequent binge eating: weight losses were similar in binge eaters and non–binge eaters (Delinsky, Latner, & Wilson, 2006). When asked what components of treatment they found to be most helpful and effective, members rated most highly the provision of continuing care and group support (Latner, Stunkard, Wilson, & Jackson, 2006).

A seeming exception to the positive results of continuing care comes from a study in Germany by Liebbrand and Fichter (2002). Ten weeks of inpatient treatment was followed up for 18 months with either monthly phone consultation with professional clinicians or no further professional treatment contact. Both groups maintained their weight losses, with a mean of 8.0 kg at 18 months, with no group differences. However, the authors suggested that the positive outcome, even in the control group receiving no further treatment, may have resulted from three possible features: (1) the distribution of detailed written therapy manuals to support long-term behavior modification, (2) the ongoing professional contact through repeated assessments, and (3) the fact that several of the cohorts in the control group "developed stronger informal structures of mutual support or founded obesity self-help groups on the basis of the cognitive-behavioral principles they had learned during therapy. . . . Social support by their peer group may have influenced the treatment outcome of the subjects more than monthly contacts with the therapist" (Liebbrand & Fichter, 2002, p. 1287). This last development supports research suggesting that individuals trying to maintain lost weight both desire and appreciate continuing self-help support (DePue, Clark, Ruggiero, Medeiros, & Pera, 1995; Latner et al., 2006). The good maintenance of weight lost in this control group suggests that such continuing support works.

The Italian study discussed previously (Dalle Grave et al., 2005) found good weight maintenance in individuals who participated in a continuing-care treatment involving a relatively nonintensive maintenance period of contacts every 2–4 months (after an initial period of more intensive treatment). These results suggest that continuing care can be effective without intensive ongoing intervention, and a study comparing two intensity levels of long-term behavior modification and nutritional counseling tested this experimentally (Melin et al., 2003). Following a very-low-calorie diet, patients were randomized to more intensive (43 sessions) or less intensive (27 sessions) ongoing treatment spread over the course of the subsequent 2 years. Compliance, dropout rate, weight reduction, and weight maintenance at 2 years were similar between the groups (6.8 kg maintained in the more intensive group, and 8.6 kg in the less intensive group).

Though the evidence is still limited, the aforementioned studies suggest that continuing care may be effective even when therapeutic contacts take place less frequently or are administered by nonprofessionals. Given the high prevalence of obesity, it is likely that the only feasible way that continuing care can become available to the population on a large scale is through self-help (Latner, 2001). In the present epidemic of obesity, "any effort to reduce the cost of the treatment would free resources to tackle larger groups of patients" (Dalle Grave et al., 2005, p. 272).

In addition to the obvious practical implications of self-help in the provision of continuing care, self-help may have additional advantages, as well. Self-help creates a sense of empowerment, which in turn may enhance self-efficacy, self-esteem, and the belief that one's efforts can cause positive change (Segal, Silverman, & Temkin, 1995). Taking responsibility for one's own problems, with the help of supportive peers, is an empowering and essential characteristic of members of self-help groups (Borkman, 1990). Furnham and McDermott (1994) found that lay persons rated self-reliance as the most effective strategy for addressing obesity. Having an internal locus of control, or believing that one's own efforts determine one's control over weight, predicts greater maintenance of weight loss (Nir & Neumann, 1995; Williams et al., 1996).

Giving recipients of help the chance to be providers of help (or turning "helpees" into "helpers") may also have particular benefits to the helper: greater feelings of independence, social usefulness, charitableness, control, and status (Riessman, 1990). Several aspects of self-help groups work to increase self-efficacy and self-reliance, such as receiving emotional support and positive reinforcement, taking on leadership responsibilities, and role modeling (Katz, 1993). Self-efficacy and coping skills, in turn, may be important predictors of weight-loss maintenance (Byrne, 2002). A recent review of the role of social support in weight-control interventions concluded that the evidence thus far suggests beneficial effects on long-term health-behavior change (Verheijden, Bakx, van Weel, Koelen, & van Staveren, 2005; see also Chapter 10, this volume). Finally, many of the principles of obesity treatment are straightforward, lending themselves well to "translation" (e.g., see Chapter 12, this volume) into lay language and adaptation across a wide range of people.

ANATOMY OF A SELF-HELP
CONTINUING CARE PROGRAM

To better address the obstacles to continued motivation, it may be valuable to examine the components of a continuing-care program that has shown success at producing long-term weight loss. Several strategies used by TBMP specifically address some of the obstacles discussed here and may be useful in making other self-help and professionally run treatment programs more effective. In addition, an analysis of this specific continuing-care program may reveal ways in which it might be improved.

Screening Procedures

In addition to providing continuing care, TBMP uses a screening procedure to identify potential successful members. Screening procedures can involve complex ethical and practical issues, such as the risk of excluding some patients who would succeed or those who are most in need of treatment (Brownell, Marlatt, Lichtenstein, and Wilson, 1986). However, although few reliable predictors of success in weight-loss programs have been identified thus far, a screening procedure may make it possible to focus treatment on members most likely to succeed (Brownell & Jeffery, 1987). TBMP's first screening device is the stipulation that program applicants must be between 20 and 100 pounds above normal weight, thus including primarily individuals with mild to moderate obesity. The second is a requirement that candidates fulfill certain essential program requirements in the first 5 weeks. (A comparable "screening phase" prior to treatment has been described by Brownell and colleagues, 1986.) Regarding the first screening tool, there is evidence that lower initial body weight is a correlate of successful weight loss (Jeffery, Wing, & Stunkard, 1978) and maintenance (Stuart & Guire, 1978). Individuals with a high percentage of body fat have been identified as high-risk patients (Dubbert & Wilson, 1983). Other variables that predict weight loss and maintenance are program attendance, early weight loss, and self-monitoring (Wilson, 1995). Full membership is earned after the 5-week screening phase only if three requirements are met: consistent attendance, weight loss, and self-monitoring. Most applicants succeed at meeting the requirements: only 10–15% do not pass the screening phase (Latner et al., 2000, 2002). In the remaining participants, the early reinforcement of these necessary behaviors may facilitate later weight loss and maintenance.

The screening phase may also identify those individuals who are "overly zealous" initiators of treatment, who overestimate the benefits and underestimate the costs of weight loss and maintenance. (For those who pass the screening phase, TBMP addresses this problem partly by adding more benefits than are usually present and by changing the individual's environment, as discussed later.) There may be some individuals who readily and frequently join weight-loss programs without realizing the effort required. For example, individuals with a history of frequent dieting are less successful at weight maintenance (Pasman, Saris, & Westerterp-Plantenga, 1999). The use of a waiting list may also help to weed out unmotivated individuals, who may lack patience and decide not to enroll when they find out about the long list.

One of the screening requirements is that a specific amount of weight be lost at the start of treatment, and specific monthly weight-loss goals are assigned thereafter during treatment. The initial weight-loss requirement has historically been 15% of the total weight-loss goal in the first 5 weeks of treatment, a substantial loss considering that a member's total goal must place him or her within the range of normal weight, according to insurance company standards of height and weight (Metropolitan Life Insurance Company, 1983). As a result, this requirement has recently been reduced for those with a total goal of 55 or more pounds to a standard total goal of 8 pounds in the first 5 weeks of treatment. Such large initial weight losses may be helpful in sustaining weight loss over longer periods of time (Wadden & Frey, 1997).

Group Support

Generic features of group support are even more helpful when they are available on a consistent basis. New TBMP members are matched with experienced members, who serve as "mentors" and contact them to give support between meetings. Meetings end with each individual announcing a positive consequence of his or her weight loss (e.g., "I no longer need to take blood pressure medication," or "I can cross my legs again"). This simple strategy may help prevent individuals from taking for granted some of the benefits of weight loss; it might also encourage them to try to identify and remember additional benefits over time. In joining, members make a public commitment to lose and maintain their weight. In addition, members often develop close friendships with other group members. These factors are likely to increase social pressure on members to continue to attend meetings and to make the effort necessary to achieve their goals.

Specific features of TBMP, such as its local reputation and atmosphere, may be important motivating factors as well. According to members' reports and media reports on the program, the group is well known in the Philadelphia area as the one weight-loss program that is most effective. The program also has a reputation of being exclusive and selective. There is a long waiting list. It is free of charge and offers long-term care, a quality that weight-loss maintainers consider essential for maintenance programs (DePue et al., 1995). Membership in the program is therefore often seen as extremely desirable, which makes individuals more willing to work hard to enter and remain in such a program.

Finally, the atmosphere within the group is encouraging and motivating. Each group usually has several members present who have achieved normal weight, providing visual incentive for new or struggling members. In addition, only successful members (who attend regularly and meet their weight-loss goals) are permitted to continue in the program. So although group members may at times be struggling, there are never members present who have given up entirely or have ceased to lose or maintain their weight. In joining, members are thus identifying themselves with a group of winners. These role models may give new members a tremendous confidence in the potential success of the program and greater faith in their own self-efficacy. That the leadership works without salary or any other financial incentive and that membership itself is free of charge may be strong guarantees of the leaders' good faith when they represent themselves as successful program graduates for new members to emulate.

Behavior Modification

During weekly sessions, program members meet in groups of approximately 10 and learn skills such as self-monitoring of food and calorie intake, making healthy food choices, and developing regular exercise habits. Group leaders are experienced members who meet monthly with the program director and annually for a day-long workshop to receive training in leadership skills and behavior modification techniques.

The behavior modification techniques taught and reviewed in weekly meetings at TBMP are based on the same strategies that have been used in weight-loss programs since the early 1970s, based on the original manual by Stuart and Davis (1968). These techniques were reported to be effective, at least in the short term, in a review by Albert Stunkard in 1972 (Penick & Stunkard, 1972), just 1 year before he helped the program's founder, David Zelitch, implement them at Trevose. They include careful description and monitoring of those behaviors to be controlled (i.e., caloric intake, exercise), modification and control of the discriminatory stimuli governing eating (i.e., learning to eat in one place), development of techniques to control the act of eating (i.e., eating more slowly), and prompt reinforcement of behaviors that delay or control eating (i.e., points on monitoring sheet, pleasurable activities).

Strategies to Address Maintenance and Waning Motivation

Behavior modification techniques appear to be effective as long as they are used. TBMP places strong emphasis on the importance of maintenance behaviors, and it teaches members that maintenance requires lifelong effort. (In other treatments, this emphasis is often neglected, Cooper & Fairburn, 2002.) Individuals do not usually have sufficient incentive to continue using these techniques after they are no longer participating in a structured program. As the reinforcers for using behavioral techniques during weight loss level off or their salience fades, the costs remain constant or increase.

The major antidote to this problem is to provide regular continuing treatment. Continuing contact gives patients the chance to boost their morale and motivation in a joint effort with concerned leaders and fellow members (Perri, 1998). Maintaining a high level of motivation is a common discussion topic at weekly meetings, and it is often addressed through problem solving, modeling by experienced members, and behavioral strategies. The program's monthly newsletter ("The Modifier") also frequently deals with the topic of boosting motivation.

In addition, the Trevose program provides a number of additional contingencies, both reinforcing and punishing, that may result in continued participation and use of the behavioral techniques. Right at the beginning of membership, members learn about these contingencies, and it is emphasized that they are strictly implemented throughout membership. First, reinforcement is given at every stage in the program for successful weight loss and maintenance. Successful members regularly graduate to higher levels of membership, maintenance, and, eventually, leadership positions. These continued incentives may counteract the usual process of declining motivation during maintenance (the period when treatment and social support are typically discontinued). The first reinforcement comes from passing the 5-week screening phase. This entitles applicants to graduate to full membership. Subsequently, four distinct levels of maintenance can be achieved when weight loss has been maintained for specific periods of time, culminating in "independence level," the attainment of which is considered a high honor in the program. At each graduation, members receive a letter praising them for their achievement. Attaining maintenance-level status permits members to participate as staff, assistant leaders, or leaders in the program, and, if they wish, to start their own groups in their communities. Maintenance levels confer additional advantages, such as second chances to meet weight-loss goals. These lessen the threat of immediate dismissal from the program.

At independence level, members are not required to regularly attend meetings, but they are encouraged to participate as group leaders or volunteers in other capacities. They are also strongly encouraged to begin attending regularly again if a weight regain occurs. This strategy was tested and failed to improve maintenance following a 6-month treatment program (Wing et al., 1996), but it may have been useful as a component of the very effective long-term Swedish program (Bjorvell & Rossner, 1985).

The addition of tangible positive reinforcements in return for continued participation sets up an approach-oriented process in which behaviors are motivated by the desire to attain positive goals. Rothman (2000) describes approach-oriented behaviors as more likely to occur than behaviors driven by an avoidance-oriented process, as discussed previously. In most programs maintenance typically is driven merely by the desire to avoid negative consequences, which is insufficient.

Members are also confronted with the threat of immediate and permanent dismissal from the program (withdrawal of both present reinforcement and the possibility of future reinforcement) if their assigned goals for weight loss and attendance are not met. Individuals are permitted to join the group only once. According to members' reports, this "fear-based" incentive is a powerful motivator early in membership, and later on in membership the positive reinforcements are viewed as the more powerful motivating force (if so, this would represent a reversal of the Rothman, 2000, model). The possibility of dismissal makes it clear to members that the only way to achieve access to the group and its benefits are through the requisite behaviors of behavior modification and weight loss. They cannot pay money to obtain access nor enter under a different name (although according to leaders' reports, this has been occasionally attempted).

Tangible incentives have been offered in previous studies in order to enhance adherence to behavioral weight-loss programs, and they have met with little success. For example, Jeffery and colleagues (1993) attempted to modify the consequences of participants' weight loss by paying them up to $25 each week to lose weight. These incentives did not improve weight loss or maintenance compared with standard behavioral treatment. As concluded by Jeffery and colleagues (1993), these results do not necessarily imply that monetary or other tangible incentives are not effective; they suggest that incentives of the type and magnitude used in their study were not sufficiently useful. However, it is possible that the incentives offered for successful participation in TBMP are of greater magnitude, more personally meaningful, or longer lasting.

A Salutary Environment

It is possible that TBMP creates a miniature environment, its own community and culture, which counteracts or protects people from the broader toxic environment. This salutary environment implements a different system of values, rewards, and incentives for a certain healthy set of behaviors. These behaviors are different from the ones conditioned by the toxic environment.

CONCLUSIONS AND FUTURE DIRECTIONS

Several obstacles present challenges to the long-term implementation of self-help continuing care, and research is needed on ways to address these. As discussed earlier, attendance in treatment, both professional and self-help, often wanes after approximately 6 months (Jeffery et al., 2000). The challenge of how to retain people in treatment is a difficult one. Some individuals who drop out of treatment do so because they are satisfied with treatment's results or have the self-efficacy to continue on their own (Dalle Grave et al., 2005). These individuals may not need continuing care. However, many individuals drop out for logistical reasons (e.g., 51% in Dalle Grave et al., 2005), such as living far from treatment, financial problems, or work conflicts. Self-help programs may be more equipped to resolve these logistical problems than professional treatments. For example, most or all group members may agree that evenings or weekends are the most convenient time to convene, whereas many professionals are not as readily available during evening or weekend hours. Financial difficulties in paying for treatment are also much more easily resolved in volunteer-led support groups that meet in public locations or community organizations, where contributions to support overheads (if any) are small and up to the individual.

Another challenge to self-help continuing care is that studies examining the naturalistic administration of self-help may sacrifice internal validity (randomization, control groups) for external validity (generalizability and clinical representativeness). Therefore, it is difficult to draw causal inferences from studies of continuing care in its natural settings (e.g., Latner et al., 2000; Dalle Grave et al., 2005). On the other hand, studies with tight controls and randomization into treatment groups sacrifice real-world applicability, making it difficult to draw practical conclusions about the effectiveness of treatment for actual patients (e.g., Leibbrand & Fichter, 2002; Flechtner-Mors et al., 2000).

In addition, the few randomized controlled studies of continuing care, as well as those studies that evaluate the extended length of treatment (see Chapter 10, this volume) have examined only professional contact, reducing the feasibility of large-scale implementation and application of their results. Controlled trials of continuing care administered in a self-help format are needed. These could be implemented by randomizing participants into either a standard time-limited or continuing-treatment condition. At the beginning of treatment, groups might need to be professionally led, but very early in treatment, one to two volunteers would be recruited from each group and trained in the principles of group facilitation and behavior modification. Gradually these facilitators (or their successors, over time) could take charge of the group and lead its ongoing maintenance, so that the continuing-treatment condition would receive maintenance support in the form of self-help.

Another challenge to implementing self-help continuing-care treatment is the applicability to individuals from different cultural and ethnic backgrounds. Although the studies of continuing care are few in number, most of them come from different countries: Sweden, Germany, Italy, and the United States. The weight maintenance achieved across these geographically diverse studies (which also used diverse treatment methods) suggests that the utility of continuing care may be generalizable across cultures. However, research is needed among different cultural groups and communities to examine the effectiveness of self-help as a venue for continuing support. It is possible, for example, that in more individualistic Western societies, self-reliance and internal locus on control are helpful strategies, consistent with the value systems commonly promoted by self-help groups. On the other hand, individuals from cultures with a more collectivist orientation may have different expectations about the extent to which they should rely on professional versus peer guidance. How individuals from collectivist cultures feel about and respond to self-help treatment for obesity remains an important empirical question. Other issues in treatment research with ethnic minorities, such as interdependence, spirituality, and discrimination (Hall, 2001), may also be relevant in the self-help treatment of obesity. An essential part of testing the portability of a self-help, continuing-care model of obesity treatment will involve examining its effectiveness across diverse cultures.

REFERENCES

Bjorvell, H., & Rossner, S. (1985). Long-term treatment of severe obesity: Four-year follow-up of results of combined behavioural modification programme. *British Medical Journal, 291,* 379–382.

Bjorvell, H., & Rossner, S. (1990). A ten-year follow-up of weight change in severely obese subjects treated in a behavioural modification-like program. *International Journal of Obesity, 14*(Suppl. 2), 88.

Borkman, T. J. (1990). Experiential, professional, and lay frames of reference. In T. J. Powell (Ed.), *Working with self-help* (pp. 3–30). Silver Spring, MD: NASW Press.

Brownell, K. D., & Horgen, K. B. (2004). *Food fight: The inside story of the food industry, America's obesity crisis, and what we can do about it.* New York: McGraw-Hill.

Brownell, K. D., & Jeffery, R. W. (1987). Improving long-term weight loss: Pushing the limits of treatment. *Behavior Therapy, 18,* 353–374.

Brownell, K. D., Marlatt, G. A., Lichtenstein, E., & Wilson, G. T. (1986). Understanding and preventing relapse. *American Psychologist, 7,* 765–782.

Byrne, S. M. (2002). Psychological aspects of weight maintenance and relapse in obesity. *Journal of Psychosomatic Research, 53,* 1029–1036.

Cooper, Z., & Fairburn, C. G. (2002). A new cognitive-behavioral approach to the treatment of obesity. In T. A. Wadden & A. J. Stunkard (Eds.), *Obesity: Theory and therapy* (3rd ed.). New York: Guilford Press.

Cooper, Z., Fairburn, C. G., & Hawker, D. M. (2003). *Cognitive-behavioral treatment of obesity: A clinician's guide.* New York: Guilford Press.

Dalle Grave, R., Melchionda, N., Calugi, S., Centis, E., Tufano, A., Fatati, G., et al. (2005). Continuous care in the treatment of obesity: An observational multicenter study. *Journal of Internal Medicine, 258,* 265–273.

Davidson, M. H., Hauptman, J., DiGiralamo, M., Foreyt, J. P., Halsted, C. H., Heber, D., et al. (1999). Weight control and risk factor reduction in obese subjects treated for 2 years with Orlistat: A randomized controlled trial. *Journal of the American Medical Association, 281,* 235–242.

Delinsky, S. S., Latner, J. D., & Wilson, G. T. (2006). Binge eating and weight loss in a self-help behavior modification program. *Obesity Research, 14,* 1244–1249.

DePue, J. D., Clark, M. M., Ruggiero, L., Medeiros, M. L., & Pera, V. (1995). Maintenance of weight loss: A needs assessment. *Obesity Research, 3,* 241–248.

Diabetes Prevention Program Research Group. (2002). Reduction in the incidence of type 2 diabetes with lifestyle intervention or metformin. *New England Journal of Medicine, 346,* 393–403.

Dubbert, P. M., & Wilson, G. T. (1983). Failures in behavior therapy for obesity: Causes, correlates, and consequences. In E. B. Foa & P. M. Emmelkamp (Eds.), *Failures in behavior therapy* (pp. 263–288). New York: Wiley.

Finch, E. A., Linde, J. A., Jeffery, R. W., Rothman, A. J., King, C. M., & Levy, R. L. (2005). The effects of outcome expectations and satisfaction on weight loss and maintenance: Correlational and experimental analyses—a randomized trial. *Health Psychology, 24,* 608–616.

Flechtner-Mors, M., Ditschuneit, H. H., Johnson, T. D., Suchard, M. A., & Adler, G. (2000). Metabolic and weight loss effects of long-term dietary intervention in obese patients: Four-year results. *Obesity Research, 8,* 399–402.

Furnham, A., & McDermott, M. R. (1994). Lay beliefs about the efficacy of self-reliance, seeking help and external control as strategies for overcoming obesity, drug addiction, marital problems, stuttering and insomnia. *Psychology and Health, 9,* 397–406.

Hall, G. C. N. (2001). Psychotherapy research with ethnic minorities: Empirical, ethical, and conceptual issues. *Journal of Consulting and Clinical Psychology, 69,* 502–510.

Jeffery, R. W., Drewnowski, A., Epstein, L. H., Stunkard A. J., Wilson, G. T., Wing, R. R., et al. (2000). Long-term maintenance of weight loss: Current status. *Health Psychology, 19*(Suppl.), 5–16.

Jeffery, R. W., French, S. A., & Rothman, A. J. (1999). Stage of change as a predictor of success in weight control in adult women. *Health Psychology, 18,* 543–546.

Jeffery, R. W., Kelly, K. M., Rothman, A. J., Sherwood, N. E., & Boutelle, K. N. (2004). The weight loss experience: A descriptive analysis. *Annals of Behavioral Medicine, 27,* 100–106.

Jeffery, R. W., Wing, R. R., & Stunkard, A. J. (1978). Behavioral treatment of obesity: The state of the art. *Behavior Therapy, 9,* 189–199.

Jeffery, R. W., Wing, R. R., Thorson, C., Burton, L. R., Raether, C., Harvey, J., et al. (1993). Strengthening behavioral interventions for weight loss: A randomized trial of food provision and monetary incentives. *Journal of Consulting and Clinical Psychology, 61,* 1038–1045.

Katz, A. H. (1993). *Self-help in America: A social movement perspective.* New York: Twayne.

Klem, M. L., Wing, R. R., McGuire, M. T., Seagle, H. M., & Hill, J. O. (1997). A descriptive study of individuals successful at long-term maintenance of substantial weight loss. *American Journal of Clinical Nutrition, 66,* 239–246.

Lance, H., Peltonen, M., Agren, L., & Torgerson, J. S. (2003). A dietary and behavioural program for the treatment of obesity: A 4-year clinical trial and a long-term posttreatment follow-up. *Journal of Internal Medicine, 254,* 272–279.

Latner, J. D. (2001). Self-help in the long-term treatment of obesity. *Obesity Reviews, 2,* 87–97.

Latner, J. D., Stunkard, A. J., Wilson, G. T., & Jackson, M. L. (2006). The perceived effectiveness of continuing care and group support in the long-term self-help treatment of obesity. *Obesity Research, 14,* 464–471.

Latner, J. D., Stunkard, A. J., Wilson, G. T., Jackson, M. L., Zelitch, D. S., & Labouvie, E. (2000). Effective long-term treatment of obesity: A continuing care model. *International Journal of Obesity, 24,* 893–898.

Latner, J. D., Wilson, G. T., Stunkard, A. J., & Jackson, M. L. (2002). Self-help and long-term behavior therapy for obesity. *Behaviour Research and Therapy, 40,* 805–812.

Liebbrand, R., & Fichter, M. M. (2002). Maintenance of weight loss after obesity treatment: Is continuous support necessary? *Behaviour Research and Therapy, 40,* 1275–1289.

Melin, I., Karlstrom, B., Lappalainen, R., Berglund, L., Mohsen, R., & Vessby, B. (2003). A programme of behaviour modification and nutrition counselling in the treatment of obesity: A randomised 2-year clinical trial. *International Journal of Obesity and Related Metabolic Disorders, 27,* 1127–1135.

Metropolitan Life Insurance Company. (1983). 1983 Metropolitan height and weight tables. *Statistical Bulletin of the Metropolitan Life Foundation, 64,* 3–9.

Nir, Z., & Neumann, L. (1995). Relationship among self-esteem, internal–external locus of control, and weight change after participation in a weight reduction program. *Journal of Clinical Psychology, 51,* 482–490.

Pasman, W., Saris, W. H. M., & Westerterp-Plantenga, M. S. (1999). Predictors of weight maintenance. *Obesity Research, 7,* 43–50.

Penick, S. B., & Stunkard, A. J. (1972). The treatment of obesity. *Advances in Psychosomatic Medicine, 7,* 217–228.

Perri, M. G. (1998). The maintenance of treatment effects in the long-term management of obesity. *Clinical Psychology: Science and Practice, 5,* 526–543.

Pinel, J. P. J., Assanand, S., & Lehman, D. R. (2000). Hunger, eating, and ill health. *American Psychologist, 55,* 1105–1116.

Pi-Sunyer, F. X. (1996). A review of long-term studies evaluating the efficacy of weight loss in ameliorating disorders associated with obesity. *Clinical Therapeutics, 18,* 1006–1035.

Pi-Sunyer, F. X., Aronne, L. J., Heshmati, H. M., Devin, J., & Rosenstock, J. (2006). Effect of rimonabant, a cannabinoid-1 receptor blocker, on weight and cardiometabolic risk factors in overweight or obese patients. *Journal of the American Medical Association, 295,* 761–775.

Riessman, F. (1990). Restructuring help: A human services paradigm for the 1990s. *American Journal of Community Psychology, 18*, 221–230.

Rothman, A. J. (2000). Toward a theory-based analysis of behavioral maintenance. *Health Psychology, 19*(Suppl.), 64–69.

Sarlio-Lahteenkorva, S., Rissanen, A., & Kaprio, J. (2000). A descriptive study of weight loss maintenance: 6- and 15-year follow-up of initially overweight adults. *International Journal of Obesity, 24*, 116–125.

Segal, S. P., Silverman, C., & Temkin, T. (1995). Measuring empowerment in client-run self-help agencies. *Community Mental Health Journal, 31*, 215–227.

Stuart, R. B., & Davis, B. (1968). *Slim chance in a fat world: Behavioral control of obesity.* Champaign, IL: Research Press.

Stuart, R. B., & Guire, K. (1978). Some correlates of the maintenance of weight lost through behavior modification. *International Journal of Obesity, 2*, 225–235.

Verheijden, M. W., Bakx, J. C., van Weel, C., Koelen, M. A., & van Staveren, W. A. (2005). Role of social support in lifestyle-focused weight management interventions. *European Journal of Clinical Nutrition, 59*(Suppl.), S179–S186.

Wadden, T. A., Butryn, M. L., & Byrne, K. J. (2004). Efficacy of lifestyle modification for long-term weight control. *Obesity Research, 12* (Suppl.), 151S–162S.

Wadden, T. A., Foster, G. D., & Letizia, K. A. (1994). One-year behavioral treatment of obesity: Comparison of moderate and severe caloric restriction and the effects of weight maintenance therapy. *Journal of Consulting and Clinical Psychology, 62*, 165–171.

Wadden, T. A., & Frey, D. L. (1997). A multicenter evaluation of a proprietary weight loss program for the treatment of marked obesity: A five-year follow up. *International Journal of Eating Disorders, 22*; 203–212.

Williams, G. C., Grow, V. M., Freedman, Z. R., Ryan, R. M., & Deci, E. L. (1996). Motivational predictors of weight loss and weight-loss maintenance. *Journal of Personality and Social Psychology, 70*, 115–126.

Wilson, G. T. (1995). Behavioral and psychological predictors of treatment outcome in obesity. In D. B. Allison & F. X. Pi-Sunyer (Eds.), *Obesity treatment* (pp. 183–189). New York: Plenum Press.

Wing, R. R., Jeffery, R. W., Burton, L. R., Thorson, C., Sperber-Nissinoff, K., & Baxter, J. E. (1996). Food provision vs. structured meal plans in the behavioral treatment of obesity. *International Journal of Obesity, 20*, 56–62.

PART V

PRACTICAL STRATEGIES AND CONSIDERATIONS

The final section of this book addresses specific weight and eating problems from a practical point of view. Behavioral treatment of obesity is demystified in Chapter 12, which provides a breakdown and clear description of the weight-control strategies used in this treatment, as well as evidence for their use. Chapter 13 addresses practical strategies for families with children at risk of overweight. The techniques reviewed in this chapter are designed to prevent weight problems and to teach families practical ideas for maintaining a healthy home environment over the long term. Chapter 14 addresses techniques that parents can use to help their children who are already overweight. Like Chapter 12, this chapter translates many of the behavioral strategies used in professional treatment for parents to implement at home.

Night-eating syndrome is an increasingly researched problem, and the development of effective treatment is in the early stages. Chapter 15 applies cognitive-behavioral principles that have been used effectively with other eating disorders to the self-help treatment of night eating. In Chapter 16, cognitive-behavioral principles are also described for the treatment of binge eating, a behavior characterizing bulimia nervosa and binge-eating disorder. These principles are expanded on with a specific focus on appetite in order to address the appetite-related disturbances that are common in these disorders.

In addition to its physical ramifications, obesity is often accompanied by the pain of frequent bias, discrimination, and stigma against overweight individuals. Chapter 17 reviews the evidence on different strategies for most effectively coping with this stigma.

12

Behavioral Obesity Treatment Translated

DELIA SMITH WEST, STACY A. GORE,
and NATALIE K. LUEDERS

Behavioral therapy for obesity has evolved and developed over the years, with significant changes in the duration, and the nature of the strategies and the targeted behaviors emerging (Foster, Makris, & Bailer, 2005; Jeffery et al., 2000). Empirical evaluations of which components are associated with better weight losses have allowed behavioral therapy to be refined and elaborated, such that there are now several elements that are considered central in research-based behavioral obesity treatments for adults. The addition of these behavioral strategies has been shown to enhance weight-loss outcomes in formal nutrition education programs (Wing, Epstein, Nowalk, Koeske, & Hagg, 1985), as well as for individuals who are losing weight on their own or in community programs (Wing & Hill, 2001) and as an adjunct to medical interventions and pharmacotherapy (Wadden et al., 2005).

Research-based behavioral weight-control programs have been demonstrated effective in producing weight losses of 7–10% in adults (Wing, 2002). Weight losses of this magnitude produce a range of improvements in health, including reduced blood pressure and improved cholesterol profile (Dattilo & Kris-Etherton, 1996; Pi-Sunyer, 1996), enhanced blood glucose control and prevention of type 2 diabetes among high-risk individuals (Diabetes Prevention Program Research Group, 2002b), and improved quality of life and decreased symptoms of depression (Wadden, Steen, Wingate, &

Foster, 1996). Further, weight losses of 7–10% of body weight can be achieved (Wing, 2002), although weight maintenance remains the most challenging aspect of obesity treatment, with average long-term weight losses of 4% (Jeffery et al., 2000). Thus most behavioral treatment experts recommend a goal of 7–10% reduction in body weight for clients engaged in weight-loss efforts, with an expectation that about one-third will maintain this magnitude of weight loss for extended periods of 3 years or more (Diabetes Prevention Program Research Group, 2004) and that the majority will regain weight (Jeffery et al., 2000). Self-monitoring, frequent contact over an extended period of time, social support, problem solving, and goal setting are the key behavioral strategies that complement dietary restriction and physical activity in effective behavioral weight-control programs. This chapter briefly reviews scientific support for these elements of behavioral weight-loss therapy and offers suggestions on how these strategies can be effectively administered.

THEORETICAL FOUNDATION OF BEHAVIORAL THERAPY FOR OBESITY

Behavioral obesity treatment strategies are founded on social-cognitive theory (Bandura, 1986) and are designed to help individuals identify the behaviors that promote excessive calorie consumption or sedentary behavior, modify or replace these behaviors, and structure their environment to support the new, more health-promoting behaviors. A key component in the application of social-cognitive-theory-based principles is the identification of antecedents or "triggers" for behaviors that are contrary to effective weight management and of the consequences of these behaviors (Wing, 1992). The conceptual rationale for focusing on the antecedents, behaviors, and consequences is that the desired weight-loss behaviors (and the weight-gain-prevention behaviors) occur in a context, and therefore effective methods of altering these behaviors must address the larger social and environmental context if they are to be sustained and incorporated into the individual's lifestyle.

SELF-MONITORING

Self-monitoring is perhaps the single most important behavioral strategy incorporated into effective programs. It is the one intervention component that is consistently associated with success in studies of weight loss and long-term weight maintenance (Streit, Stevens, Stevens, & Rossner, 1991). Individuals who have successfully maintained weight losses for extended time periods report that they continue to monitor their dietary intake. Self-monitoring is effective regardless of whether individuals lost weight on their own or with the help of a structured program (Wing et al., 2004; Wing & Klem, 2002). Even partial self-monitoring, in which individuals fail to record everything or are inconsistent in their recording, can be effective in promoting weight control (Baker & Kirschenbaum, 1998).

Self-Monitoring of Dietary and Exercise Behavior

Self-monitoring in behavioral obesity therapy involves the daily recording of all food and beverage intake, with portion size and calorie level (and fat grams) of foods typically recorded, and logging all physical activity, including the type of activity and number of minutes (or caloric expenditure equivalent). A variety of methods of recording dietary intake and physical activity can be used, with little evidence that one is superior to another. Individuals can record food intake and exercise in a pen-and-paper diary or spiral notebook, but more "hi-tech" methods, including Palm Pilots or Web-based diaries, can also be used with equal success (Yon, Johnson, Harvey-Berino, & Gold, 2006; see also Chapter 7, this volume). Recording can also be simplified to accommodate individuals with low literacy. Such methods include lists or pictures of foods that an individual can check off as those items are consumed (particularly useful when a finite number of servings of a specific food are targeted) or food cards that can be moved from one envelope to another after the food has been consumed; see also Chapter 13, this volume. In addition to information regarding type of food and portion size consumed, diaries can also include time of day, other activities performed while eating, precursors to eating, and mood before, during, and after eating. Physical activity is usually recorded in terms of type of exercise or activity completed and the number of minutes spent participating in the exercise or the calories expended in the exercise. Situational information similar to that recorded in relation to food intake can also be recorded.

It is likely that self-monitoring is useful for several reasons. As has been demonstrated in a range of behavior-change arenas, the act of observing a behavior changes it (Korotitsch & Nelson-Gray, 1999). In the case of monitoring food intake, this phenomenon seems to work to the advantage of weight-loss efforts, causing decreased caloric intake (Kumanyika et al., 2000). Individuals become more cognizant of their food intake when they see it recorded in black and white, and they report that they reconsider whether they really want to eat a high-calorie food or large portion size when they think about having to write it down. The presence of a food diary on a kitchen table or in their pocket or purse may serve as a reminder of their weight-loss goals. Self-monitoring of food consumption provides an objective, tangible record that can either be consistent or discordant with the individual's goals for weight loss. Self-monitoring may achieve greater adherence to dietary recommendations by promoting perceptions of a discrepancy between personal weight-loss goals and an objective assessment of current behavior (such as a diary with food intake that does not promote weight loss), which, in turn may increase motivation to adhere to dietary recommendations or calorie goals (DiLillo, Siegfried, & West, 2003). Wanting to behave in a socially desirable manner (i.e., decreasing caloric intake to look good to or to please the weight-loss counselor) may also play a role.

Self-monitoring of food intake allows an individual to see a more accurate and objective picture of his or her current dietary behavior rather than relying on his or her memory about eating habits. Indeed, individuals are often surprised at their food consumption when they start keeping a food diary and see an objective record of their intake. Given that there are rather strong data that self-monitoring of food intake is inaccurate and usually underestimates food consumption (Drougas, Reed, & Hill, 1992), the power of the food diary is even more impressive. Efforts to improve accuracy of monitoring, such as training in recognizing portion sizes, weighing and measuring foods, and reading food labels, can all improve the utility of the self-monitoring record. Information about calorie and fat content is usually provided to participants to facilitate accurate self-monitoring. A variety of books on the subject are available widely, and those that are easy to transport (pocket or purse size) and have a broad range of prepared foods included (such as convenience foods or restaurant fare) tend to be the most useful. Online calorie information can also be very helpful. However, it must be emphasized that accuracy in quantifying food intake is only one of the salient factors that contribute to the efficacy of self-monitoring in promoting weight loss.

Perhaps most important for a behavioral weight-loss program, self-monitoring recordings provide useful information when trying to make targeted changes in eating and exercise behavior. These diaries can be used by individuals and their counselors to gain insight into eating patterns, such as times of day that are especially problematic or triggers for eating. This information can then be used to set specific, personalized goals for changing behavior to reduce caloric intake or increase exercise. For example, activities that are incompatible with eating can be identified and scheduled during times of day in which the individual is more likely to engage in snacking. Additionally, diaries allow individuals to evaluate progress toward behavior-change goals. With regard to physical activity, similar opportunities for identifying barriers to exercise and environmental cues that increase physical activities can be identified.

Several key components will improve the usefulness of self-monitoring. Recording food intake or exercise as soon as possible after the behavior rather than waiting to fill out diaries at the end of the day or week increases their accuracy and decreases the likelihood that memory will distort the behaviors. The more immediately the self-monitoring is done, the greater the potential for reactivity to modify behavior through the rest of the day or the following day. If an individual waits for an extended time period to record, there is less opportunity for reactivity to influence behavior. As has been stated earlier, these diaries serve as the basis of behavior change efforts, and their accuracy will allow better behavioral analysis. Therefore, diaries should be reviewed on a regular basis to identify and encourage positive changes in eating and exercise habits and to conduct problem solving when difficulties are encountered. This important review process is best accomplished at first by a weight-loss professional or counselor who brings an objective eye with the goal of assisting the individual in developing skills in behavioral analysis that he or she can apply to his or her own self-monitoring record.

Self-Monitoring of Weight

Another particularly valuable type of self-monitoring is the practice of regular weighing. The majority of successful dieters report weighing themselves at least weekly (Wing & Klem, 2002), and daily weighing has been shown to facilitate weight maintenance (McGuire, Wing, Klem, & Hill, 1999; Wing et al., 2006). From a behavioral perspective, frequent weighing may seem contradictory to the principle of focusing on behaviors over which the individual has direct control. However, regular weighing serves as an objective measure of the effects of behavior change. For both individual and counselor, weekly weighing is a barometer of progress. Therefore, if the individual's weight remains stable or rises during the weight-loss phase of treatment, changes may need to be made to decrease calorie intake and increase expenditure. Conversely, watching the scale decrease can be very encouraging and indicates that the individual is on the right track. After the individual has reached weight-loss goals, regular weighing can also be helpful in preventing weight regain. Modest weight gains can be caught early and can serve as a trigger to institute behaviors that prevent a more dramatic weight gain or relapse, such as returning to recording food intake or meal replacement and increasing physical activity.

Regular weighing is often incorporated into behavioral weight-loss treatment by having individuals weigh-in when they attend weekly treatment sessions. Although group support is important, weigh-ins are usually conducted individually in order to protect an individual's privacy. In addition, many individuals find public weighing extremely anxiety provoking, and this practice may serve as a barrier to attending group treatment, especially when they believe they have gained weight. Conducting weighing in the presence of a counselor also provides an opportunity to model an adaptive response to the results. Individuals are not scolded for weight gains, nor are weight gains seen as a sign of failure but as useful information with which to guide short-term behavior goals. Similarly, cautionary notes can be sounded when weight losses are not accompanied by appropriate behavior changes. Typically, individuals are asked to weigh themselves once per day at home, identifying a consistent time of day in which to weigh. Weight is recorded on a graph to identify the long-term trends and to ensure that weight changes are kept in a broader context. This attenuates the impact of day-to-day fluctuations that often occur and provides an indication of progress toward personal goals.

LENGTH OF PROGRAM AND NATURE OF CONTACT

Another factor that plays a role in the level of success that overweight individuals achieve is the amount of contact with their weight-loss counselors. Most behavioral obesity programs involve weekly meetings with a weight-loss professional, either individually or in a group setting. These meetings provide opportunities to learn new skills, to evaluate progress toward behavioral goals, and to review weekly diaries. In addition, problem solving and goal setting for the following week can prepare the individual for upcoming challenges and encourage continued progress toward long-term weight-loss goals. In general, the longer the weight-loss program, the longer individuals adhere to behavior changes and the greater weight loss achieved (Perri, Nezu, Patti, & McCann, 1989). Further, extending treatment appears to hold off the weight regain that often follows the conclusion of treatment (Perri et al., 1989). However, attendance at treatment sessions seems to decline substantially over time, and expecting weekly individual participation over an extended period may be unrealistic (Jeffery et al., 2000). Tapering off contact instead of stopping abruptly after the initial weight-loss program may provide an appropriate balance, maximizing individual participation and decreasing the amount of weight regain often observed. Thus many weight-loss programs involve meeting weekly for 4–6 months of weight-loss induction and reducing contact during a maintenance phase of 6–18 months (Diabetes Prevention Program Research Group, 2002b; Perri & Corsica, 2002). Using this structure, weight-loss goals are ideally met in the intensive phase of treatment (e.g., the first 6 months). When contact decreases to biweekly or monthly meetings, the individual continues to practice weight-loss techniques such as self-monitoring, weighing, and problem solving, as well as following dietary and exercise goals, on his or her own, using the support of the now less frequent meetings to facilitate the adoption of these behavioral skills into the individual's personal behavioral repertoire. The maintenance phase will also give individuals the opportunity to identify which behaviors they wish to continue at the conclusion of the weight-loss program. This maintenance phase of treatment can allow the individual to gain more confidence in his or her ability to continue newly acquired behaviors while still having access to a weight-loss professional or counselor (see also Chapter 11, this volume). In addition, new skills, such as relapse prevention techniques, can be practiced. Ideally, when individuals begin to regain weight during the maintenance phase, they will be able to reinstitute behaviors they learned in the program, thereby preventing serious relapses.

Because of the cost-effectiveness of group delivery and the additional social support offered, most behavioral obesity programs are implemented in a group setting, with 10–20 individuals included in the group, with meetings usually lasting 60–90 minutes. Groups are usually closed, meaning that once a group has been constituted, new people do not drop in or join the group, and the group remains together throughout at least the weight-loss-induction phase of treatment (the first 6 months). This allows group cohesion to build and develop over time. Some programs will combine several weight-loss induction groups during the weight-loss-maintenance phase. Despite the benefits of group administration, it is often not practical to deliver behavioral obesity treatment in a group format (scheduling is a common barrier), or specific individuals may be more inclined to individual treatment. One of the most successful behavioral weight-loss research studies to date, the Diabetes Prevention Program (DPP), delivered a lifestyle obesity treatment program individually to overweight men and women at high risk for type 2 diabetes (Diabetes Prevention Program Research Group, 2002a).

Empirical support exists for delivering program content in formats other than in person. Internet delivery of behavioral weight-control programs has been shown to be effective (Harvey-Berino, Pintauro, Buzzell, & Gold, 2004) and may offer fewer barriers to participating in in-person programs (see also Chapter 7, this volume). There are also some indications that phone-delivered weight-loss programs may be successful (Donnelly, Stewart, Menke, & Smith, 2005); however, mail-based or correspondence programs have produced negligible weight losses in studies to date (Jeffery et al., 2003).

SOCIAL SUPPORT

Social support is consistently identified by individuals as one of the major facilitators of their weight-loss efforts (Jeffery et al., 2000) and is often cited as critical in their decision to seek assistance with weight-loss efforts. Social support can be incorporated into weight loss programs in a variety of ways, and attention to increasing social support is associated with increased success in weight loss and weight maintenance (Wing & Jeffery, 1999). The delivery of weight-loss programs in a group setting is common, because group members can provide emotional support, offer suggestions on techniques they have found useful, and act as sources of accountability to other individuals working toward similar goals. One study that examined the delivery of a behavioral weight program in a group format compared with individual sessions demonstrated greater weight losses among individuals who received the program in the group (Renjilian et al., 2001), presumably because of the greater social support provided by the group.

Some weight-loss programs have attempted to increase social support by recruiting participants with their friends so that individuals will have "built-in" social support when entering a weight-loss program. Recruiting individuals with friends who are also attempting to lose weight and including opportunities to build social support within a weight-loss group by having team projects and team contests have both been demonstrated to increase weight loss and improve weight maintenance (Wing & Jeffery, 1999). Friendly competitions to achieve behavioral goals (e.g., minutes of exercise, number of self-monitoring diaries completed, etc.) or weight-loss goals (number of pounds, total team weight loss, etc.) between teams have been shown to spark greater adherence and motivation and are usually offered with some form of modest incentive (Wing & Jeffery, 1999).

Most behavioral weight-control program curricula include a discussion of how to use social support to help reach weight-loss goals. Family and friends can act as either barriers or prompts to positive behaviors. Participants may learn how to better involve their social network in their weight-loss efforts or how to negotiate conflicts between their newly acquired behaviors and their families or friends. Individuals who report greater social support among their families and friends lose more weight in programs, and, therefore, efforts to develop and buttress this social support are a key focus of behavioral weight-loss programs (Elfhag & Rossner, 2005).

PROBLEM SOLVING

A formal problem-solving approach is included in most behavioral obesity programs to help individuals address barriers to success and plan for high-risk situations that might precipitate a lapse or relapse. This five-step process has been shown to be an effective approach to long-term weight maintenance (Perri et al., 2001) and is a central strategy in successful lifestyle interventions such as the Diabetes Prevention Program (DPP; Diabetes Prevention Program Research Group, 2002a). The first step is to foster the adoption of a problem-solving orientation, which posits that problems are a normal aspect of behavior change and that individuals can cope with problems such that those problems do not derail them from achieving their goals. The second step is to define the problem, using descriptions of the situation that focus on problem behaviors and clarify the individual's goal.

The third step involves the generation of alternative solutions to this problem, or brainstorming. The more creative and broader the range of solutions to the problem that can be generated, the greater the chances that an effective solution for the individual will be included on the list. Individuals often need to be encouraged to avoid censoring themselves during the brainstorming step, because they have a tendency to jump to considering the barriers to the solution. They should be urged to brainstorm unfettered by evaluation during this step in order to make the problem solving most productive. In the fourth step, an evaluation of the consequences or likely outcomes of the different solutions is conducted. This evaluation guides the selection of a solution that looks most likely to accomplish the individual's goals (and to minimize negative consequences). The final step is to implement the problem solution and then to evaluate whether it was effective. Ideally, the individual outlines a plan for evaluating whether he or she would consider the outcome of the problem solving effective prior to implementing the solution.

Problem solving can be conducted with individuals or in group settings. When done in a group, it allows soliciting input from multiple group members about problems that are common to group members or bringing together suggestions from the larger group to address challenges faced by a single individual. Often the solution an individual selects represents a combination of several of the solutions generated in the brainstorming phase, and this is fine. In guiding the process of problem solving, the weight-loss counselor can be helpful in shaping the problem definition to ensure that it is crafted in a fashion that is amenable to behavioral solutions and in facilitating the generation of numerous alternative solutions so that there is rich range of options from which to select. However, caution is recommended in the selection of the "best" solution. Individuals who select their own solutions rather than having one prescribed or being given the solution by their counselors appear to be most likely to follow through with the solution. Counselors can prompt appropriate evaluation of the pros and cons of the different strategies but are advised to leave the selection of the solution up to the individual.

GOAL SETTING

Goal setting is another integral component of behavioral obesity therapy, with short-term and long-term goals beneficial in achieving successful behavior changes and associated weight loss (Bandura & Simon, 1977). Short-term goals are most helpful in guiding proximal or daily behaviors and would include such things as daily calorie intake goals, physical activity goals (type, duration, which days, etc.), or even going to the supermarket to purchase healthy, low-calorie snacks or calling a friend to set up a walking date. Long-term goals are more helpful for maintaining motivation for behavior change than for guiding specific behavior changes and usually focus on weight-loss goals, but they can also include such things as health, emotional, relationship, professional, and other goals. Short-term goals tend to be more effective when they are objectively stated in behavioral terms ("I will exercise 3 days this week" vs. "I will do better with my exercise"). Descriptions of the goal that are specific and detailed enough to describe how the goal will be accomplished ("I will go walking for 20 minutes on Monday, Wednesday, and Friday mornings") are more likely to facilitate achievement of the goal. Similarly, identifying goals that are realistic and obtainable (i.e., able to be accomplished) contributes to more successful outcomes. For example, a sedentary individual who sets a goal of running a marathon by the end of the month is less likely to be successful than if that same sedentary individual were to set a goal of walking for 20 minutes on Monday, Wednesday, and Friday mornings. Care must be taken to help individuals evaluate whether the goal is realistic and obtainable in the short run, for they are often so very enthusiastic about reaching their long-term goals that they fail to identify realistic short-term goals that build to the eventual outcome they desire.

Recommended calorie and physical activity goals are usually outlined for participants in behavioral weight-control programs, and the focus of short-term goal setting for individuals tends to be on identifying manageable strategies to accomplish these calorie intake and physical activity levels. The graded nature of some program targets provides for a mid-range goal—one that the short-term goals lead toward but that is not quite as overarching as the motivational long-term goal. For all levels of goals, it is preferable to have them stated in objective or behavioral terms to facilitate assessment of whether the goal has been achieved. By way of example, it is very hard to evaluate whether one's goal to "get healthier" has been accomplished. This fairly ambiguous goal lends itself to emotional evaluation rather than to an objective assessment of whether progress has been made, especially when an individual is discouraged or in a negative mood. This can lead to further discouragement and abandoning of behavior change efforts. Reframing the same long-term goal to be "I would like to reduce my blood pressure and improve my cholesterol levels" allows the goal to be monitored and evaluated more objectively. Even better would be a clarification of the degree of change that the individual desires or with which he or she would be satisfied. Objectiveness and specification facilitate the recognition that progress has been made and that one isn't a total failure in behavior-change efforts, and they may protect against abandonment of behavior change efforts. The ability to set objective, detailed, reasonable, and achievable goals is a skill that often requires practice to master. Behavioral obesity programs introduce this skill early in the program and continue to apply and refine this skill throughout treatment.

Despite the significant health improvements and enhancements to quality of life that typically accompany a 7–10% weight loss, it is often the case that individuals who embark on weight-loss efforts have more ambitious long-term personal weight-loss goals and may be disappointed with the more modest weight losses that are likely to be achieved even in state-of-the-art behavioral obesity treatments. Efforts to dissuade individuals from unrealistic goals and to promote more appropriate weight-loss goals do not appear to be helpful in boosting overall weight losses (Foster et al., 2004). Indeed, it may be those individuals with the unrealistically high weight-loss goals who lose the most weight in programs (Linde, Jeffery, Levy, Pronk, & Boyle, 2005).

DIETARY INTERVENTION

Changes to dietary intake are central to successful weight loss and sustained weight maintenance. Calorie restriction has been shown to be essential to achieving weight loss (Harvey-Berino, 1999). The addition of fat restriction can increase the amount of weight lost (Pascale, Wing, Butler, Mullen, & Bononi, 1995), but in and of itself it is insufficient to produce weight losses of the magnitude achieved with reduced caloric consumption. The general goal is to reduce calorie intake sufficiently to promote weight losses that average 1 to 2 pounds per week. In empirically validated programs such as the DPP (Diabetes Prevention Program Research Group, 2002a), the typical calorie intake goal for individuals weighing 250 pounds or less is 1,200–1,500 kcal per day (10,000/week), and it is 1,500–1,800 kcal per day for individuals over 250 pounds (12,000/week). Individuals are taught to use their self-monitoring diaries to allow them to plan out the day and the week to stay within their calorie goals. The broadening of the focus to include the week allows for some flexibility from day to day to account for special occasions, lapses, and other "overindulgences" without abandoning calorie goals. Guidance is given to distribute these calories with less than 30% from fat and less than 10% from saturated fat so as to contribute to lowering cardiovascular risk, given that most overweight individuals are vulnerable to cardiovascular disease. Some successful programs have specifically focused on intake of fruits and vegetables and low-fat dairy products, in addition to calorie goals, to facilitate the consumption of foods low in calories and high in nutrients (Premier Collaborative Research Group, 2003). There is growing evidence that increasing intake of foods low in calorie density, such as fruits and vegetables, whole grains, and soups, may produce greater weight losses than trying to eat smaller portion sizes of calorie-rich foods (Rolls, Roe, Beach, & Kris-Etherton, 2005).

Using the analogy of a checking account can often help individuals to adhere to the calorie goals. They have a finite "calorie budget" and can spend it in a variety of ways, although there is a strong recommendation that the "bills" of good nutrition be paid prior to spending on "luxuries" of high-calorie foods. The key to this budget analogy is that the individual has no credit! The goal is to stay in the black and not the red. If the prescribed calorie goals are not effective in producing weight loss, they can be revised. This process is usually one of first ensuring that portion size and calorie estimates of foods are accurate and then making slight adjustments downward until the desired weight loss is achieved. Once an individual has achieved the desired weight loss and moves into weight maintenance, the reverse process occurs. Adjustments upward are made to the calorie goal in the "checking account" until equilibrium is achieved that offers weight stability. Modifications to decrease the calorie goal are made if weight creeps back up over the desired weight range.

Portion-Controlled Meals

One strategy that has been effective in assisting adherence to calorie goals and increasing weight losses is the use of portion-controlled meals or meal replacements. Weight losses can be increased by approximately 3 kg when these products are incorporated in weight-loss programs (Heymsfield, van Mierlo, van der Knaap, Heo, & Frier, 2003). Individuals are encouraged to substitute the portion-controlled meal or meal replacement for conventional self-selected foods for two meals (usually breakfast and lunch) and one snack per day during the weight-loss-induction period, transitioning to one meal replacement or portion-controlled meal and one snack during weight maintenance (Ditschuneit & Flechtner-Mors, 2001). The addition of structure and the decreased need to make decisions in the moment about what and how much to eat appear to be the critical elements, as structured meal plans that outline what to eat and the amount (and that even provide a shopping list) produce weight losses comparable to actually giving the individuals the same meal ingredients (Wing et al., 1996). The foremost issue in using these meal replacements may be identifying the meal replacements, prepackaged meals, or meal plans that are most acceptable to the client and therefore likely to be incorporated into his or her lifestyle and maintained. Reinstituting more frequent use of meal replacements or structured meals can be useful when small weight regains are noted.

Meal Patterns

Many overweight individuals skip breakfast. However, individuals who are successful at long-term weight loss report that they regularly eat breakfast (Wyatt et al., 2002). Therefore, one strong recommendation a weight-loss counselor can make is to plan and eat a reasonable breakfast. A further common recommendation is to avoid long periods without eating anything, because this can make an individual vulnerable to overeating either high-calorie foods or excessive portions. Although there is nothing inherently destructive about eating in the evening, it is often a time that individuals struggle with sticking to their eating plans. Therefore, evening snacking often merits specific discussion using a problem-solving approach to deal with unplanned overconsumption of high-calorie foods.

PHYSICAL ACTIVITY

Successful behavioral weight-loss programs target both dietary changes and increases in physical activity. A majority of overweight and obese individuals are sedentary, and the addition of exercise to a weight-control program significantly increases weight losses (Elfhag & Rossner, 2005; Jeffery et al., 2000) and may have a specific role to play in promoting weight maintenance (Pronk & Wing, 1994). The primary focus is on planned physical activity, which can include aerobic exercise and other lifestyle exercise, such as walking. Lifestyle exercises are as effective in promoting weight loss as aerobic activities such as running or high-impact dance (Andersen et al., 1999). Walking is the most common form of physical activity encouraged for overweight individuals in weight-control research programs such as the DPP (Diabetes Prevention Program Research Group, 2002a), although other aerobic activities are also effective in facilitating weight loss. The levels of physical activity needed to promote or sustain weight loss have been the source of some controversy. The Surgeon General's Report recommends 30 minutes a day on more days than not (U.S. Department of Health and Human Services, 1996), a goal traditionally translated into 150 minutes per week and one that is recommended by other weight-loss and health experts (Jakicic et al., 2001; National Heart, Lung, and Blood Institute, 1998). However, studies of individuals who have been successful at long-term weight loss indicate that they report engaging in substantially higher levels of physical activity (Jakicic, Winters, Lang, & Wing, 1999; Jeffery, Wing, Sherwood, & Tate, 2003), with 200–250 minutes per week of physical activity reported by these individuals. Research-based behavioral weight-control programs such as the DPP outline exercise goals of 150 minutes per week, but it is becoming increasingly clear that the more physical activity that an individual incorporates into his or her day, the greater are his or her the chances of weight loss and successful weight maintenance.

Increasing Adherence to Physical Activity Goals

Graded physical activity goals that gradually increase the number of days and the duration of activity are critical to developing activity habits among sedentary individuals. Graded goals challenge the individual to increase to a level of exercise that promotes weight loss, fitness, and long-term weight management while promoting safety. For example, many programs recommend an initial short-term exercise goal of 10 minutes three times per week for a previously sedentary individual. After this goal is achieved, frequency and/or duration of exercise is increased weekly until the long-term exercise prescription of 30 minutes per day 5 days a week is achieved.

Physical activity can be attained in a variety of ways, allowing for customization to an individual's preferences and lifestyle (see also Chapter 3, in this volume). Home-based physical activity programs that an individual can perform on his or her own have been shown to be sustained for longer periods than supervised exercise programs that rely on travel to a facility and on the supervision of another individual (Perri, Martin, Leermakers, Sears, & Notelovitz, 1997). Physical activity can be accumulated over the day, with four bouts of 10 minutes of physical activity accumulated over the course of the day equally as effective in producing weight loss as a single daily bout of 40 minutes (Jakicic, Wing, Butler, & Robertson, 1995). Therefore, individuals can select whether shorter bouts or longer bouts best fit their lifestyle, increasing the likelihood that they successfully incorporate exercise into their day and adhere to the exercise goals. Pedometers are often provided to give individuals an easy way to assess the amount of lifestyle activity they are accumulating during the day. A long-term goal of 10,000 steps is provided (Le Masurier, Sidman, & Corbin, 2003), with short-term goals that focus on increasing daily step totals by 250 until the target of 10,000 has been reached. Research has demonstrated that directly giving individuals treadmills for their homes will both increase their physical activity level and produce greater weight losses (Jakicic et al., 1999), presumably because barriers to exercise are reduced. Although giving people treadmills can be beyond the budget of many behavioral weight-loss programs, the principle of reducing barriers to physical activity by providing equipment is often generalized to such practices as giving the aforementioned pedometers, exercise videotapes or audiotapes, strength-training tubes or weights, and the like. Further, these studies suggest that programs make very strong recommendations to their participants about the benefits of acquiring appropriate exercise equipment to facilitate achieving and sustaining physical activity goals.

Self-monitoring records can be very helpful in establishing and maintaining these new physical activity habits. Individuals are encouraged to total their daily exercise (and step) efforts for the week and to graph them over time as a way to monitor progress and maintain motivation. Individuals are often very surprised at the progress that they make in becoming less sedentary and more active in a relatively short time. Weekly self-monitoring records allow individuals and their counselors to identify patterns that can help target and refine efforts to incorporate activity. For example, if one were to observe that an individual who exercises in the morning is consistently able to achieve the targeted minutes but who exercises less often or for a shorter time on days when he or she exercises in the afternoon, this would direct the counselor and individual to consider planning morning activity. Alternatively, an individual who noted that stress was associated with excess snacking after work might find that going out for a walk right after getting home from work was effective in both reducing the overeating and finding a time that worked well into his or her lifestyle.

Social support can play a particularly powerful role in facilitating adherence to physical activity goals. Having an "exercise buddy" or a personal trainer with whom an individual has scheduled an exercise date is likely to increase follow-through with planned exercise (Jeffery, Wing, Thorson, & Burton, 1998). This finding may reflect greater accountability, enhanced motivation, or greater enjoyment in the activity when done with a friend. Whatever may be responsible for the superior activity levels among individuals with an exercise partner, it is clearly a strategy on which many behavioral weight-control programs seek to capitalize. Motivational campaigns that include team training for walking a half marathon or a local race can put an extra spark into social support for physical activity.

MOTIVATION

Although education about dietary intake and physical activity is a central part of all behavioral weight-loss programs, most participants will express the sentiment that "they know what they need to do, it's just doing it that's the problem." Therefore, attention to sustained motivation for behavior-change efforts becomes a very important component of most behavioral obesity treatment programs (Jeffery et al., 2000). Some strategies to enhance or sustain motivation have already been discussed, such as using self-monitoring to track progress, employing short- and long-term goals, and developing social support networks around the desired behavior changes. Behavioral programs frequently address the issue of rewarding oneself for achieving goals along the way. This strategy reinforces behavior changes and helps to maintain motivation. However, this particular practice has not been empirically examined to determine how effective participants are in appropriately rewarding themselves or how significantly this process affects overall weight loss and weight maintenance. Nonetheless, one of the fundamental aspects of the motivational nature of goals is having an opportunity to recognize and celebrate accomplishments. For the most part, individuals do a better job of recognizing achievements than of celebrating or reinforcing goal attainment. Generating a list of ways in which a person can "reward" himself or herself, particularly with non-food-related rewards, is often difficult for participants in obesity treatment programs. Further, when generating ideas for non-food-related rewards, participants often think in terms of purchased rewards, such as buying flowers or a new CD, getting nails manicured, or buying a new power tool and often omit from their list intangible rewards (such as enjoying some quiet time, making a phone date with a friend or family member, going dancing, reading a book, watching a favorite movie, etc.) that can help keep the costs of self-rewarding from being prohibitive. Another strategy that has shown promise in promoting improved outcomes by focusing on motivation is the approach outlined in motivational interviewing (Miller & Rollnick, 2002). When individuals receive empathetic and nonjudgmental counseling that explores personally relevant reasons for weight loss and lifestyle behavior changes and that draws a discrepancy between current behaviors that are divergent from these personal goals while also exploring any ambivalence about behavior change, individuals appear to demonstrate better attendance at obesity treatment sessions and more frequent self-monitoring, as well as greater overall weight losses (Smith, Heckemeyer, Kratt, & Mason, 1997). A motivational interviewing approach can be utilized successfully by weight-loss professionals (West, DiLillo, Greene, Kratt, & Kirk, 2003) and by nonprofessionals seeking to facilitate dietary change (Resnicow et al., 2001).

ADAPTING BEHAVIORAL WEIGHT CONTROL FOR MINORITY POPULATIONS

Some minority groups have smaller average weight losses than the 7–10% reported in research-based behavioral obesity treatment programs, and they may benefit from adaptations to the general behavioral weight-reduction intervention outlined. For example, some well-designed clinical trials with behavioral obesity programs report that African Americans lose significantly less weight than Whites (Kumanyika, Obarzanek, Stevens, Hebert, & Whelton, 1991; Wing & Anglin, 1996). However, more recent research suggests that differences between weight losses achieved by black and white women are not apparent when participants are of comparable socioeconomic status (Hong, Li, Wang, Elshoff, & Heber, 2005) or if participants are followed for an extended time period (Diabetes Prevention Program Research Group, 2004). For example, the DPP enrolled a large number of overweight individuals from 16 sites across the United States, including a significant proportion (46%) of overweight individuals from minority groups that are vulnerable to diabetes (including African Americans, Hispanic Americans, and Native Americans), and delivered a state-of-the art behavioral weight-loss intervention (Diabetes Prevention Program Research Group, 2002a). Although at the end of the 6-month weight-loss-induction phase, whites were significantly more likely to have achieved the study goal of a 7% weight-loss than individuals in minority groups, by the end of the study (about 3.5 years) there were no significant differences between the ethnic groups (Diabetes Prevention Program Research Group, 2004). For example, the majority of African Americans who lost 7% by the end of the weight-loss program maintained it throughout the study (approximately 35% had lost 7% at the end of treatment, and 30% maintained it). This suggests that the trajectory of weight loss may differ between ethnic minority groups and Whites, with either a deferred weight loss induction phase or better weight maintenance among minorities (Kumanyika et al., 2002). However, it is prudent to note that the 7–10% average weight losses achieved in the initial 6 months of a behavioral weight-control program may be attenuated among members of ethnic minority groups.

Methods for tailoring or adapting behavioral weight-control programs to be culturally relevant for minority populations have been well described (Kumanyika, 2002). Surface aspects of the program materials can be adapted for the target populations. For example, dietary recommendations that are congruent with traditional or preferred foods can be incorporated, role models who are relevant and admired within the community can be identified and included, and physical activity options outlined can reflect activities that are both acceptable and accessible to individuals within the community. Logistics can also be addressed to tailor behavioral interventions to specific populations. Language modifications and delivery in a convenient community locale are two such accommodations that tend to increase participation and effectiveness of a behavioral program. Treatment delivery by staff familiar with or indigenous to the target community is another frequent adaptation. Standards of physical attractiveness and cultural norms about weight loss, concerns about the role of the individual in the family or in the community, and the specific role of women can emerge as keynote themes that may need to be addressed when tailoring interventions to specific minority communities. Other elemental concerns exist that may require attention in the development of a successful weight-loss program, particularly one designed for disadvantaged minority communities, including issues surrounding food insecurity (uncertainty about being able to obtain enough food, often due to financial limitations), neighborhood availability of healthy foods, and venues for safe physical activity.

However, even with the tailoring or adaptations that have been described, the fundamental elements of an effective behavioral program remain the same. The core behavioral weight-loss strategies for minority populations remain self-monitoring, caloric restriction, and increased physical activity. Further, no data are currently available that compare a culturally tailored behavioral weight-control program with a standard state-of-the-art behavioral weight-control program with the same population to determine whether using a culturally tailored weight-control program produces better weight-loss outcomes. Indeed, many programs that provide details of culturally tailored obesity-related interventions fail to provide outcome data to evaluate the efficacy of the program. Nonetheless, it has been noted that using interventions that engage the target community in the design and implementation of the program so that it is culturally competent and acceptable does appear to substantially affect the level of participation (Yancy et al., 2004). That is, with culturally appropriate interventions, more members of the targeted population become engaged, and more are retained.

SUMMARY

Behavioral weight-control methods utilized in controlled trials have evolved over time, and there now exists a standard core of best practices that might be recommended for obesity treatment. Critical components include a strong focus on self-monitoring, use of calorie-restricted dietary guidelines, and implementation of graded physical activity goals that progress to a minimum level of 150 minutes per week but that produce substantial benefits at higher levels. Emerging evidence points to the benefits of structured meals or meal replacements and opportunities to distribute physical activity bouts over the course of the day in enhancing adherence to dietary and exercise treatment recommendations. Extended, regular contact with weight-loss counselors or interventionists enhances weight-loss outcomes and is therefore considered emblematic of behavioral obesity treatment programs, as are the strategies of problem solving and goal setting. Attention to motivation and social support is also a key feature of empirically supported behavioral weight-loss therapies. Using these methods, research teams have produced weight losses on the order of 7–10%, which have been associated with substantial and clinically significant improvements in a range of health parameters. Tailoring of behavioral obesity programs to be culturally competent can assist in engaging individuals in obesity treatment and may facilitate adoption of dietary and activity patterns conducive to weight loss.

REFERENCES

Andersen, R. E., Wadden, T. A., Bartlett, S. J., Zemel, B., Verde, T. J., & Franckowiak, S. C. (1999). Effects of lifestyle activity vs. structured aerobic exercise in obese women: A randomized trial. *Journal of the American Medical Association, 281,* 335–340.
Baker, R. C., & Kirschenbaum, D. S. (1998). Weight control during the holidays: Highly consistent self-monitoring as a potentially useful coping mechanism. *Health Psychology, 17,* 367–370.
Bandura, A. (1986). *Social foundations of thought and action: A social cognitive theory.* Englewood Cliffs, NJ: Prentice-Hall.
Bandura, A., & Simon, K. (1977). The role of proximal intentions in self-regulation of refractory behavior. *Cognitive Therapy Research, 1,* 177–193.
Dattilo, A., & Kris-Etherton, P. (1996). Effects of weight reduction on blood lipids and

lipoproteins: A meta-analysis. *American Journal of Clinical Nutrition, 56*, 320–328.

Diabetes Prevention Program Research Group. (2002a). The Diabetes Prevention Program (DPP): Description of lifestyle intervention. *Diabetes Care, 25*, 2165–2171.

Diabetes Prevention Program Research Group. (2002b). Reduction in the incidence of type 2 diabetes with lifestyle intervention or metformin. *New England Journal of Medicine, 346*, 393–403.

Diabetes Prevention Program Research Group. (2004). Achieving weight and activity goals among Diabetes Prevention Program lifestyle participants. *Obesity Research, 12*, 1426–1435.

DiLillo, V. G., Siegfried, N. J., & West, D. S. (2003). Incorporating motivational interviewing into behavioral obesity treatment. *Cognitive and Behavioral Practice, 10*, 120–130.

Ditschuneit, H. H., & Flechtner-Mors, M. (2001). Value of structured meals for weight management: Risk factors and long-term weight maintenance. *Obesity Research, 9*(Suppl. 4), 284S–289S.

Donnelly, J., Stewart, E., Menke, L., & Smith, B. (2005). Comparison of phone vs. clinic to achieve HLBI guidelines for weight loss. *Obesity Research, 13*(Suppl. 9), A36–A37.

Drougas, H. J., Reed, G., & Hill, J. O. (1992). Comparison of dietary self-reports with energy expenditure measured using a whole-room indirect calorimeter. *Journal of the American Dietetic Association, 92*, 1073–1077.

Elfhag, K., & Rossner, S. (2005). Who succeeds in maintaining weight loss? A conceptual review of factors associated with weight-loss maintenance and weight regain. *Obesity Reviews, 6*, 67–85.

Foster, G. D., Makris, A. P., & Bailer, B. A. (2005). Behavioral treatment of obesity. *American Journal of Clinical Nutrition, 82*, 230S–235S.

Foster, G. D., Phelan, S., Wadden, T. A., Gill, D., Ermold, J., & Didie, E. (2004). Promoting more modest weight losses: A pilot study. *Obesity Research, 12*, 1271–1277.

Harvey-Berino, J. (1999). Calorie restriction is more effective for obesity treatment than dietary fat restriction. *Annals of Behavioral Medicine, 21*, 35–39.

Harvey-Berino, J., Pintauro, S., Buzzell, P., & Gold, E. C. (2004). Effect of Internet support on the long-term maintenance of weight loss. *Obesity Research, 12*(2), 320–329.

Heymsfield, S. B., van Mierlo, C. A., van der Knaap, H. C., Heo, M., & Frier, H. I. (2003). Weight management using a meal replacement strategy: Meta- and pooling analysis from six studies. *International Journal of Obesity and Related Metabolic Disorders, 27*, 537–549.

Hong, K., Li, Z., Wang, H.-J., Elshoff, R., & Heber, D. (2005). Analysis of weight loss outcomes using VLCD in black and white overweight and obese women with and without metabolic syndrome. *International Journal of Obesity, 29*, 436–442.

Jakicic, J., Clark, K., Coleman, E., Donnelly, J., Foreyt, J., Melanson, E., et al. (2001). Appropriate intervention strategies for weight loss and prevention of weigh regain for adults. *Medicine and Science in Sports and Exercise, 33*, 2145–2155.

Jakicic, J. M., Wing, R. R., Butler, B. A., & Robertson, R. J. (1995). Prescribing exercise in multiple short bouts versus one continuous bout: Effects on adherence, cardiorespiratory fitness, and weight loss in overweight women. *International Journal of Obesity and Related Metabolic Disorders, 19*, 893–901.

Jakicic, J. M., Winters, C., Lang, W., & Wing, R. R. (1999). Effects of intermittent exercise and use of home exercise equipment on adherence, weight loss, and fitness in overweight women: A randomized trial. *Journal of the American Medical Association, 282*, 1554–1560.

Jeffery, R. W., Drewnowski, A., Epstein, L. H., Stunkard, A. J., Wilson, G. T., Wing, R. R., et al. (2000). Long-term maintenance of weight loss: Current status. *Health Psychology, 19*(Suppl. 1), 5–16.

Jeffery, R. W., Sherwood, N. E., Brelje, K., Pronk, N. P., Boyle, R., Boucher, J. L., et al. (2003). Mail and phone interventions for weight loss in a managed-care setting: Weigh-To-Be one-year outcomes. *International Journal of Obesity and Related Metabolic Disorders, 27,* 1584–1592.

Jeffery, R. W., Wing, R. R., Sherwood, N., & Tate, D. (2003). Physical activity and weight loss: Does prescribing higher physical activity goals improve outcome? *American Journal of Clinical Nutrition, 78,* 684–689.

Jeffery, R. W., Wing, R. R., Thorson, C., & Burton, L. R. (1998). Use of personal trainers and financial incentives to increase exercise in a behavioral weight-loss program. *Journal of Consulting and Clinical Psychology, 66,* 777–783.

Korotitsch, W., & Nelson-Gray, R. (1999). An overview of self-monitoring research in assessment and treatment. *Psychological Assessment, 11,* 415–425.

Kumanyika, S. K. (2002). Obesity treatment in minorities. In T. A. Wadden & A. J. Stunkard (Eds.), *Handbook of obesity treatment* (pp. 416–446). New York: Guilford Press.

Kumanyika, S., Espeland, M., Bahnson, J., Bottom, J., Charleston, J., Folmar, S., et al. (2002). Ethnic comparison of weight loss in the trial of nonpharmacologic interventions in the elderly. *Obesity Research, 10,* 96–106.

Kumanyika, S. K., Obarzanek, E., Stevens, V. J., Hebert, P. R., & Whelton, P. K. (1991). Weight-loss experience of black and white participants in NHLBI-sponsored clinical trials. *American Journal of Clinical Nutrition, 53*(Suppl. 6), 1631S–1638S.

Kumanyika, S. K., Van Horn, L., Bowen, D., Perri, M. G., Rolls, B. J., Czajkowski, S. M., et al. (2000). Maintenance of dietary behavior change. *Health Psychology, 19*(Suppl. 1), 42–56.

Le Masurier, G. C., Sidman, C. L., & Corbin, C. B. (2003). Accumulating 10,000 steps: Does this meet current physical activity guidelines? *Research Quarterly for Exercise and Sport, 74,* 389–394.

Linde, J. A., Jeffery, R. W., Levy, R. L., Pronk, N. P., & Boyle, R. G. (2005). Weight loss goals and treatment outcomes among overweight men and women enrolled in a weight loss trial. *International Journal of Obesity and Related Metabolic Disorders, 29,* 1002–1005.

McGuire, M. T., Wing, R. R., Klem, M. L., & Hill, J. O. (1999). Behavioral strategies of individuals who have maintained long-term weight losses. *Obesity Research, 7,* 334–341.

Miller, W. R., & Rollnick, S. (2002). *Motivational interviewing: Preparing people for change.* New York: Guilford Press.

National Heart, Lung, and Blood Institute. (1998). Clinical guidelines on the identification, evaluation, and treatment of overweight and obesity in adults: The evidence report. *Obesity Research, 6*(Suppl. 2), 51S–209S.

Pascale, R. W., Wing, R. R., Butler, B. A., Mullen, M., & Bononi, P. (1995). Effects of a behavioral weight loss program stressing calorie restriction versus calorie plus fat restriction in obese individuals with NIDDM or a family history of diabetes. *Diabetes Care, 18,* 1241–1248.

Perri, M. G., & Corsica, J. A. (2002). Improving the maintenance of weight lost in behavioral treatment of obesity. In T. Wadden & A. Stunkard (Eds.), *Handbook of obesity treatment* (pp. 357–379). New York: Guilford Press.

Perri, M. G., Martin, A. D., Leermakers, E. A., Sears, S. F., & Notelovitz, M. (1997). Effects of group- versus home-based exercise in the treatment of obesity. *Journal of Consulting and Clinical Psychology, 65,* 278–285.

Perri, M. G., Nezu, A. M., McKelvey, W. F., Shermer, R. L., Renjilian, D. A., & Viegener, B. J. (2001). Relapse prevention training and problem-solving therapy in the long-term management of obesity. *Journal of Consulting and Clinical Psychology, 69,* 722–726.

Perri, M. G., Nezu, A. M., Patti, E. T., & McCann, K. L. (1989). Effect of length of treatment on weight loss. *Journal of Consulting and Clinical Psychology, 57*, 450–452.

Pi-Sunyer, F. (1996). A review of long-term studies evaluating the efficacy of weight loss in ameliorating disorders associated with obesity. *Clinical Therapeutics, 18*, 1006–1035.

Premier Collaborative Research Group. (2003). Effects of comprehensive lifestyle modification on blood pressure control: Main results of the PREMIER clinical trial. *Journal of the American Medical Association, 289*, 2083–2093.

Pronk, N. P., & Wing, R. R. (1994). Physical activity and long-term maintenance of weight loss. *Obesity Research, 2*, 587–599.

Renjilian, D. A., Perri, M. G., Nezu, A. M., McKelvey, W. F., Shermer, R. L., & Anton, S. D. (2001). Individual versus group therapy for obesity: Effects of matching participants to their treatment preferences. *Journal of Consulting and Clinical Psychology, 69*, 717–721.

Resnicow, K., Jackson, A., Wang, T., De, A., McCarty, F., Dudley, W., et al. (2001). A motivational interviewing intervention to increase fruit and vegetable intake through Black churches: Results of the Eat for Life trial. *American Journal of Public Health, 91*, 1686–1693.

Rolls, B., Roe, L., Beach, A., & Kris-Etherton, P. (2005). Provision of foods differing in energy density affects long-term weight loss. *Obesity Research, 13*, 1052–1060.

Smith, D. E., Heckemeyer, C. M., Kratt, P. P., & Mason, D. A. (1997). Motivational interviewing to improve adherence to a behavioral weight-control program for older obese women with NIDDM: A pilot study. *Diabetes Care, 20*, 52–54.

Streit, K. J., Stevens, N. H., Stevens, V. J., & Rossner, J. (1991). Food records: A predictor and modifier of weight change in a long-term weight loss program. *Journal of the American Dietetic Association, 91*, 213–216.

U.S. Department of Health and Human Services. (1996). *Physical activity and health: A report of the Surgeon General*. Atlanta, GA: U.S. Department of Health and Human Services, Centers for Disease Control and Prevention, National Center for Chronic Disease Prevention and Health Promotion.

Wadden, T. A., Berkowitz, R. I., Womble, L. G., Sarwer, D. B., Phelan, S., Cato, R. K., et al. (2005). Randomized trial of lifestyle modification and pharmacotherapy for obesity. *New England Journal of Medicine, 353*, 2111–2120.

Wadden, T. A., Steen, S. N., Wingate, B. J., & Foster, G. D. (1996). Psychosocial consequences of weight reduction: How much weight loss is enough? *American Journal of Clinical Nutrition, 63*(Suppl. 3), 461S–465S.

West, D., DiLillo, V., Greene, P., Kratt, P., & Kirk, K. (2003). Motivational interviewing enhances weight loss and glycemic improvements among overweight women with type 2 diabetes. *Annals of Behavioral Medicine, 25*, S40.

Wing, R. (1992). Behavioral treatment of severe obesity. *American Journal of Clinical Nutrition, 55*(Suppl. 2), 545S–551S.

Wing, R. (2002). Behavioral weight control. In T. Wadden & A. Stunkard (Eds.), *Handbook of obesity treatment* (pp. 301–316). New York: Guilford Press.

Wing, R., & Anglin, K. (1996). Effectiveness of a behavioral weight control program for blacks and whites with NIDDM. *Diabetes Care, 19*, 409–413.

Wing, R., Epstein, L. H., Nowalk, M., Koeske, R., & Hagg, S. (1985). Behavior change, weight loss and physiological improvements in type 2 diabetic patients. *Journal of Consulting and Clinical Psychology, 53*, 111–122.

Wing, R., Hamman, R. F., Bray, G. A., Delahanty, L., Edelstein, S. L., Hill, J. O., et al. (2004). Achieving weight and activity goals among diabetes prevention program lifestyle participants. *Obesity Research, 12*, 1426–1434.

Wing, R., & Hill, J. O. (2001). Successful weight loss maintenance. *Annual Review of Nutrition, 21*, 323–341.

Wing, R., & Jeffery, R. W. (1999). Benefits of recruiting participants with friends and increasing social support for weight loss and maintenance. *Journal of Consulting and Clinical Psychology, 67*, 132–138.

Wing, R., Jeffery, R. W., Burton, L. R., Thorson, C., Nissinoff, K. S., & Baxter, J. E. (1996). Food provision vs. structured meal plans in the behavioral treatment of obesity. *International Journal of Obesity and Related Metabolic Disorders, 20*, 56–62.

Wing, R., & Klem, M. L. (2002). Characteristics of successful weight maintainers. In C. G. Fairburn & K. D. Brownell (Eds.), *Eating disorders and obesity: A comprehensive handbook* (2nd ed., pp. 588–598). New York: Guilford Press.

Wing, R., Tate, D. F., Gorin, A. A., Raynor, H. A., & Fava, J. L. (2006). A self-regulation program for maintenance of weight loss. *New England Journal of Medicine, 355*, 1563–1571.

Wyatt, H. R., Grunwald, G. K., Mosca, C. L., Klem, M. L., Wing, R. R., & Hill, J. O. (2002). Long-term weight loss and breakfast in subjects in the National Weight Control Registry. *Obesity Research, 10*, 78–82.

Yancy, A. K., Kumanyaka, S. K., Ponce, N. S., McCarthy, W., Fielding, J., Leslie, J., et al. (2004). Population-based interventions engaging communities of color in healthy eating and active living: A review. *Preventing Chronic Disease*. Retrieved November 18, 2006 from *http://www.cdc.gov/pcd/issues/2004/jan/03_0012.htm*

Yon, B. A., Johnson, R. K., Harvey-Berino, J., & Gold, B. C. (2006). The use of a personal digital assistant for dietary self-monitoring does not improve the validity of self-reports of energy intake. *Journal of the American Dietetic Association, 160*, 1256–1259.

13

Prevention of Overweight with Young Children and Families

MEREDITH S. DOLAN *and* MYLES S. FAITH

There is a striking irony concerning the topic of "childhood obesity prevention" that is apparent to most pediatricians. This irony is perplexing, and for those who treat obese children, it can be clinically frustrating. On the one hand, there may be no medical topic that is currently "hotter" in the public press, drawing attention from major medical journals, receiving robust research funding, and garnering international attention, than the prevention of childhood obesity. On the other hand, parents whose children are at high risk for obesity often do not perceive a problem or potential future health risks. These parents may believe that their children will "grow out" of their excess baby fat or may not define "obesity" using the same definitions that the medical field promotes. Thus, although health professionals advocate the body mass index (BMI; see the next section) as the standard for defining obesity, parents often rely on different standards, such as perceptions of child activity levels, whether or not the child is just "big boned," and whether or not a child is teased about body weight (Baughcum, Burklow, Deeks, Powers, & Whitaker, 1998). Consequently, the topic of obesity prevention is not on the minds of many parents whose children are at elevated risk.

The main purpose of this chapter is to provide guidance for health care professionals, parents, and other family members pertinent to the prevention of excess weight gain in children at risk for obesity. It is well known that BMI during childhood is strongly related to BMI in adulthood and that child overweight is predictive of adult morbidity and mortality (Barlow &

Dietz, 1998). Paralleling the increased prevalence of childhood obesity, pediatricians are seeing more comorbidities in children, such as Type 2 diabetes, hypertension, impaired glucose tolerance, sleep apnea, and joint problems. These factors suggest the importance of focusing obesity prevention efforts on younger generations, given that childhood obesity often persists into adulthood and that, once established, obesity is extremely difficult to treat.

Obesity *prevention* differs from the issue of obesity *treatment* in several regards. First, the children addressed in this chapter are not clinically obese per se (defined later), although obesity typically runs in their families. Second, guidance for child obesity prevention should address parent or caregiver perceptions about their child's weight status, given that their children are not yet obese; consequently, self-help strategies should aim to raise parental awareness of the criteria for high risk for obesity. Third, the topic of child obesity prevention pays somewhat closer attention to infants and young children, rather than the periods of later childhood and adolescence, which are typically targeted for childhood obesity treatment. This chapter draws on several literatures, including epidemiological studies that document behavioral and lifestyle risk factors for childhood obesity, family and school intervention studies for weight-gain prevention, and focus group research addressing caregiver perceptions of childhood obesity. As discussed elsewhere (Kumanyika & Obarzanek, 2003; Faith, Calamaro, et al., 2004), few controlled obesity prevention studies have been published. Hence, there is a need for further research to guide clinical practice.

This chapter is organized into five sections: defining "at-risk children"; assessing parent and caregiver readiness to change; identifying critical periods for intervention; identifying target behaviors for obesity prevention; and discussing general behavior-change strategies. Each of these sections covers a variety of topics that are geared to enable pediatricians, other health professionals, parents, and other family members to initiate behavior change. Recognition and awareness of the health risks associated with pediatric obesity is a critical first step toward child obesity prevention and, therefore, is a central focus of this chapter. While reviewing the pertinent scientific literature, the aim is to provide concrete and practical suggestions for the reader.

DEFINING AT-RISK CHILDREN

Is My Child At Risk for Becoming Overweight?

Parents of young children do not always recognize that their children are at increased risk for becoming obese in later childhood or adolescence. Because not all children are at increased risk, it is important to provide guidelines to help parents grasp this topic and to better understand whether their children are more vulnerable to becoming overweight as they age. There are several criteria for identifying children who are at high risk: (1) a familial history of obesity, (2) a child BMI in the "at risk for overweight" range, and (3) rapid BMI gain, as documented in growth charts. With respect to family history, parental obesity is one of the most reliable predictors of obesity in children. A seminal study by Whitaker et al. (Whitaker, Wright, Pepe, Seidel, & Dietz, 1997) illustrates this point, showing that a child's probability of becoming an obese adult increased as a function of the number of obese parents. For example, compared with a 5-year-old child who has two normal-weight parents, a 5-year-old child with two obese parents is 15 times more likely to become an obese adult. Thus parents can first and foremost look to their own obesity status and that of their own parents to understand the obesity risk for their children.

BMI can be computed for children as young as 2 years of age and converted to percentiles using standard growth charts (Ogden, Kuczmarski, et al., 2002). Separate BMI growth charts have been developed for boys and girls, and they provide age-specific norms (available at *www.cdc.gov/ growthcharts*). Figures 13.1 and 13.2 provide growth charts for boys and girls, respectively, and are publicly available at *www.cdc.gov/growthcarts*.

To calculate BMI, a child's weight in kilograms is divided by the square of his or her height in meters (BMI = kg/m^2). It can also be computed as the child's weight in pounds divided by the square of his or her height in inches and then multiplied by 703 (BMI = $[lb/in^2] \times 703$). Next, a child's BMI is plotted against his or her age on the gender-specific growth chart to determine his or her BMI percentile. Child overweight is defined as a BMI greater than or equal to the 95th percentile for age. Children with BMIs falling between the 85th and 95th percentiles are defined as "at risk for overweight," a fact that should be noteworthy to their parents, because these children may not appear to be excessively large on visual inspection.

With respect to rapid BMI gain, a child who has experienced a recent large increase in BMI may need to receive a medical evaluation. What constitutes a "large change" in BMI has not been defined, although an annual increase of 3–4 BMI units indicates a large increase in fat mass among most children (Barlow & Dietz, 1998). This estimate is based on the fact that within any given BMI percentile range, BMI increases 1 unit per year and that the BMI at the 85th percentile is about 3 to 4 units higher than that at the 50th percentile (Must, Dallal, & Dietz, 1991). There is also evidence from prospective epidemiological studies that rapid weight gain during the first 4 months of life (expressed as 100 g/month) is a risk factor for obesity at age 7 (Stettler, Zemel, Kumanyika, & Stallings, 2002). Compared with infants who were not rapid weight gainers during the first 4 months of life, infants who gained weight rapidly were 1.38 times more likely to be obese at age 7 years. In other words, every 100 g increase in weight between birth

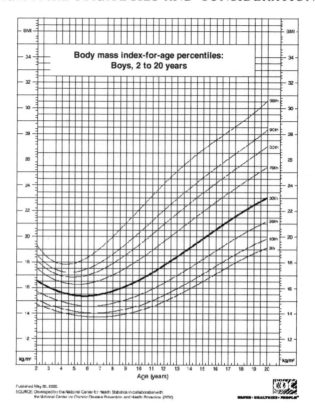

FIGURE 13.1. National Center for Health Statistics 2000 BMI-for-age growth chart (boys 2 to 20 years).

and 4 months was associated with a 38% increased risk for obesity at 7 years of age. Thus examination of annual changes in a child's BMI percentile is also informative for assessing whether a child is at increased risk for becoming obese.

Is "Obesity in the Eye of the Beholder?"

A common misbelief of parents is that a chubby child is a healthy child (Baughcum et al., 1998), whereas little concern is given to the potential for obesity-associated comorbities (Young-Hyman, Herman, Scott, & Schlundt, 2000). Some caregivers may not have a sense of urgency to improve the diet and exercise habits of an at-risk child because associated health problems may not develop for years or decades. More frequently, parents appear to take action only when their child presents with health symptoms, when there is a family history of obesity-related illness, or when their child is be-

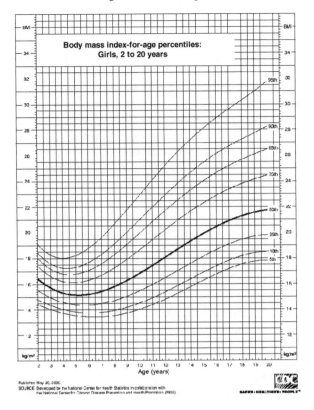

FIGURE 13.2. National Center for Health Statistics 2000 BMI-for-age growth chart (girls 2 to 20 years).

ing teased by peers or family members or to prevent their child from being teased in the future.

One of the biggest challenges for childhood obesity prevention is that many parents do not appear to define or conceptualize obesity in terms of BMI cutoffs, growth charts, or other factors listed in the previous section (Faith, Goldstein, & Pietrobelli, 2002). This important observation primarily comes from focus group studies with parents from low-income families who were enrolled in the federal Supplemental Program for Women, Infants, and Children (WIC; Baughcum, Chamberlin, Deeks, Powers, & Whitaker, 2000). For example, Baughcum et al. (1998) conducted focus groups with more than 600 low-income mothers of young children to assess their attitudes concerning child feeding. Their focus group revealed three major themes, including: (1) belief that a heavy child is a healthy child, (2) fear that the child is not getting enough to eat, and (3) the use of food to influence a child's behavior. Similarly, Jain et al. (2001) reported that mothers of children who were overweight and at risk for overweight did not acknowledge the definition of child overweight based on the standard growth charts. Instead, these mothers judged their children's weight status by weight-related teasing and by their ability to partake in physical activity when considering obesity status. These mothers defined obesity as a condition that caused severe functional impairment or immobility, and, strikingly, they reported that they had never known a young child whom they considered obese. Finally, a study published in the *British Medical Journal* conducted surveys with 277 mothers concerning their perceptions of their children's weight. Out of a total of 55 children who were overweight or obese, 33% of their mothers believed that their children's weight was "about right"(Jeffery, Voss, Metcalf, Alba, & Wilkin, 2005).

Clinically, these issues can pose major barriers when considering self-help strategies for child obesity prevention, to the extent that parents might not perceive a problem and therefore may not be motivated to make changes. Thus, for parents with children at increased risk for obesity, a crucial consideration is how their consciousness or knowledge of this risk status may be elevated. Unfortunately, there are no data to guide clinicians on this matter, although several approaches may be useful. First, awareness of increased risk status can be raised by informing parents and caregivers of the criteria for child obesity, including family history of overweight or obesity, a BMI between the 85th and 95th percentiles, and a recent large increase in BMI. Many parents are unaware of these issues, in part because a sizable number of pediatricians do not evaluate BMI and share this information with parents (Barlow, Dietz, Klish, & Trowbridge, 2002).

Open-ended questions can be useful in eliciting parents' thoughts on childhood obesity. We have used such questions clinically in family treatment groups for overweight children to generate discussion and self-reflection by parents. Although these questions have not been empirically validated, we have found them useful at times and when talking with certain families. Examples of such questions include: "Could you tell me about your child's health?" "How is your child's diet and weight?" "How much TV does your child watch on a daily basis and what do you think about it?" "How much activity does your child get each day and what do you think about it?" Questions can be posed in a relaxed and nonjudgmental manner to minimize parent or caregiver defensiveness and to ease conversations.

Ethnicity and Socioeconomic Differences in "Acceptance" of Obesity

The issue of ethnic and racial disparities in obesity prevalence is important to the issue of obesity prevention. The prevalence of obesity among black and Mexican American adolescents increased more than 10% between the years 1988 and 1994 and 1999 and 2000 compared with a nonsignificant change in prevalence among non-Hispanic white adolescents (Ogden, Flegal, Carrol, & Johnson, 2002). Based on these obesity trends, it has been observed that the black and Mexican American subcultures have a greater acceptance of larger body sizes. Kimm et al. (Kimm, Barton, Berhane, Ross, Payne, & Schreiber, 1997) administered a questionnaire to 2,205 black and white girls, ages 9–10 years, to examine the relationship between obesity and measures of self-esteem. Results showed a significant negative association between adiposity and ratings of physical appearance and global self-worth among both ethnicities, but the slopes were steeper among white girls. Consequently, white girls showed a significant inverse association between adiposity and social acceptance, whereas there were no differences in social acceptance across adiposity ranges in black girls.

Similarly, Strauss (2000) conducted a longitudinal study on ethnic differences in childhood self-esteem and found that overweight Hispanic females and overweight white females exhibited significantly lower self-esteem than did their normal-weight counterparts, whereas there were no differences in reported self-esteem between overweight and normal-weight black girls. Another study examined 219 Mexican children between 6 and 12 years of age, of whom 24.2% were obese, and reported no differences in self-esteem measures among obese and nonobese children. Also, the obese children in this study were no more likely to be rejected or isolated by their peers than were their nonobese counterparts (Brewis, 2003). These results suggest that there may be greater cultural acceptance of larger body sizes among Hispanic and black children than among white children. Similarly, greater acceptance of obesity might be present among their parents.

In addition to cultural differences, socioeconomic differences in attitudes and acceptance of obesity may be an issue when advising parents and children on the importance of prevention. The rising increase in obesity prevalence has been attributed to a modern transition in diet and exercise, with diets high in fat and added sugar and low in fiber combined with increased sedentary activity, especially in urban settings (Popkin, 2001). Whereas obesity used to be associated with affluent communities in the United States, it is now more prevalent among individuals of lower socioeconomic status (James, Leach, Kalamara, & Shayeghi, 2001). Several studies have reported the relationship between income and obesity in adults (Sobal & Stunkard, 1989; Rosmond, Lapidus, & Bjorntorp, 1996; Rosmond & Bjorntorp, 1999; Wardle, Waller, & Jarvis, 2002), although few studies have examined the same association in children and adolescents. Wang (2001) conducted an international study on the association between socioeconomic status and obesity in children and adolescents ages 6–18 years. The final sample included 6,110 children from the United States, 3,028 from China, and 6,883 from Russia. Whereas the child obesity prevalence was higher in the affluent families in both China and Russia, income was inversely related to obesity in American children (Wang, 2001). Another study reported that low household income and low parental education level accounted for approximately one-third of the obesity prevalence in a nationally representative sample of more than 15,000 adolescents in the United States (Goodman, Slap, & Huang, 2003).

These reported obesity trends in minority groups and families from lower socioeconomic strata have clinical relevance. It may be especially important for pediatric practitioners to increase these families' awareness of child obesity and its comorbidities, given that their children are at increased risk.

ASSESSING PARENTS AND CAREGIVERS OF AT-RISK CHILDREN: READY, WILLING, AND ABLE?

"Readiness to change" refers to a parent or caregiver's level of commitment to implementing dietary, exercise, and behavioral changes necessary to create a less "obesigenic" home environment. In addition, greater successes can be achieved by getting commitment from as many family members as possible, including siblings and grandparents. Results from childhood obesity treatment studies clearly indicate that parental involvement is a key component of successful weight loss in children (Epstein, Valoski, Wing, & McCurley, 1994; see also Chapter 14, this volume). Reduction in parent BMI is a significant predictor of reduction in child BMI (Wrotniak, Epstein, Paluch, & Roemmich, 2004), and interventions that treat only parents in child behavior-change strategies do better than treatments that solely target the child (Golan, Weizman, & Fainaru, 1998). Based on these findings, it is reasonable to predict that parent readiness to change may be an important factor in childhood obesity prevention strategies.

Parents may or may not be ready to implement changes, in part depending on the extent to which they perceive elevated obesity risk to be a problem. Clinical experience suggests that parents with at-risk children may feel that other priorities take precedence over child obesity prevention. Parents often feel that the efforts involved in pediatric obesity prevention are too demanding considering their already hectic schedules. Therefore, it is important to communicate to parents that the key to developing a healthier lifestyle is to make small, gradual changes. Instead of completely altering the child's environment at once, it is generally best to begin with one behavior change, such as decreasing television viewing time or increasing the availability of fruits and vegetables (see some strategies later in the chapter). The caregiver should evaluate the child's progress with one goal before adding another.

There has been no systematic research to date addressing readiness to change among parents of children who are at increased risk for obesity. For example, there are no validated instruments that assess the extent to which a parent or caregiver perceives elevated obesity risk as a health problem that merits family behavior change. In addition, readiness-to-change questionnaires have had limited success in predicting outcome in the adult weight-loss literature (Wadden & Letizia, 1992; U.S. Department of Health and Human Services, 2000).

Even though readiness-to-change questionnaires may not be useful in predicting successful outcomes, they sometimes can help raise parent awareness of the range of behaviors that could be targeted for intervention and can help evaluate their self-perceptions. For example, a sample self-assessment checklist using this approach is provided in Figure 13.3. Again, we note that this figure has not been empirically validated.

Readiness to change can be assessed behaviorally by challenging the parent to keep a food, physical activity, or TV log for at least 3 days during a single week (see Figure 13.4). Given that self-monitoring is a fundamental behavior-change strategy, parents who can monitor a single target behavior for at least 3 days can demonstrate to themselves that they are prepared to make personal changes that may enable prevention of excess weight gain in their children. In addition, children can also be encouraged to self-monitor a target behavior to gauge their readiness to change. Examples of self-monitoring exercises aimed at minimizing excess child weight gain include writing down everything that the child eats, keeping a physical activity log, or recording how many hours the child watches television each day. Children, especially those who lack adequate reading and writing skills, may need assistance with self-monitoring. The guidelines offered in Table 13.1 can facilitate self-monitoring procedures.

1. How ready are you to change TV and screen time at home?

     1   2   3   4   5   6   7

2. How ready are you to decrease your family's fast-food visits or make healthier choices at fast-food restaurants?

     1   2   3   4   5   6   7

3. How ready are you to eliminate high fat high sugar snack foods from your house?

     1   2   3   4   5   6   7

4. How ready are you to decrease the amount of sugar-sweetened beverages and fruit juice that your child consumes?

     1   2   3   4   5   6   7

5. How ready are you to begin cooking healthier meals for your family?

     1   2   3   4   5   6   7

6. How ready are you to help your child get more physical activity?

     1   2   3   4   5   6   7

FIGURE 13.3. Self-assessment checklist for parents to examine their own readiness to implement individual lifestyle changes for their child. Responses correspond to a scale of 1 to 7 (1 = *extremely unready*; 7 = *extremely ready*).

Day of the week: _____   Date: ___/___/___

(Circle one TV for every 30 minutes of television that you watch today.)

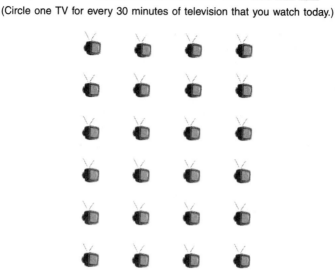

FIGURE 13.4. Sample television monitoring form.

TABLE 13.1. Guidelines to Help Children Learn to Self-Monitor Behaviors

1. Choose a target behavior for the child to improve, such as eating more fruits and vegetables, decreasing television viewing time, drinking more water, or increasing play time. (The following steps target reduced TV viewing.)
2. Create a worksheet or buy a notebook for the child to begin self-monitoring. For children who are unable to write, allow them to use stickers or drawings to monitor their activity. For example, instruct them to draw a picture of a television for every show that they decide not to watch during the day. Figure 13.4 illustrates an example of a self-monitoring worksheet used to encourage decreased television viewing time.
3. Hold a conversation with the child about the purpose of this monitoring activity. Explain that your family is going to make some healthy changes and that this involves limiting the amount of time that the entire family watches television.
4. Encourage as many family members as possible in the monitoring activity, asking everyone to monitor his or her own TV viewing time. The child's success is dependent on support and encouragement from other family members.
5. Encourage family members to log their TV viewing time as soon as possible. If they do not have immediate access to their journals, instruct them to document their behavior on a scrap piece of paper and transfer the information to their journals as soon as possible.
6. Schedule a daily meeting, perhaps at dinner time, to discuss each family member's activity log. Discuss barriers pertaining to decreasing TV viewing time and brainstorm methods to overcome these barriers.
7. To make monitoring more entertaining, hold a contest. For example, whoever watches the least amount of TV during the week or comes up with the most creative alternative to watching TV gets to choose the featured board game for family game night!

ARE THERE "CRITICAL PERIODS" FOR OBESITY ONSET AND OBESITY PREVENTION?

The three main critical periods for the development of obesity during childhood are the prenatal period, infancy, and the period of "adiposity rebound," which usually occurs between the ages of 5 and 7 years. Prenatal predictors of child obesity include maternal overweight (Laitinen, Power, & Jarvelin, 2001), as well as birth weight (Ravelli, Stein, & Susser, 1976; Barker, Robinson, Osmond, & Barker, 1997), a marker of prenatal nutrition status. During the first year of life, the main risk factors for child obesity include bottle feeding (as opposed to breast feeding; Kramer, 1981) and a high rate of weight gain (Ong, Ahmed, Emmett, Preece, & Dunger, 2000; Stettler, Kumanyika, Katz, Zemel, & Stallings, 2003). In addition, an early onset of adiposity rebound has been associated with a greater risk of obesity later in life (Whitaker, Pepe, Wright, Seidel, & Dietz, 1998). Adiposity rebound, which usually occurs between 5 and 7 years of age, is the point at which children attain their minimum amount of fat mass (following a period of increasing height) before fat mass increases gradually into adulthood. Obese children experience adiposity rebound at earlier ages than nonobese children. Other risk factors associated with child obesity include lower socioeconomic status (Laitinen et al., 2001; Wang, 2001), low levels of physical activity (Sallis et al., 1992), increased television viewing (Gortmaker et al., 1996), restrictive parental feeding styles (Faith, Scanlon, Birch, Francis, & Sherry, 2004), increased fast-food consumption (Gillis & Bar-Or, 2003), and increased sugar-sweetened beverage consumption (Gillis & Bar-Or, 2003).

TARGET BEHAVIORS FOR OBESITY PREVENTION

This section reviews potential target behaviors for obesity prevention initiatives, including specific parental feeding practices and more general behavioral-change principles.

Parental Feeding Practices

Breast Feeding versus Bottle Feeding

Prospective epidemiological studies have reported a lower prevalence of child and adolescent overweight among infants who were breast-fed than among those who were bottle-fed (Kramer, 1981) and among infants who were breast-fed for longer than for shorter durations (Liese et al., 2001; Armstrong & Reilly, 2002). Several mechanisms could explain why breast feeding seems to protect against child and adolescent overweight. One mechanism relates to child self-regulation of food intake. Laboratory and field studies suggest that young children generally are able to self-regulate their energy intake over time to maintain energy balance (Birch & Deysher, 1986; Birch & Fisher, 1998). Thus, if children overeat at one meal, they generally "compensate" by eating less at the next meal and vice versa. It appears that children are more adept than adults at recognizing internal hunger and satiety cues and thus regulating food intake. However, there is evidence that restrictive feeding practices may interfere with children's ability to recognize these internal signals. Overly restrictive feeding may teach children to eat in response to external or environmental cues, rather than internal feelings of hunger and fullness.

It is suggested that breast feeding better teaches children to recognize hunger and satiety cues and to learn healthier self-regulation patterns. By contrast, bottle feeding may discourage such practices, as these mothers tend to exert more control over their infants' consumption patterns. For example, parents of bottle-fed infants may be able to see the remaining infant formula in the bottle and hence encourage their infants to finish the bottle at each feeding, whereas mothers of breast-fed infants allow the infant to stop feeding when he or she pulls away from the breast. Bottle-fed infants are typically placed on a regular eating schedule, feeding every 3 to 4 hours. In contrast, mothers who breast feed their infants typically rely on infants' hunger cues to let them know when to nurse. Taveras et al. (2004) found that mothers who breast fed their infants for longer durations reported less restrictive child-feeding practices at 1 year than mothers who exclusively bottle fed their infants. Thus it is possible that bottle feeding promotes child obesity by disrupting children's natural ability to compensate their caloric intake through feelings of hunger and fullness.

Given this information, breast feeding is one strategy that may help prevent excess weight gain or obesity later in childhood. Even if they are unable or unwilling to breast feed their infants, mothers are encouraged to attend to an infant's communications of hunger and satiety to help guide the scheduling of feedings. Acredolo, Goodwyn, and Gentieu (2002) provide a practical book for new parents on this topic. Parents are discouraged from automatically feeding their infant every time he or she cries and are advised to attend to other possible problems, including fatigue, teething, or lack of attention. In addition, infants do not necessarily consume consistent amounts of breast milk or formula every day. Therefore, parents should attend to clues that the infant is finished feeding, such as a decreased sucking rate or pulling his or her head away from the bottle or breast.

Restrictive Feeding Practices

Parents often believe that the most effective way to improve their children's eating habits is to restrict intake of foods high in fat and sugar, by limiting either portion sizes or how often these foods are offered. There may be merits to restriction and, certainly, reducing children's total caloric intake is essential for treatment of obese children. On the other hand, there may be drawbacks to *excessive* restriction. There is evidence that restricting children's access to desirable foods may be counterproductive by *increasing* their liking for and intake of those foods (Fisher & Birch, 1999). Stated differently, restricted foods may become "forbidden fruits" that are more intensely craved and consumed when given the chance (Fisher & Birch, 1999; Liem, Mars, & De Graaf, 2004; also see Chapter 14, this volume). Indeed, a recent review of the literature found that parental restriction of children's food intake—but no other parenting style—was consistently associated with increased food intake and weight status in children (Faith, Berkowitz, et al., 2004). One study found that the association between restrictive feeding and excess weight gain during childhood was present in children with a familial predisposition to obesity but not in those with a familial predisposition to thinness (Faith, Berkowitz, et al., 2004).

These findings suggest that, when limiting access to certain high-fat, high-sugar foods at home, parents should be careful about being overly restrictive or controlling with their child. The use of positive parenting styles, including reinforcement of healthy foods, may be desirable approaches to use with high-risk children who are not currently obese. Because caregivers have control over the availability of foods in the home, they can stock their pantries and refrigerators with plenty of whole grains, low-fat dairy products such as yogurt or string cheese, fresh fruits and vegetables, and lean meats (see also Chapter 14, this volume). Instead of restricting specific food items, parents should ensure that children consume a well-balanced diet with foods from all food groups. That the parent is responsible for what the child eats and the child is responsible for how much food he or she eats has been described as "division of responsibility" in parent–child feeding relations (Satter, 1987). Table 13.2 provides guidelines for parenting styles from an expert panel review (Barlow & Dietz, 1998).

Television Viewing

Television viewing is an independent risk factor for child overweight (Dietz & Gortmaker, 1985; Proctor et al., 2003). This behavior may affect child weight status by displacing more vigorous physical activity or by encouraging increased energy intake during viewing or through television commercials (Halford, Gillespie, Brown, Pontin, & Dovey, 2004). The average child watches between 3 and 4 hours of TV each day (Huston & Wright, 1999) compared with the maximum 2 hours per day recommended by the American Academy of Pediatrics (American Academy of Pediatrics, 2003).

Reducing TV viewing can potentially be perceived by the child as a punishment. Therefore, it is desirable for the entire family to partake in fun alternative activities, such as family game night, arts and crafts, making a

TABLE 13.2. Suggested Parenting Guidelines for Pediatric Obesity Treatment

- Find reasons to praise the child's behavior.
- Never use food as a reward.
- Parents can ask for "rewards" from children in exchange for the changes in their own behavior.
- Establish daily family meal and snack times.
- Parents or caregivers should determine what food is offered and when, and the child should decide whether to eat and how much to eat.
- Offer only healthy options.
- Remove temptations.
- Be a role model.
- Be consistent.

Note. Data from Barlow and Dietz (1998).

scrapbook, or other family activities. The general behavioral practices reviewed in the next section should be used to reduce TV viewing. Table 13.3 provides a sample list of TV-free activities for families.

Clinical experience suggests that efforts to reduce screen time should be directed to the entire family, not just the at-risk child. It is difficult to restrict the television time of one child without doing so for his or her siblings. In addition, it is usually preferable to set realistic goals in which TV time is "faded" (gradually reduced) rather than implementing drastic TV reductions at once. For example, TV viewing time may be reduced by 30 minutes per day for the first month, followed by 1 hour per day during the second month, and so forth. By the third month, the family might strive to watch a maximum of 2 hours of television per day, as recommended by the American Academy of Pediatrics (Committee on Public Health, 2001). Table 13.4 provides some practical guidelines to help reduce children's television viewing time (Calamaro & Faith, 2004).

TABLE 13.3. Ideas for Alternative Activities to Television Viewing

- Have family members take turns reading short stories or poems every evening.
- Play charades or have a family game night.
- Help children plant their own vegetable or herb garden.
- Set up a healthy outdoor picnic.
- Have children decorate your driveway with sidewalk chalk.
- Make dinner together as a family.
- Lay down on a blanket outside and try to identify constellations. See who can count the highest number of shooting stars!
- Take a family walk every evening after dinner.
- Have children write a letter to a friend or family member.
- Allow children to invite friends over to partake in an arts and crafts project, such as finger painting or making homemade play dough.
- Make a scrapbook.
- Take a trip down Memory Lane with family photo albums.
- Have a family slumber party in the living room, taking turns telling scary stories.

TABLE 13.4. Strategies to Help Reduce Children's Television Viewing Time

1. Children should watch no more than 1–2 hours of TV per day.
2. Family members can use simple charts to monitor their TV viewing time.
3. The TV should be turned off when there are no viewers in the room.
4. The TV should be turned off during meal or snack time.
5. Televisions should not be installed in the child's bedroom.
6. Caregivers should model the TV viewing practices that they would like their children to adopt.
7. Caregivers and children should be encouraged to use their creativity to come up with alternate activities to television viewing.

Beverage Consumption

Excess intake of sugar-sweetened beverages and fruit juice may promote excess weight gain in growing children and adolescents. The mechanism for this association is unknown, but potential causes include the high glycemic index of sugared beverages and children's inability to regulate perfectly the calories consumed from these beverages (Ludwig, Peterson, & Gortmaker, 2001). The result is a positive energy balance that can promote weight gain.

Many parents are aware that 100% fruit juice, not to be confused with "fruit drink" or "fruit beverage," is a good source of vitamins and minerals. However, many parents do not place limits on the amount of fruit juice that their children consume, and so, similar to soda consumption, excess fruit juice intake may lead to excess child weight gain due to the extra calories. Dennison, Rockwell, and Baker (1997) reported that the energy intake of preschool-age children who drank 12 fluid ounces or more per day of fruit juice was greater than that of children who consumed 12 or less fluid ounces per day (1,665 kcal vs. 1,399 kcal, respectively). In addition, children who consumed at least 12 fluid ounces per day of fruit juice had a higher prevalence of obesity than those who drank less than 12 fluid ounces per day. There is no nutritional need for fruit juice for infants less than 6 months of age, as breast milk or formula should serve as their primary source of nutrition. The American Academy of Pediatrics recommends a maximum fruit juice intake of 4–6 ounces for children 1–6 years old and 8–12 ounces for children 8–12 years old (Committee on Nutrition, 2001).

Fast-Food Consumption

Consumption of fast food by 2- to 17-year-old children and adolescents increased fivefold between the late 1970s and the mid-1990s, from 2 to 10% of total energy intake (Guthrie, Lin, & Frazao, 2002). Bowman, Gortmaker, Ebbeling, Pereira, and Ludwig (2004) reported that children who ate fast food consumed significantly more total fat, more saturated fat, more added sugars, more sugar-sweetened beverages, less fiber, and fewer fruits and nonstarchy vegetables than children who did not eat fast food.

This study also found that fast-food consumers ate an average of 187 kcals more per day than nonconsumers. The palatability of foods high in fat and added sugars may lead to increased energy intake (Rolls, 2000), and may displace children's intakes of low-energy-dense foods such as fruits and vegetables (Gillis & Bar-Or, 2003; see also Chapter 16, this volume). Each of these factors can promote weight gain, especially in children with a predisposition for obesity. In fact, Gillis and Bar-Or (2003) found that obese children ate significantly more food away from home than nonobese children.

Parents and caregivers often visit fast-food restaurants because of the fast service and convenience and the decreased need for meal planning. Reducing the number of visits to these restaurants, perhaps by reserving them for special occasions, may be especially important for children at high risk for obesity. Parents and caregivers are advised to plan home-cooked meals, which involves making a structured grocery list with all of the necessary ingredients each week before going shopping. Indeed, results from adult weight-loss studies indicate that structured shopping lists can enhance weight loss (Wing et al., 1996).

GENERAL BEHAVIOR CHANGE STRATEGIES

This final section reviews general behavior-change strategies that can be used to modify the behaviors reviewed in the prior section. These include exposure, role modeling, and reinforcement techniques.

Exposure

Repeated exposure to novel or less preferred foods is necessary to increase children's acceptance of those foods. Sullivan et al. (Sullivan & Birch, 1990) found that 8–15 exposures to an initially novel food item was necessary to achieve increased acceptance among 3- to 6-year-old children. Single exposures are rarely sufficient to shape children's food preferences (Birch & Marlin, 1982; see also Chapter 14, this volume). For most children, it does not take many exposures to enhance the appeal of energy-dense foods such as cookies or ice cream. However, getting a child to accept low-energy-dense foods, namely vegetables, is more challenging.

Many parents force their children to eat disliked foods by using bribery: "If you eat your vegetables, you can have a brownie." This is not recommended (Barlow & Dietz, 1998) because the food that serves as the reward (the brownie) may become more appealing to the child, whereas the vegetables may become even less appealing. As an alternative practice, it may be more effective to encourage the child to at least try everything on his or her plate before leaving the table.

Another method of increasing a child's exposure to a target food is to incorporate the food into a creative game or contest. We have used this method extensively in group treatments with young children. Examples include a "Name That Food" game, in which each child takes a turn tasting and guessing different foods while wearing a blindfold. Another game is to hold a family contest to see who can eat the most servings of fruits and vegetables during a particular week.

The effectiveness of exposure strategies may partially explain the positive correlation between parent and child food preferences. Vereecken, Keukelier, and Maes (2004) reported that the consumption frequency of a food item by mothers was associated with that of their children. Borah-Giddens and Falciglia (1993) found that foods that had never been offered to a child were more likely to be disliked by their mothers. This may be concerning if parents do not provide fruits and vegetables because they do not like those foods. To increase a child's exposure to a variety of healthy foods, parents could have their child choose one new healthy food item each week to add to the grocery list.

Role Modeling

Observational learning plays a large role in determining children's eating and exercise behaviors. A child is more likely to make healthy choices if he or she observes parents (Contento et al., 1993), teachers (Hendy & Raudenbush, 2000), and friends (Hendy & Raudenbush, 2000) making healthy choices. Parents, therefore, are encouraged to incorporate a variety of healthy behaviors into their lives, such as increasing their own fruit and vegetable intake, monitoring food portion sizes, finding alternatives to television viewing, and exercising 30–60 minutes each day, to serve as role models for their children. Parents are discouraged from expressing their own body dissatisfaction in front of their children, as previous research has shown that mothers and daughters have corresponding degrees of weight concern (Hill, Weaver, & Blundell, 1990; Steiger, Stotland, Ghadirian, & Whitehead, 1995). Children's eating behaviors and attitudes toward food correspond closely with those of their parents (Brown & Ogden, 2004), and parents or adult caregivers have the most control over what food is available to the child. Therefore, parents are encouraged to make active behavioral changes for themselves and to the home environment. Indeed, Golan, Fainaru, and Weizman (1998) showed that obese children achieved greater weight loss and behavioral change when parents, as opposed to the children themselves, were responsible for implementing the intervention. These results suggest that role modeling also plays a key role in child obesity prevention.

Positive Reinforcement

The use of positive reinforcement by parents is a critical behavior-change strategy when shaping healthy food choices and physical activity in children. Many parents have the misconception that they must be prepared to "buy off" or "bribe" their children with an endless supply of gifts in order to achieve enduring behavior change. However, parent attention and praise or "special time" with parents are among the most powerful reinforcements for children. These reinforcements can be overlooked by parents who may not recognize how important these strategies are for shaping child behavior. Hence, parent training in most child obesity treatment studies focuses extensively on the use of "positive parenting" techniques to shape behavior, while discouraging the use of punishment, parent demands, or related strategies that can escalate parent–child tensions surrounding eating. One popular self-help book that describes positive parenting techniques, although not in the context of obesity prevention per se, is *Family First* (McGraw, 2004).

CONCLUSIONS

Pediatric obesity has been associated with feeding practices and events that occur in infancy and early childhood. For this reason, child obesity prevention efforts should target a younger age range than treatment interventions. In this chapter, we reviewed the risk factors for child obesity and parenting strategies that aim to change children's behaviors but that may contribute to excess weight gain. Clinical practice and research suggest that these are modifiable risk factors that could play a role in child obesity prevention. For more information on prevention of child obesity, Table 13.5 provides a list of additional Internet and book resources that address the topic.

TABLE 13.5. References to Guide Parents in Improving Children's Eating and Exercise Habits

Websites

- *www.eatright.org* (American Dietetic Association)
- *www.cdc.org* (Centers for Disease Control and Prevention)
- *www.diabetes.org* (American Diabetes Association)
- *www.kidshealth.org* (The Nemours Foundation)
- *www.dole5aday.com* (Dole Food Company)

Books

- Kirschenbaum, D. S., Johnson, W. G., & Stalonas, P. M., Jr. (1987). *Treating childhood and adolescent obesity*. New York: Pergamon Press.
- LeBow, M. D. (1995). *Overweight teenagers*. New York: Plenum Press.
- Piscatella, J. C. (1999). *Fat-proof your child*. New York: Workman.
- Dietz, W. H., & Stern, L. (1999). *American Academy of Pediatrics guide to your child's nutrition: Feeding children of all ages*. New York: Villard Books.
- Sothern, M. (2001). *Trim kids*. New York: HarperCollins.
- Cooper, K. H. (1999). *Fit kids*. Nashville, TN: Broadman & Holman.
- Epstein, L. H., & Squires, S. (1988). *The stoplight diet for children*. Boston: Little, Brown.

Prior to intervention implementation, the first step in preventing child obesity is increasing parental awareness of the issue and the potential associated health risks. This involves identifying families with children who are at high risk for obesity by evaluating family history of overweight and plotting children's BMIs on standard growth charts. Once children are identified as being at risk for obesity, the next challenges for health care professionals are raising parental concern levels in a supportive and nonthreatening way and addressing cultural differences in the acceptance of larger body sizes. Table 13.6 provides guidelines for pediatric practitioners on proper evaluation of child obesity, parental guidance instructions, and strategies to advocate child obesity prevention in the community.

TABLE 13.6. American Academy of Pediatrics Recommendations for the Prevention of Pediatric Overweight and Obesity

Health supervision

- Identify and track patients at risk by virtue of family history, birth weight, or socioeconomic, ethnic, cultural, or environmental factors.
- Calculate and plot BMI once a year for all children and adolescents.
- Use changes in BMI to identify rate of excessive weight gain relative to linear growth.
- Encourage, support, and protect breast feeding.
- Encourage parents and caregivers to promote healthy eating patterns by offering nutritious snacks, such as vegetables and fruits, low-fat dairy foods, and whole grains; encouraging children's autonomy in self-regulation of food intake and setting appropriate limits on choices; and modeling healthy food choices.
- Routinely promote physical activity, including unstructured play at home, in school, in child-care settings, and throughout the community.
- Recommend limitation of television and video time to a maximum of 2 hours per day.
- Recognize and monitor changes in obesity-associated risk factors for adult chronic disease, such as hypertension, dyslipidemia, hyperinsulinemia, impaired glucose tolerance, and symptoms of obstructive sleep apnea syndrome.

Advocacy

- Help parents, teachers, coaches, and others who influence youth to discuss health habits, not body habits, as part of their efforts to control overweight and obesity.
- Enlist policy makers from local, state, and national organizations and schools to support a healthful lifestyle for all children, including proper diet and adequate opportunity for regular physical activity.
- Encourage organizations that are responsible for health care and health care financing to provide coverage for effective obesity prevention and treatment strategies.
- Encourage public and private sources to direct funding toward research into effective strategies to prevent overweight and obesity and to maximize limited family and community resources to achieve healthful outcomes for youth.
- Support and advocate for social marketing intended to promote healthful food choices and increased physical activity.

Note. Data from American Academy of Pediatrics (2003).

The majority of child obesity research has been treatment-focused, with few studies examining obesity prevention strategies. There is a need for further research on effective ways to raise the consciousness and motivation levels among families with at risk children to make behavioral and environmental changes toward a healthier lifestyle. In addition, more clinical studies, involving young children and their families, are necessary to determine the most practical and effective approaches to child obesity prevention.

REFERENCES

Acredolo, L. P., Goodwyn, S., & Gentieu, P. (2002). *Baby signs for mealtimes*. New York: Harper Festival.

American Academy of Pediatrics. (2003). Prevention of pediatric overweight and obesity. *Pediatrics, 112*(2), 424–430.

Armstrong, J., & Reilly, J. J. (2002). Breastfeeding and lowering the risk of childhood obesity. *Lancet, 359*(9322), 2003–2004.

Barker, M., Robinson, S., Osmond, C., & Barker, D. J. (1997). Birth weight and body fat distribution in adolescent girls. *Archives of Disease in Childhood, 77*(5), 381–383.

Barlow, S. E., & Dietz, W. H. (1998). Obesity evaluation and treatment: Expert committee recommendations. *Pediatrics, 102*(3), e29.

Barlow, S. E., Dietz, W. H., Klish, W. J., & Trowbridge, F. L. (2002). Medical evaluation of overweight children and adolescents: Reports from pediatricians, pediatric nurse practitioners, and registered dietitians. *Pediatrics, 110*(1), 222–228.

Baughcum, A. E., Burklow, K. A., Deeks, C. M., Powers, S. W., & Whitaker, R. C. (1998). Maternal feeding practices and childhood obesity: A focus group study of low-income mothers. *Archives of Pediatrics and Adolescent Medicine, 152*(10), 1010–1014.

Baughcum, A. E., Chamberlin, L. A., Deeks, C. M., Powers, S. W., & Whitaker, R. C. (2000). Maternal perceptions of overweight preschool children. *Pediatrics, 106*(6), 1380–1386.

Birch, L. L., & Deysher, M. (1986). Caloric compensation and sensory specific satiety: Evidence for self-regulation of food intake by young children. *Appetite, 7*, 323–331.

Birch, L. L., & Fisher, J. O. (1998). Development of eating behaviors among children and adolescents. *Pediatrics, 101*(3), 539–549.

Birch, L. L., & Marlin, D. W. (1982). I don't like it; I never tried it: Effects of exposure on two-year-old children's food preferences. *Appetite, 3*, 353–360.

Borah-Giddens, J., & Falciglia, G. A. (1993). A meta-analysis of the relationship in food preferences between parents and children. *Journal of Nutrition Education, 25*(3), 102–107.

Bowman, S. A., Gortmaker, S. L., Ebbeling, C. B., Pereira, M. A., & Ludwig, D. S. (2004). Effects of fast-food consumption on energy intake and diet quality among children in a national household survey. *Pediatrics, 113*(1), 112–118.

Brewis, A. (2003). Biocultural aspects of obesity in young Mexican school children. *American Journal of Human Biology, 15*(3), 446–460.

Brown, R., & Ogden, J. (2004). Children's eating attitudes and behavior: A study of the modeling and control theories of parental influence. *Health Education Research, 19*(3), 261–271.

Calamaro, C. J., & Faith, M. S. (2004). Preventing childhood overweight. *Nutrition Today, 39*(5), 194–199.

Committee on Public Health. (2001). Children, adolescents, and television. *Pediatrics,* 107, 423–426.

Committee on Nutrition. (2001). The use and misuse of fruit juice in pediatrics. *Pediatrics,* 107(5), 1210–1213.

Contento, I. R., Basch, C., Shea, S., Gutin, B., Zybert, P., Michela, J. L., et al. (1993). Relationship of mothers' food choice criteria to food intake of preschool children: Identification of family subgroups. *Health Education Quarterly,* 20(2), 243–259.

Dennison, B. A., Rockwell, H. L., & Baker, S. L. (1997). Excess fruit juice consumption by preschool-aged children is associated with short stature and obesity. *Pediatrics,* 99(1), 15–22.

Dietz, W. H., & Gortmaker, S. L. (1985). Do we fatten our children at the television set? Obesity and television viewing in children and adolescents. *Pediatrics, 75,* 807–812.

Epstein, L. H., Valoski, A., Wing, R. R., & McCurley, J. (1994). Ten-year outcomes of behavioral family-based treatment for childhood obesity. *Health Psychology, 13*(5), 373–383.

Faith, M. S., Berkowitz, R. I., Stallings, V. A., Kerns, J., Storey, M., & Stunkard, A. J. (2004). Parental feeding attitudes and styles and child body mass index: Prospective analysis of a gene–environment interaction. *Pediatrics, 114,* e429–e436.

Faith, M. S., Calamaro, C. J., Peitrobelli, A., Dolan, M. S., Allison, D. B., & Heymsfield, S. B. (2004). *Prevention of pediatric obesity: Examining the issues and forecasting research directions.* Totowa, NJ: Humana Press.

Faith, M. S., Goldstein, R., & Pietrobelli, A. (2002). Defining obesity and weight disturbance in children: Researchers, health professionals, and parents. *Pediatric Nutrition, 4,* 14–17.

Faith, M. S., Scanlon, K. S., Birch, L. L., Francis, L. A., & Sherry, B. (2004). Parent–child feeding strategies and their relationships to child eating and weight status. *Obesity Research, 12,* 1711–1722.

Fisher, J. O., & Birch, L. L. (1999). Restricting access to palatable foods affects children's behavioral response, food selection, and intake. *American Journal of Clinical Nutrition, 69*(6), 1264–1272.

Gillis, L. J., & Bar-Or, O. (2003). Food away from home, sugar-sweetened drink consumption and juvenile obesity. *Journal of the American College of Nutrition, 22*(6), 539–545.

Golan, M., Fainaru, M., & Weizman, A. (1998). Role of behaviour modification in the treatment of childhood obesity with the parents as the exclusive agents of change. *International Journal of Obesity, 22*(12), 1217–1224.

Golan, M., Weizman, A. A., & Fainaru, M. (1998). Parents as the exclusive agents of change in the treatment of childhood obesity. *American Journal of Clinical Nutrition, 67,* 1130–1135.

Goodman, E., Slap, G. B., & Huang, B. (2003). The public health impact of socioeconomic status on adolescent depression and obesity. *American Journal of Public Health, 93,* 1844–1850.

Gortmaker, S. L., Must, A., Sobol, A. M., Peterson, K., Colditz, G. A., & Dietz, W. H. (1996). Television viewing as a cause of increasing obesity among children in the United States, 1986–1990. *Archives of Pediatrics and Adolescent Medicine, 150*(4), 356–362.

Guthrie, J. F., Lin, B.-H., & Frazao, E. (2002). Role of food prepared away from home in the American diet, 1977–78 versus 1994–96: Changes and consequences. *Journal of Nutrition Education and Behavior, 34*(3), 140–150.

Halford, J. C., Gillespie, J., Brown, V., Pontin, E. E., & Dovey, T. M. (2004). Effect of television advertisements for foods on food consumption in children. *Appetite, 42*(2), 221–225.

Hendy, H. M., & Raudenbush, B. (2000). Effectiveness of teacher modeling to encourage food acceptance in preschool children. *Appetite, 34*(1), 61–76.

Hill, A. J., Weaver, C., & Blundell, J. E. (1990). Dieting concerns of 10-year-old girls and their mothers. *British Journal of Clinical Psychology, 29*(Pt. 3), 346–348.

Huston, A. C., & Wright, J. C. (1999). How young children spend their time: Television and other activities. *Developmental Psychology, 35*(4), 912–925.

Jain, A., Sherman, S. N., Chamberlin, L. A., Carter, Y., Powers, S. W., & Whitaker, R. C. (2001). Why don't low-income mothers worry about their preschoolers being overweight? *Pediatrics, 107*(5), 1138–1146.

James, P. T., Leach, R., Kalamara, E., & Shayeghi, M. (2001). The worldwide obesity epidemic. *Obesity Research, 9*(Suppl. 4), 228S–233S.

Jeffery, A. N., Voss, L. D., Metcalf, B. S., Alba, S., & Wilkin, T. J. (2005). Parents' awareness of overweight in themselves and their children: Cross-sectional study within a cohort (Earlybird 21). *British Medical Journal, 330*, 23–24.

Kimm, S. Y. S., Barton, B. A., Berhane, K., Ross, J. W., Payne, G. H., & Schreiber, G. B. (1997). Self-esteem and adiposity in black and white girls: The NHLBI growth and health study. *Annals of Epidemiology, 7*, 550–560.

Kramer, M. S. (1981). Do breast-feeding and delayed introduction of solid foods protect against subsequent obesity? *Journal of Pediatrics, 98*(6), 883–887.

Kumanyika, S. K., & Obarzanek, E. (2003). Pathways to obesity prevention: Report of a National Institutes of Health workshop. *Obesity Research, 11*, 1263–1274.

Laitinen, J., Power, C., & Jarvelin, M. R. (2001). Family social class, maternal body mass index, childhood body mass index, and age at menarche as predictors of adult obesity. *American Journal of Clinical Nutrition, 74*(3), 287–294.

Liem, D. G., Mars, M., & De Graaf, C. (2004). Sweet preferences and sugar consumption of 4- and 5–year-old children: Role of parents. *Appetite, 43*(3), 235–245.

Liese, A. D., Hirsch, T., von Mutius, E., Keil, U., Leupold, W., & Weiland, S. K. (2001). Inverse association of overweight and breast feeding in 9- to 10-year-old children in Germany. *International Journal of Obesity and Related Metabolic Disorders, 25*(11), 1644–1650.

Ludwig, D. S., Peterson, K. E., & Gortmaker, S. L. (2001). Relation between consumption of sugar-sweetened drinks and childhood obesity: A prospective, observational analysis. *Lancet, 357*(9255), 505–508.

McGraw, P. C. (2004). *Family first.* New York: Simon & Schuster.

Must, A., Dallal, G. E., & Dietz, W. H. (1991). Reference data for obesity: 85th and 95th percentiles of body mass index and triceps skinfold thickness. *American Journal of Clinical Nutrition, 53*, 839–846.

Ogden, C. L., Flegal, K. M., Carrol, M. D., & Johnson, C. L. (2002). Prevalence and trends in overweight among U.S. children and adolescents, 1999–2000. *Journal of the American Medical Association, 288*(14), 1728–1732.

Ogden, C. L., Kuczmarski, R. J., Flegal, K. M., Mei, Z., Guo, S., Wei, R., et al. (2002). Centers for Disease Control and Prevention 2000 growth charts for the United States: Improvements to the 1977 National Center for Health Statistics version. *Pediatrics, 109*(1), 45–60.

Ong, K. K., Ahmed, M. L., Emmett, P. M., Preece, M. A., & Dunger, D. B. (2000). Association between postnatal catch-up growth and obesity in childhood: Prospective cohort study. *British Medical Journal, 320*, 967–971.

Popkin, B. M. (2001). The nutrition transition and obesity in the developing world. *Journal of Nutrition, 131*(3), 871S–873S.

Proctor, M., Moore, L., Gao, D., Cuppler, L., Bradle, M., Hood, M., et al. (2003). Television viewing and change in body fat from preschool to early adolescence: The Framingham children's study. *International Journal of Obesity and Related Metabolic Disorders, 27*, 827–833.

Ravelli, G. P., Stein, Z. A., & Susser, M. W. (1976). Obesity in young men after famine expo-sure *in utero* and early infancy. *New England Journal of Medicine, 295*(7), 349–353.

Rolls, B. J. (2000). The role of energy density in the overconsumption of fat. *Journal of Nutrition, 130,* 268S–271S.

Rosmond, R., & Bjorntorp, P. (1999). Psychosocial and socio-economic factors in women and their relationship to obesity and regional body fat distribution. *International Journal of Obesity and Related Metabolic Disorders, 23,* 138–145.

Rosmond, R., Lapidus, L., & Bjorntorp, P. (1996). The influence of occupational and so-cial factors on obesity and body fat distribution in middle-aged men. *International Journal of Obesity and Related Metabolic Disorders, 20,* 599–607.

Sallis, J. F., Simons-Morton, B. G., Stone, E. J., Corbin, C. B., Epstein, L. H., Faucette, N., et al. (1992). Determinants of physical activity and interventions in youth. *Medicine and Science in Sports and Exercise, 24*(Suppl. 6), S248–S257.

Satter, E. (1987). *How to get your child to eat . . . But not too much.* Palo Alto, CA: Bull.

Sobal, J., & Stunkard, A. J. (1989). Socioeconomic status and obesity: A review of the liter-ature. *Psychology Bulletin, 105,* 260–275.

Steiger, H., Stotland, S., Ghadirian, A. M., & Whitehead, V. (1995). Controlled study of eating concerns and psychopathological traits in relatives of eating-disordered probands: Do familial traits exist? *International Journal of Eating Disorders, 18*(2), 107–118.

Stettler, N., Kumanyika, S. K., Katz, S. H., Zemel, B. S., & Stallings, V. A. (2003). Rapid weight gain during infancy and obesity in young adulthood in a cohort of African Americans. *American Journal of Clinical Nutrition, 77*(6), 1374–1378.

Stettler, N., Zemel, B. S., Kumanyika, S. K., & Stallings, V. A. (2002). Infant weight gain and childhood overweight status in a multicenter, cohort study. *Pediatrics, 109,* 194–199.

Strauss, R. S. (2000). Childhood obesity and self-esteem. *Pediatrics, 105*(1), 15–20

Sullivan, S. A., & Birch, L. L. (1990). Pass the sugar, pass the salt: Experience dictates pref-erence. *Developmental Psychology, 26*(4), 546–551.

Taveras, E. M., Scanlon, K. S., Birch, L. L., Rifas-Shiman, S. L., Rich-Edwards, J. W., & Gillman, M. W. (2004). Association of breastfeeding with maternal control of infant feeding at age 1 year. *Pediatrics, 114*(5), 577–583.

U.S. Department of Health and Human Services. (2000). *The practical guide to the identifi-cation, evaluation, and treatment of overweight and obesity in adults.* Bethesda, MD: National Institutes of Health, National Heart, Lung, and Blood Institute.

Vereecken, C. A., Keukelier, E., & Maes, L. (2004). Influence of mother's educational level on food parenting practices and food habits of young children. *Appetite, 43*(1), 93–103.

Wadden, T. A., & Letizia, K. A. (1992). Predictors of attrition and weight loss in patients treated by moderate to severe caloric restriction. In T. A. Wadden & T. B. Van Itallie (Eds.), *Treatment of the seriously obese patient* (pp. 383–410). New York, Guilford Press.

Wang, Y. (2001). Cross-national comparison of childhood obesity: The epidemic and the relationship between obesity and socioeconomic status. *International Journal of Epi-demiology, 30*(5), 1129–1136.

Wardle, J., Waller, J., & Jarvis, M. J. (2002). Sex differences in the association of socioeco-nomic status with obesity. *American Journal of Public Health, 82,* 1299–1304.

Whitaker, R. C., Pepe, M. S., Wright, J. A., Seidel, K. D., & Dietz, W. H. (1998). Early adi-posity rebound and the risk of adult obesity. *Pediatrics, 101*(3), E5.

Whitaker, R. C., Wright, J. A., Pepe, M. S., Seidel, K. D., & Dietz, W. H. (1997). Predicting obesity in young adulthood from childhood and parental obesity. *New England Jour-nal of Medicine, 337,* 869–873.

Wing, R. R., Jeffery, R. W., Burton, L. R., Thorson, C., Nissinoff, K. S., & Baxter, J. E.

(1996). Food provision vs. structured meal plans in the behavioral treatment of obesity. *International Journal of Obesity and Related Metabolic Disorders, 20*(1), 56–62.

Wrotniak, B. H., Epstein, L. H., Paluch, R. A., & Roemmich, J. N. (2004). Parent weight change as a predictor of child weight change in family-based behavioral obesity treatment. *Archives of Pediatrics and Adolescent Medicine, 158*(4), 342–347.

Young-Hyman, D., Herman, L. J., Scott, D. L., & Schlundt, D. G. (2000). Care giver perception of children's obesity-related health risk: A study of African American families. *Obesity Research, 8*, 241–248.

14

Treatment of Overweight Children
Practical Strategies for Parents

KATHRYN E. HENDERSON *and* MARLENE B. SCHWARTZ

Marilyn accompanied her son, Josh, into their pediatrician's office for Josh's annual physical. Dr. Henry checked Josh's weight and frowned. "Marilyn, you've got to do something about Josh's weight. He's blowing up. What foods have you been serving at home? Are you allowing him to spend all his time watching TV or on the computer?" Marilyn felt simultaneously ashamed of Josh's body and angry at his pediatrician for blaming her and criticizing her son.

John arrived home from work to find his daughter, Stacey, in tears. He asked what was wrong, and she, somewhat reluctantly, related that she had been teased about her weight at school that day. John wasn't sure what to say. He thought Stacey needed to lose weight and had, in fact, seen her teased before. He felt a little embarrassed that his daughter was overweight and could not understand why this was the case, given his own athletic background. He secretly hoped that the teasing would help motivate her to lose weight.

Emma arrived home to discover her daughter, Katie, in the kitchen snacking on cookies and milk. Emma reminded Katie that cookies were not on the list of approved foods for her weight-loss program. Katie looked embarrassed. Emma responded with, "I'm doing this for your own good. I was overweight as a teenager and suffered terribly because of it. I just don't want you to go through what I went through."

All three vignettes present, unfortunately, the real experiences of parents and children struggling with a child's weight. They also present a range of issues that we discuss in this chapter. We want to note at the outset that there is surprisingly little empirical literature on self-help treatment for childhood obesity. Thus specific recommended strategies outlined in this chapter are largely extrapolated from professionally led treatments, data on general factors involved in determining eating and exercise behaviors, and clinical experience detailed in the literature and of our own.

THE GREAT CHALLENGE FOR PARENTS

Parents with overweight children face a number of unique challenges. They must acknowledge and actively address current behaviors, even though there may not yet be any measurable medical consequences. They also need to express their concern about their child's health without becoming overbearing in the arena of food and weight. Many parents worry that focusing on eating and weight may cause their child to develop an eating disorder (in point of fact, the research shows this to be unlikely; Butryn & Wadden, 2005). Finally, parents struggle with how to promote weight loss while also maintaining the child's self-esteem.

Once parents have decided on weight loss as a goal, how to go about it presents a challenge. Contradictory nutritional information abounds. "Experts" promote, in turn, high-protein/low-carb diets, high-carb/low-fat diets, and macronutritionally balanced diets (Dansinger, Gleason, Griffith, Selker, & Schaefer, 2005; Ludwig, 2000; Samaha et al., 2003; Tsai & Wadden, 2005; Willet, 2002). Parents may turn to popular diets or programs they have tried themselves. Unfortunately, the effectiveness of most of these approaches has been inadequately tested in adults and never tested at all in children.

Further, parents may put forth all the heroic efforts that can be mustered, but such efforts pale in comparison with the opposing forces of our current environment. The International Obesity Task Force (IOTF) has proclaimed that "the current obesity pandemic reflects the profound changes to society over the past 20–30 years that have created an environment that promotes a sedentary lifestyle and the consumption of a high fat, energy dense diet" (IOTF, 2002). There is now general consensus among obesity experts that the "toxic environment" is a major contributor to the obesity epidemic (Brownell, 2005; Brownell & Horgen, 2004; Critser, 2003; Nestle, 2002; Schlosser, 2001). Some of the environmental factors that are specific to children include the rise in competitive foods (i.e., foods that do not comprise the school lunch or breakfast) sold in schools, decreases in physical education and in walking to school, and significant increases in the amount of sedentary entertainment options (Booth, Pinkston, & Poston, 2005; Kaur, Hyder, & Poston, 2003).

A further challenge that parents face is in deciding how to manage food for the rest of the family. It is enormously difficult for the overweight child to decrease his or her consumption of nutritionally poor foods when brothers and sisters continue to eat these foods at home. On the other hand, parents anticipate—often correctly—that siblings and other family members will protest any limits placed on their own consumption. Even worse, siblings may openly "blame" the overweight child for the imposed deprivation.

Genetic factors contribute greatly to weight and obesity (Bar-Or et al., 1998; Bouchard, 1997). Thus an overweight child is reasonably likely to have an overweight parent. When overweight parents—or those with a history of overweight—take on the weight struggle with their child, complicated feelings can arise on both sides. On the one hand, parents can perhaps more easily empathize with their child if they, too, have struggled. On the other, parents can feel pressured to protect their child from the teasing and stigma that they have faced and can overfocus on weight and implement very restrictive food rules.

Finally, sustained weight loss can be difficult to achieve. The adult literature shows that the average patient regains one-third of lost weight in the year following treatment, with increasing regain over subsequent years; by the 5-year follow-up, over 90% of patients have regained their lost weight (Kramer, Jeffery, Forster, & Snell, 1989). The limited data on children are more encouraging and suggest that they can be successful in both the short and long term (Epstein, Valoski, Wing, & McCurley, 1994; Epstein, Valoski, Kalarchian, & McCurley, 1995; Epstein, Myers, Raynor, & Saelens, 1998; Jelalian & Saelens, 1999). One study has produced good weight maintenance as far as the 10-year follow-up point (Epstein et al., 1994). Thus parents should feel encouraged to work with their children on healthy changes. In fact, because most successful treatments of childhood overweight are family-based and involve having the parents implement many of the treatment components, one might predict that self-help with parent guidance has a reasonable chance of success.

In summary, the task of addressing overweight in one's child can be complicated, confusing, difficult, and painful. Much effort can be invested for little apparent "reward." Mixed messages are pervasive, and emotions can run high. However, there is reason to be optimistic about weight-loss interventions during childhood. Parents need all the support and resources that can be made available to assist them in this challenging task.

SETTING GOALS

Most essential is maintaining the happiness and overall well-being of the child. Numerous authors have reported that obesity in children and adolescents, and in girls in particular, is associated with an increased risk for general psychosocial problems and distress (Banis et al., 1988; Dietz, 1998; Mellin, Neumark-Sztainer, Story, Ireland, & Resnick, 2002). Identified areas of concern have included depression (Erickson, Robinson, Haydel, & Killen, 2000; Sheslow, Hassink, Wallace, & DeLancey, 1993), self-esteem (French, Story, & Perry, 1995; Braet, Mervielde, & Vandereycken, 1997; Martin, Housley, McCoy, & Greenhouse, 1988; Sallade, 1973), and body esteem (Hendry & Gillies, 1978; Mendelson & White, 1982, 1985; Mendelson, White, & Mendelson, 1996), although the data are not entirely consistent in finding these associations. One important finding has been that self-esteem in domains other than physical appearance acted as a protective factor for overall self-esteem in overweight children (Israel & Ianova, 2002). This finding speaks to the need for parents to continue to focus on the whole child, not just his or her weight. Maintenance and improvement of self-esteem and body esteem are important goals.

Also important are maintaining of family harmony in the context of setting goals for the overweight child and establishing a philosophy of family teamwork to address the problem. One issue previously noted is whether or not to impose dietary changes on other family members who do not necessarily struggle with weight. Most treatments for overweight children involve a strong stimulus control component (Epstein & Wing, 1987). That is, the environment should support the child's efforts by eliminating temptations and encouraging the targeted behavior changes. The implication for families is that the entire family needs to embrace the lifestyle changes. In fact, the literature on childhood obesity is strongly consistent in its implementation of a range of behavioral strategies for the entire family (Epstein et al., 1994). An oft-heard protest from families that we have treated is, "But why should my other children be deprived of treat foods because of the weight problem of the one child?" Our standard response is, "In fact, frequent consumption of high-sugar, high-fat, low-nutrition foods is not healthy for any child, regardless of weight." A parent might say, "But my other child needs to *gain* weight—I need to be feeding him potato chips, cookies, and the like." We respond to this concern with, "To our knowledge, few pediatricians would recommend gaining weight through consumption of potato chips and cookies. Rather, they would recommend emphasizing high-nutrition foods with higher caloric density, such as nuts and nut butters, dried fruit, and more whole-milk-based dairy products such as yogurt or cheese."

Many parents find themselves at a loss as to both when and how to proceed in establishing specific weight goals. In fact, research suggests that parents do not accurately estimate their child's weight status (Carnell, Edwards, Croker, Boniface, & Wardle, 2005; also see Chapter 13, this volume). It is important to realize that for children, BMI is not interpreted in the same manner as it is for adults—the cutoffs of 25 for overweight and 30 for obesity are not used. Instead, BMI should be plotted on the age-and sex-specific growth charts provided by the Centers for Disease Control. A BMI above the 85th percentile is considered "at risk for overweight" and above the 95th percentile is considered "overweight." In addition to this index, the Expert committee recommendations on the evaluation and treatment of overweight children and adolescents (Barlow & Dietz, 1998) suggest that parents consider the child's current status on a variety of health indices, including the trend or rate of weight gain, the child's family medical history, and the child's psychosocial adjustment. A good relationship with a sensitive pediatrician is crucial in making these determinations.

In setting specific weight goals, Barlow and Dietz (1998) differentiate between recommendations for weight *maintenance* and those for weight *loss*. They suggest weight maintenance as the first goal. Maintaining a steady weight during increases in height leads to a percentile drop on the BMI charts, although no change in actual weight took place. It is important to emphasize this outcome as a success and to avoid disappointment in not seeing the number on the scale change. For children who are over 7 years old and over the 95th percentile for BMI or who are between the 85th and 95th percentiles but also experiencing comorbid medical complications, a slow and gradual weight loss is recommended.

The importance of specific weight goals notwithstanding, it is actually most important to keep the focus on the behavior-change component. Notably, weight is *not* a behavior; eating and physical activity *are* behaviors. Behaviors are things over which a child can conceivably have control, whereas an outcome such as weight is influenced by a broad array of factors, including genetics (Grilo & Pogue-Greile, 1991) and available resources (Booth, Pinkston, & Poston, 2005). Further, these behaviors have positive implications beyond mere weight loss; thus a focus only on weight loss fails to appreciate the full effects of the child's efforts. With these points in mind, we therefore recommend tracking specific changes in eating behaviors, physical activity behaviors, and attitudes toward these behaviors.

Because of the critical importance of childhood and adolescence to growth and development, all weight-management efforts should be closely supervised by a child's pediatrician. This will ensure that nutritional needs are being met. Pediatrician monitoring will also provide an opportunity to track outcomes beyond mere changes in weight—for example, better control over blood sugar, reductions in hypertension and hypocholesteremia, and generally improved fitness—thereby creating additional positive reinforcement for the lifestyle changes. The sensitivity of the pediatrician is crucial. Weight bias and stigma are pervasive in our culture (Puhl & Brownell, 2001), and health care professionals are not immune to this bias (Schwartz, Chambliss, Brownell, Blair, & Billington, 2003). It is important that the pediatrician make extra effort to understand the difficulty of weight loss and the often painful experience of childhood overweight and to appreciate and focus on the whole child rather than only on the weight problem. Many patients have noted to us how meaningful it was for their physician to recall and inquire about other details in their lives, such as success in school or artistic talents. Parents should feel free to be assertive with the pediatrician in insisting that their child be dealt with in a kind and sensitive manner.

CREATING A SUPPORTIVE ENVIRONMENT

Golan and Weizman (2001) reviewed the literature on family-based treatments of childhood obesity and subsequently outlined a broad conceptual framework for such treatment. They noted that an essential step in tackling the weight challenge is to create a home environment supportive of the behaviors. It is critical that parents help children understand the importance of the proposed changes and also that they acknowledge how difficult making changes can be and predict with their child that frustration may arise. We suggest that parents plan a regular time to check in with their child with respect to how he or she is feeling about the changes and his or her progress and that the tone of such conversations be supportive and understanding.

We emphasize here the importance of establishing and maintaining a theme of *collaboration* between parent and child. During each step of intervention it should be clear that the parent is "on the child's side" and that the parent is eliciting and considering the child's thoughts and feelings in making decisions about how to move forward.

As noted previously, research shows consistently that overweight children are more likely to have poor body image than their normal-weight counterparts. Concrete strategies for improving and maintaining a more positive body image are available, some more programmatically than others (National Eating Disorders Association, 1999). School-based media literacy or "ad-busting" programs have been developed to teach children to question rigid cultural ideals of attractiveness (such as those available from the Media Literacy Clearinghouse, 2006). Research shows that exposure to fashion magazines and other media portraying the cultural ideal of thinness has a negative effect on body satisfaction, at least in the short run (e.g., Yamamiya, Cash, Melnyk, Posavac, & Posavac, 2005). Keeping only positive reading and viewing materials in the home may provide some protection against these kinds of influences. Parents can also support a positive body image by focusing on other functions of the body than outward appearance. For example, one might note the body's ability to play all day and to get the child wherever she or he needs to go. A parent can also encourage a child to enjoy clothing as an expression of his or her preferences and personality. Overweight children are often encouraged to dress in "slimming" styles and dark colors, when they may indeed have a preference for sleeveless shirts or bright purple outfits. We recommend honoring a child's clothing preferences and encouraging him or her to take pride in expression through dressing his or her body. Finally, parents can communicate their acceptance of their child's body by being sure to show physical affection, sending the message that the parents are just as interested in physical contact with the overweight child as they might be with a normal-weight sibling or as other children's parents are.

In addition to media literacy in the body-image domain, it can be helpful to teach media literacy with respect to food advertisements. Children are exposed to significant numbers of food advertisements. One study found that children view 10,000 food advertisements per year on television, with 95% of them being for unhealthy foods (Horgen, Choate, & Brownell, 2001). More recently, children's media have been targeted for product placements of soft drinks and food. One extreme example of this is "advergaming," in which elaborate websites are built for the sole purpose of immersing children in a branded environment without their realizing it's a commercial (Stafford & Faber, 2004). For example, Postopia.com comprises games that feature characters from Post children's cereals. Here, it may be useful for parents to play to a child's dislike of being deceived and manipulated and point out how these games are really commercials for certain products, paid for by the manufacturers. This strategy has the potential to be especially helpful with older children and adolescents.

Children learn first and foremost by observing others' behaviors. Therefore, there is significant opportunity for parents to influence children's eating and activity behaviors simply by example. Parents should attempt to demonstrate healthy eating and exercise habits themselves, as well as to model positive feelings about their own bodies. Parents should avoid self-critical body-focused commentary. Finally, this is a particularly useful issue around which to share one's own struggles with a child. If the parent has struggled with weight, he or she can let the child know that he or she knows what the child is going through and that they are in this together.

ADDRESSING WEIGHT BIAS

Many obese children and adolescents suffer harassment and rejection at school related to their weight, and they can be subjected to merciless teasing from peers and siblings (Neumark-Sztainer et al., 2002; Pierce & Wardle, 1997; Neumark-Sztainer, Story, & Faibisch, 1998). The literature on ways of decreasing incidents of childhood bullying suggests that parents should actively respond to such events rather than ignore weight-related teasing (Fekkes, Pijpers, & Verloove-Vanhorick, 2005). Ignoring the behavior, in fact, is likely to send the message that the child deserves this treatment (see also Chapter 17, this volume). Some parents are hesitant to interfere because they worry that they will make the situation worse for their child by confronting the bully, or they may hope that the teasing will motivate their child to lose weight. Parents must put these thoughts aside; it is critical that parents provide a clear and consistent message that teasing and bullying by anyone (strangers, peers, family members) is unacceptable and will not be tolerated.

Unfortunately, research also suggests that overweight children may be stigmatized by adults, including teachers and their own parents (Latner & Schwartz, 2005). Parents must pay close attention to their own behavior and make sure that they do not make negative comments about their child's body. Here, there is an extremely important distinction between saying something to a child about behavior (e.g., "Good health involves eating fruits and vegetables every day") versus appearance (e.g., "You are too fat"). Bias due to body weight or shape is no different from racial discrimination or discrimination against children with disabilities—it is a negative attitude toward a person based on a physical characteristic.

CRAFTING A HEALTHY FOOD ENVIRONMENT

What is a healthy food environment? As noted previously, contradictory opinions abound. However, most would agree that moving toward less sugar and saturated fat, eliminating transfats, increasing consumption of vegetables and fruits, and choosing leaner protein sources, and whole grains would benefit most children (Dietz & Stern, 1999). In addition, research suggests that caloric intake decreases with the consumption of less calorie-dense foods (Rolls & Barnett, 2003; see also Chapter 16, this volume). For example, eating a large serving of vegetables will produce a feeling of fullness, whereas a small but calorie-equivalent portion of cake will not. Finally, research suggests that children do not compensate for the calories consumed in liquid form by decreasing their consumption of solid foods (DellaValle, Roe, & Rolls, 2005). Thus calorie-free beverages are a better choice for children struggling with weight. A recent meta-analysis of the soft-drink literature found that soft-drink consumption is associated with higher calorie consumption, even beyond that of the soft drinks themselves (Vartanian, Schwartz, & Brownell, in press). This research suggests that one dietary change that is clearly indicated is removing all sugared soft drinks from a child's diet (see also Chapter 13, this volume).

Once healthier food choices have been identified, the goal becomes celebrating and making available these healthy foods. One framing change that can be helpful is to conceptualize eating changes as increasing the consumption of food that is good for the body rather than restricting the "fun" foods. In this way, the changes do not follow a deprivation model and are focused on the positive. Parents often complain to us that they feel "mean" when "depriving" their children of treat foods. It is revealing that we have become so reliant as a culture on food as reward (Puhl & Schwartz, 2003). One approach to dealing with this complaint is to be creative in terms of rewarding and celebrating with children. For example, special time with a child or playing a favorite game can be framed as a reward. Most children are delighted to have time and attention from their parents.

It is also important to initiate a connection between healthy foods and good taste. Most children will have a taste for at least some fruits and vegetables. Raw carrots and green beans appeal to most children. Corn—especially "on the cob"—is perceived as novel and fun by children. Most children do like a number of fruits, and blending a variety of colors in a fruit plate or fruit basket can produce delight in groups of children. One of us (M.B.S.) has taken the bold step of arriving at her daughter's classroom on her daughter's birthday bearing an exotic "edible bouquet" made of strawberries, pineapple, grapes, and melon instead of cupcakes. The children were entranced. Such anecdotes offer support for the notion that children are often more flexible than we might predict.

A typical question on the mind of parents of overweight children is whether "treat" foods should be in the home. Some have argued that if the child does not have the opportunity for these foods at home, he or she will overeat the foods when outside the home. Others have argued, conversely, that the presence of these foods increases desire for them. A third possibility is that the presence of these foods increases desire only when they are "forbidden" or given special status; thus having free access to these foods will render them less appealing to children. The empirical data do not yet provide a resolution of this debate. Birch and Fisher (2000) found that restriction of treat foods by mothers was associated with increased weight and an increased desire for these foods in daughters; however, it is unclear which came first. One possibility is that restricting these foods increases children's desire for them. Another possibility is that some children have difficulty self-regulating intake of sweets; therefore, the mothers restrict these foods in response to the child's behavior (see also Chapter 13, this volume).

The research on the importance of stimulus control when trying to change a behavior that has specific triggers suggests that it makes sense to keep unhealthful foods out of the house so that seeing them will not trigger desire to eat them. A number of studies have shown that the more visible and easily accessible food is, the more likely we are to eat it (Wansink, 2004). This line of research supports an "out of sight, out of mind" approach.

On the other hand, specifically telling a child that he or she will never eat another cookie will likely cause a negative response. Instead, we advocate telling children that certain foods are only eaten sometimes, and then making those "sometimes" events as predictable as possible. For example, the family may decide that on birthdays they make a cake to eat, or on Sundays they bake cookies. This strategy provides a number of benefits. First, the actual food will be homemade and will not include hydrogenated oils, high-fructose corn syrup, or other processed ingredients. Second, the portions can be controlled by making a cake that is big enough for only one serving per person, or enough cookies so that each person may have a few. Third, it provides an opportunity for a fun activity for the family to create something together. If a child knows there will be opportunities to eat these foods, then they are not forbidden, but they are also eaten in reasonable quantities. With that said, defining a "reasonable quantity" is not easy. Essentially, the family must figure out how many calories per day the child should eat in order to maintain or lose weight and then factor in the key nutrients that he or she needs. Once the calories in those are calculated, anything else can be considered "discretionary calories." The website for the Food Guide Pyramid has some guidelines for this that may be useful; we present these data in Table 14.1.

Portion sizes are often on the minds of parents. In our experience, parents—and mothers especially—seem to have a very strong negative reaction to the idea of their child going hungry. Thus parents often present chil-

TABLE 14.1. Recommended Total and Discretionary Daily Calorie Levels

	Sedentary		Active	
	Total calories	Discretionary calories	Total calories	Discretionary calories
Children				
2–3 years	1,000	165	1,400	171
Females				
4–8 years	1,200	171	1,800	195
9–13	1,600	132	2,200	290
14–18	1,800	195	2,400	362
19–30	2,000	267	2,400	362
31–50	1,800	195	2,200	290
51+	1,600	132	2,200	290
Males				
4–8 years	1,400	171	2,000	267
9–13	1,800	195	2,600	410
14–18	2,200	290	3,200	648
19–30	2,400	362	3,000	512
31–50	2,200	290	3,000	512
51+	2,000	267	2,800	426

Note. Data from *MyPyramid.gov*. "Sedentary" means a lifestyle that includes only the light physical activity associated with typical day-to-day life. "Active" means a lifestyle that includes physical activity equivalent to walking more than 3 miles per day at 3 to 4 miles per hour, in addition to the light physical activity associated with typical day-to-day life.

dren with portions larger than they need. Research on the influence of portion size on consumption shows that, in both adults and children, the larger the portion, the greater the caloric intake (Rolls, Roe, Kral, Meengs, & Wall, 2004). Thus parents can assist children simply by serving reasonable portions of food. A related strategy is to serve children their food from serving dishes that remain off the table during the meal. That is, we recommend parental serving rather than "family style" self-serve. This strategy controls the initial portion served and also makes use of the influence of proximity (i.e., people are less likely to eat a food the farther away it is; Painter, Wansink, & Hieggelke, 2002).

The goal of having children increase their intake of healthier foods usually means that children must try new foods. Parents often find themselves discouraged after presenting a food once and having the child refuse it. Research shows that it takes up to 10 presentations of a new food for children to develop a preference for the food (Birch & Marlin, 1982). Thus children can "learn to like it," but parents must be persistent. Also, research shows that children must actually try the food to acquire the preference (Birch, McPhee, Shoba, Pirok, & Steinberg, 1987); thus one suggestion for easing this path is to set a house rule that all family members *must* at least try a new food, even if they don't finish it. It can also be helpful to set parameters for trying foods; for example, no dramatics are permitted when one doesn't like the food. Finally, we have found that children respond to different framings of new foods. Some children are more likely to try a new food if it is presented as "grown up" or in some other way exciting.

Parents often have questions about whether snacks are permissible for a child attempting to lose weight. In fact, behavioral weight-loss programs (e.g., Brownell, 2004) typically incorporate planned healthy snacks to promote weight loss. Children often have long days, and the stretches between breakfast and lunch and lunch and dinner can be long. If a child goes without eating for 6 hours, he or she is likely to arrive at the next meal famished. Research shows that this pattern encourages overeating at the meal (Brownell, 2004). Thus well-placed snacks can actually reduce overall caloric intake.

We recommend placing a strong emphasis on eating breakfast. As noted, eating consistently decreases the likelihood of overeating at any given meal or snack. In addition, eating breakfast is associated with lower body mass index in children, although studies are not uniformly in agreement on this point (Rampersaud, Pereira, Girard, Adams, & Metzl, 2005). Finally, eating breakfast has been associated with improved school performance (Rampersaud et al., 2005). The degree to which this relationship is causal and, if so, exactly what kind of breakfast is associated with these advantages is not known; however, the data support a strong recommendation that children eat breakfast.

The strategies we have detailed thus far can all be implemented by parents; however, other adults often influence a child's eating, and this can present a challenge. For many children, relatives such as grandparents are regular providers of meals or snacks. Other adults may wish to give the child sweets, and when the parent protests, respond with "Oh, it's only once in a while" or "It's a special occasion." This can be enormously frustrating for both the parent and child, who are working hard to make difficult changes. When embarking on a program of change, it is helpful to include close relatives in the plan and elicit their support. Outlining concern for the child's health and well-being can bring well-meaning saboteurs on board.

Other adults to consider speaking with include babysitters, nannies, and friends' parents. Research shows that children eat the healthiest meals when in their own homes—that is, they eat less healthfully when eating in restaurants or even when eating in other people's homes (Biing-Hwan, Guthrie, & Frazao, 2001). The reason may be that families will often bring out the "fun" food (e.g., soda, potato chips) when the children's friends are visiting. Eating meals at home has been associated with greater success in weight loss (Epstein et al., 1994). If one's child eats regularly at a close friend's home, it may be useful to speak with the friend's parents to let them know that the family is attempting to make some healthy lifestyle changes and to ask that they not bring out "special foods" when the child visits. Similarly, babysitters and nannies can be instructed regarding what foods you wish your child to be fed. Again, this task is much easier when changes are being made at the family level so that all children are treated equally.

Finally, the school environment can be incredibly difficult for children (Brownell & Horgen, 2004). It is the norm for schools to house vending machines, to maintain contracts with soda producers, to use food as reward in the classroom, and to celebrate with sugary, high-fat foods in the classroom (e.g., birthday cupcakes). This environment is overwhelming for a child, and the child should not be expected to learn how to manage it. Rather, a more productive, albeit labor-intensive, effort is to modify the school environment. Increasingly, schools and parents are open to ideas for improving the health of students, and many school districts have adopted policies to create a better food environment. Parents are among the most powerful advocates for children, and many major policy changes across the country were set into motion by one or two parents.

It is important for the child to be involved in the process of creating a healthy food environment. To this end, parents can involve the child in the grocery shopping, meal planning, and cooking. Many parents find that children are more likely to try new foods when they have helped to cook them. Parents can also collaborate with the child on ways to handle difficult situations, such as whether or not to buy snacks sold at school. A child who has been involved in setting the policy (e.g., buying a snack once a week) may feel better about following through.

CRAFTING A PHYSICAL ACTIVITY ENVIRONMENT

Physical activity is a useful part of any successful weight-loss plan for both adults and children (Grilo, 1994; Grilo, Brownell, & Stunkard, 1993; Elfhag & Rossner, 2005; Jakicic, 2002), and it is critically important in weight maintenance (Andersen et al., 1999; Bryner, Toffle, Ulrich, & Yeater, 1997; Kayman, Bruvold, & Stern, 1990; Marston & Criss, 1984; Jeffery et al., 1984; Hartman et al., 1993; Epstein, Wing, Koeske, & Valoski, 1984). Further, increased physical activity is solidly associated with improved health indices (e.g., blood pressure, diabetes indicators, cholesterol), as well as with all-cause mortality, independent of weight or weight loss (Barlow, Kohl, Gibbons, & Blair, 1995; Lee, Jackson, & Blair, 1998). Although there continues to be controversy regarding how much and what type of exercise is best for weight loss and weight management, compelling evidence shows that even modest levels of physical activity may be sufficient to improve health in many people (Barlow et al., 1995; Duncan, Gordon, & Scott, 1991; Lee et al., 1998; Rippe et al., 1988).

Physical Activity versus Formal Exercise

It is important to distinguish physical activity and formal exercise. A large literature has been amassed on the benefits of what is known as *lifestyle physical activity* (LPA). LPA refers to incorporating increased activity into the natural course of one's day, for example, taking the stairs instead of the elevator, walking to the store a half-mile away, parking at a distant spot in the parking lot, making family time active by taking a walk to have a talk. Considerable research has addressed the question of whether structured formal exercise is superior to LPA for weight loss or weight maintenance (Andersen et al., 1999; Dunn et al., 1999). Strong debate continues. However, given the general consensus that consistency is the key to long-term success, many experts still advocate that overweight persons aim to accumulate at least 30 minutes of some form of physical activity on at least 5 days of every week. Indeed, compliance is greater with less intensive forms of activity, supporting the encouragement of LPA. Studies have found that interventions that foster LPA may be as effective as traditional structured exercise programs in both adults and children (Andersen et al., 1999; Dunn et al., 1999; Epstein, Wing, Koeske, & Valoski, 1985; Fogelholm, Kukkonen-Harjula, Nenonen, & Parsanen, 2000; King, Haskell, Young, Oka, & Stefanick, 1995; Simkin-Silverman, Wing, Boraz, & Kuller, 2003) (see also

Chapter 3, this volume). Thus parents can feel free to be creative in helping their children incorporate activity into their lives.

Obstacles to Promoting Physical Activity

Physical activity, in whatever form, is often difficult for an overweight child. Engaging in formal exercise, such as playing a sport, takes time, and children in our current culture often have heavily scheduled lives. One way to address the time barrier is to prioritize physical activity. That is, when choosing among all of the potential extracurricular activities, at least one should be physically active, for example, swimming, dance, or a team sport. Alternatively, a parent might limit extracurriculars and spend some of the child's nonschool time regularly doing something active with the child, such as hiking or cycling. The latter is a nice opportunity for positive modeling.

Money can be an obstacle for some families. Many formal sports are quite expensive. Again, this obstacle can be overcome with LPA approaches to activity or with family-based activity such as hiking, walking, swimming, or cycling, if bicycles are available.

Safety issues have been identified by some as a primary reason for the decline in children's physical activity. That is, most parents today are not comfortable having their children walk alone to school or play freely outside unsupervised, whereas this was not the case a generation ago. Given current constraints on many parents' time, this is a significant barrier. One way to approach the problem is to work together with other families such that parents rotate walking the children to school or supervising children in the neighborhood.

Related to the issue of safety, many new communities are constructed in a way that discourages physical activity. For example, many communities lack sidewalks, rendering it unsafe for children to bike or walk to school or other activities. Many communities are far from parks and other open-play areas. Studies on the effects of the built environment on obesity have consistently demonstrated an association between obesity and area of residence, resources, television, walkability, land use, sprawl, and level of deprivation (Booth, Pinkston, & Poston, 2005; Kaur, Hyder, & Poston, 2003). The remedy, of course, needs to be sought at systemic levels.

Finally, embarrassment can be a major obstacle to exercise for the overweight child. Because overweight children have often been less active than their peers, they tend to be less skilled at popular sports. In addition, they tend to show more physical signs of exertion (e.g., sweating, breathing heavily, flushing) and can have less stamina. They also can have a history of being teased while participating in activity. Faith, Leone, Ayers, Heo, and Pietrobelli (2002) found that being teased during sports and physical activity is associated with poorer attitudes toward and reduced participation in sports. These factors combine to produce a significantly aversive conditioning effect with regard to activity. This barrier is best overcome by collaborating with your child to find fun ways to be active. A walk to a special destination or working toward a particular exercise goal can pique interest and develop pride for the child in his or her physical abilities.

Sports

As noted, organized sports can be difficult for overweight children. However, some children are interested in trying something new, and they should be encouraged to do so. Parents can collaborate with the child to discover whether he or she might prefer a team sport (e.g., soccer, basketball) or a more individual sport (e.g., swimming). Interestingly, organized sports do not necessarily provide more activity than informal playing. There is much starting and stopping in most sports, and, on a big team, children spend a fair amount of time on the bench. If the goal is to increase activity, parents may wish to investigate the amount of activity the child will get. It is also a good idea to talk with the child's coach about his or her philosophy of coaching children. Parents will want to seek out an environment in which all children get to play and the focus is on having fun and learning skills, not winning at all costs. The goal here is to instill lifelong interest in activity in the child, not to create further aversion to activity.

Making Activity a Family Goal

As with changes in eating habits, we encourage parents to make increasing activity a goal for the entire family. When choosing a means of spending family time together, try to be active rather than sedentary. For example, instead of watching a movie, go on a family hike. In having a meal together, make it an outdoor picnic that involves a nature walk to the destination. Encourage family members to walk or cycle to most destinations within reasonable distance. When driving, park a little farther away from the destination and walk the last couple of blocks. An alternate framework in which to view the change is as environmental protection. Children can become excited at the thought of contributing to such an important global project as conserving energy and fighting pollution.

Increasing Activity by Decreasing Sedentary Behavior

One reason that we have become less active overall as a society is that we have replaced active pastimes with sedentary ones. Increase activity by reversing this trend. Research shows that increased television viewing and video game use is associated with overweight in children (Caroli, Argentieri, Cardone, & Masi, 2004; Vandewater, Shim, & Caplovitz, 2004) and with poorer health behaviors and health outcomes in adults (Hu, Li, Colditz, Willett, & Manson, 2003). We recommend that parents limit television, video game, and computer time for children. One strategy is to create a "bank account" of hours for each child. For example, each child has 5 hours per week of television and can spend that however he or she wishes (of course, with some limits concerning homework completion, bedtime, etc.). Alternatively, some families prefer to set per diem limits or to not allow television viewing at all on weekdays. Devices for televisions exist that will monitor and limit each child's viewing. If children are limited in their viewing, however, parents should model this behavior and limit their own viewing. To support this transition, many families decide to have only one television in the home and not to put it in a place of prominence.

CONCLUSIONS

In this chapter, we have described some of the difficult challenges facing parents of overweight children. We have outlined specific approaches and strategies for creating a supportive environment, a healthy food environment, and a healthy physical activity environment. We have identified significant barriers to the goal of lifestyle change and have outlined some strategies for overcoming or circumventing them. Much of what we have put forth is based on broad clinical experience and the clinical literature; data on self-help weight-loss interventions for children are lacking. We encourage the research community to work toward remedying this dearth in the service of making more widely available empirically supported interventions in this area.

We also present this chapter with the strong belief that, in fact, the kinds of changes that will markedly affect the health of all children will be those made at national and global system levels rather than at the family level. Although the latter is indeed important, the emphasis on personal responsibility for weight does not reflect the reality of the etiology of obesity.

REFERENCES

Andersen, R. E., Wadden, T. A., Bartlett, S. J., Zemel, B., Verde, T. J., & Franckowiak, S. C. (1999). Effects of lifestyle activity vs. structured aerobic exercise in obese women: A randomized trial. *Journal of the American Medical Association. 281,* 335–340.

Barlow, C. E., Kohl, H. W., Gibbons, L. W., & Blair, S. N. (1995). Physical fitness, mortality, and obesity. *International Journal of Obesity, 19,* S41–S44.

Bar-Or, O., Foreyt, J., Bouchard, C., Brownell, K. D., Dietz, W. H., Ravussin, E., et al. (1998). Physical activity, genetic and nutritional considerations in childhood weight management. *Medicine and Science in Sports and Exercise, 30,* 2–10.

Banis, H. T., Varni, J. W., Wallander, J. L., Korsch, B. M., Jay, S. M., Adler, R., et al. (1988).

Psychological and social adjustment of obese children and their families. *Child Care, Health and Development, 14,* 157–173.

Barlow, S. E., & Dietz, W. H. (1998). Obesity evaluation and treatment: Expert committee recommendations. *Pediatrics, 102,* E29.

Biing-Hwan, L., Guthrie, J., & Frazao, E. (2001). American children's diets not making the grade. *Food Review, 24,* 8–17. Retrieved November 29, 2006, from *www.ers.usda.gov/publications/FoodReview/May2001/FRV24I2b.pdf*

Birch, L. L., & Fisher, J. O. (2000). Mothers' child feeding practices influence daughters' eating and weight. *American Journal of Clinical Nutrition, 71,* 1054–1061.

Birch, L. L., & Marlin, D. W. (1982). I don't like it; I never tried it: Effects of exposure on two-year-old children's food preferences. *Appetite, 3,* 353–360.

Birch, L. L., McPhee, L., Shoba, B. C., Pirok, E., & Steinberg, L. (1987). What kind of exposure reduces children's food neophobia? Looking vs tasting. *Appetite, 9,* 171–178.

Booth, K. M., Pinkston, M. M., & Poston, W. S. (2005). Obesity and the built environment. *Journal of the American Dietetic Association, 105*(Suppl. 1), S110–S117.

Bouchard, C. (1997). Genetics of human obesity: Recent results from linkage studies. *Journal of Nutrition, 127,* S1887–1890.

Braet, C., Mervielde, I., & Vandereycken, W. (1997). Psychological aspects of childhood obesity. *Journal of Pediatric Psychology, 22,* 59–71.

Brownell, K. D. (2004). *LEARN.* Dallas, TX: American Health.

Brownell, K. D. (2005). Does a "toxic" environment make obesity inevitable? *Obesity Management, 2,* 52–55.

Brownell, K. D., & Horgen, K. B. (2004). *Food fight: The inside story of the food industry, America's obesity crisis, and what we can do about it.* New York: McGraw-Hill/Contemporary Books.

Bryner, R. W., Toffle, R. C., Ulrich, I. H., & Yeater, R. A. (1997). The effects of exercise intensity on body composition, weight loss, and dietary composition in women. *Journal of the American College of Nutrition, 16,* 68–73.

Butryn, M. L., & Wadden, T. A. (2005). Treatment of overweight in children and adolescents: Does dieting increase the risk of eating disorders? *International Journal of Eating Disorders, 37,* 285–293.

Carnell, S., Edwards, C., Croker, H., Boniface, D., & Wardle, J. (2005). Parental perceptions of overweight in 3–5-year-olds. *International Journal of Obesity, 29,* 353–355.

Caroli, M., Argentieri, L., Cardone, M., & Masi, A. (2004). Role of television in childhood obesity prevention. *International Journal of Obesity, 28,* S104–S108.

Critser, G. (2003). *Fat land: How Americans became the fattest people in the world.* Boston: Houghton Mifflin.

Dansinger, M. L., Gleason, J. A., Griffith, J. L., Selker, H. P., & Schaefer, E. J. (2005). Comparison of the Atkins, Ornish, Weight Watchers, and Zone diets for weight loss and heart disease risk reduction. *Journal of the American Medical Association, 293,* 43–53.

DellaValle, D. M., Roe, L. S., & Rolls, B. J. (2005). Does the consumption of caloric and noncaloric beverages with a meal affect energy intake? *Appetite, 44,* 187–193.

Dietz, W. H. (1998). Health consequences of obesity in youth: Childhood predictors of adult disease. *Pediatrics, 101,* 518–525.

Dietz, W. H., & Stern, L. (Eds.). (1999). *Guide to your child's nutrition.* New York: Villard Books.

Duncan, J. J., Gordon, N. F., & Scott, C. B. (1991). Women walking for health and fitness: How much is enough? *Journal of the American Medical Association, 266,* 3295–3299.

Dunn, A. L., Marcus, B. H., Kampert, J. B., Garcia, M. E., Kohl, H. W., & Blair, S. N. (1999). Comparison of lifestyle and structured interventions to increase physical activity and cardiorespiratory fitness: A randomized trial. *Journal of the American Medical Association, 281,* 327–334.

Elfhag, K., & Rossner, S. (2005). Who succeeds in maintaining weight loss? A conceptual review of factors associated with weight loss maintenance and weight regain. *Obesity Reviews, 6,* 67–85.

Epstein, L. H., Myers, M. D., Raynor, H. A., & Saelens, B. (1998). Treatment of pediatric obesity. *Pediatrics, 101,* 554–570.

Epstein, L. H., Valoski, A. M., Kalarchian, M. A., & McCurley, J. (1995). Do children lose and maintain weight easier than adults? A comparison of child and parent weight changes from six months to ten years. *Obesity Research, 3,* 411–417.

Epstein, L. H., Valoski, A. M., Wing, R. R., & McCurley, J. (1994). Ten-year outcomes of behavioral family-based treatment for childhood obesity. *Health Psychology, 13,* 373–383.

Epstein, L. H., & Wing, R. R. (1987). Behavioral treatment of childhood obesity. *Psychological Bulletin, 101,* 331–342.

Epstein, L. H., Wing, R. R., Koeske, R., & Valoski, A. (1984). Effects of diet plus exercise on weight change in parents and children. *Journal of Consulting and Clinical Psychology, 52,* 429–437.

Epstein, L. H., Wing, R. R., Koeske, R., & Valoski, A. (1985). A comparison of lifestyle exercise, aerobic exercise, and calisthenics on weight-loss in obese children. *Behavior Therapy, 16,* 345–356.

Erickson, S. J., Robinson, T. N., Haydel, K. F., & Killen, J. D. (2000). Are overweight children unhappy? Body mass index, depressive symptoms, and overweight concerns in elementary school children [Comment]. *Archives of Pediatrics and Adolescent Medicine, 154,* 931–935.

Faith, M. S., Leone, M. A., Ayers, T. S., Heo, M., & Pietrobelli, A. (2002). Weight criticism during physical activity, coping skills, and reported physical activity in children. *Pediatrics, 110,* e23.

Fekkes, M., Pijpers, F. I. M., & Verloove-Vanhorick, S. P. (2005). Bullying: Who does what, when and where? Involvement of children, teachers and parents in bullying behavior. *Health Education Research: Theory and Practice, 20,* 81–91.

Fogelholm, M., Kukkonen-Harjula, K., Nenonen, A., & Parsanen, M. (2000). Effects of walking training on weight maintenance in a very-low-calorie-energy diet in premenopausal obese women: A randomized controlled trial. *Archives of Internal Medicine, 160,* 2177–2184.

French, S. A., Story, M., & Perry, C. L. (1995). Self-esteem and obesity in children and adolescents: A literature review. *Obesity Research, 3,* 479–490.

Golan, M., & Weizman, A. (2001). Familiar approach to the treatment of childhood obesity: Conceptual model. *Journal of Nursing Education, 33,* 102–107.

Grilo, C. M. (1994). Physical activity and obesity. *Biomedicine and Pharmacotherapy, 48,* 127–136.

Grilo, C. M., Brownell, K. D., & Stunkard, A. J. (1993). The metabolic and psychological importance of exercise in weight control. In A. J. Stunkard & T. A. Wadden (Eds.), *Obesity: Theory and therapy* (pp. 253–273). New York: Raven Press.

Grilo, C. M., & Pogue-Geile, M. F. (1991). The nature of environmental influences on weight and obesity: A behavior genetic analysis. *Psychological Bulletin, 110,* 520–537.

Hartman, W. M., Stroud, M., Sweet, D. M., & Saxton, J. (1993). Long-term maintenance of weight-loss following supplemented fasting. *International Journal of Eating Disorders, 14,* 87–93.

Hendry, L. B., & Gillies, P. (1978). Body type, body esteem, school, and leisure: A study of overweight, average, and underweight adolescents. *Journal of Youth and Adolescence, 7,* 181–195.

Horgen, K. B., Choate, M., & Brownell, K. D. (2001). Food advertising: Targeting children in a toxic environment. In D. G. Singer & J. L. Singer (Eds.), *Handbook of children and the media* (pp. 447–462). Thousand Oaks, CA: Sage.

Hu, F. B., Li, T. Y., Colditz, G. A., Willett, W. C., & Manson, J. E. (2003). Television watching and other sedentary behaviors in relation to risk of obesity and type 2 diabetes mellitus in women. *Journal of the American Medical Association, 289,* 1785–1791.

International Obesity Task Force. (2002). *About obesity.* Retrieved June 30, 2005 from *http://www.iotf.org/aboutobesity.asp*

Israel, A. C., & Ivanova, M. Y. (2002). Global and dimensional self-esteem in preadolescent and early adolescent children who are overweight: Age and gender differences. *International Journal of Eating Disorders, 31,* 424–429.

Jakicic, J. M. (2002). The role of physical activity in prevention and treatment of body weight gain in adults. *Journal of Nutrition, 132,* 3826S–3829S.

Jeffery, R. W. (1984). Correlates of weight loss and its maintenance over 2 years of follow-up among middle-aged men. *Preventative Medicine, 12,* 155–168.

Jeffery, R. W., Bjornson-Benson, W. M., Rosenthal, B. S., Lindquist, R. A, Kurth, C. L., & Johnson, S. L. (1984). Correlates of weight loss and its maintenance over two years of follow-up among middle aged men. *Preventive Medicine, 12,* 155–168.

Jelalian, E., & Saelens, B. E. (1999). Interventions for pediatric obesity: Treatments that work. *Journal of Pediatric Psychology, 24,* 223–248.

Kaur, H., Hyder, M. L., & Poston, W. S. (2003). Childhood overweight: An expanding problem. *Treatments in Endocrinology, 2,* 375–388.

Kayman, S., Bruvold, W., & Stern, J. S. (1990). Maintenance and relapse after weight loss in women: Behavioral aspects. *American Journal of Clinical Nutrition, 52,* 800–807.

King, A. C., Haskell, W. L., Young, D. R., Oka, R. K., & Stefanick, M. L. (1995). Long-term effects of varying intensities and formats of physical activity on participation rates, fitness, and lipoproteins in men and women aged 50 to 65 years. *Circulation, 91,* 2596–2604.

Kramer, F. M., Jeffery, R. W., Forster J. L., & Snell, M. K. (1989). Long-term follow-up of behavioral treatment for obesity: Patterns of weight regain among men and women. *International Journal of Obesity, 13,* 123–136.

Latner, J., & Schwartz, M. B. (2005). Weight bias in a child's world. In K. D. Brownell, R. M. Puhl, M. B. Schwartz, & L. Rudd (Eds.), *Bias, stigma, discrimination, and obesity* (pp. 54–67). New York: Guilford Press.

Lee, C. D., Jackson, A. S., & Blair, S. N. (1998). U.S. weight guidelines: Is it also important to consider cardiorespiratory fitness? *International Journal of Obesity, 22,* S2–S7.

Ludwig, D. S. (2000). Dietary glycemic index and obesity. *Journal of Nutrition, 130*(Suppl. 2S), 280S–283S.

Marston, A. R., & Criss, J. (1984). Maintenance of successful weight loss: Incidence and prediction. *International Journal of Obesity, 8,* 435–439.

Martin, S., Housley, K., McCoy, H., & Greenhouse, P. (1988). Self-esteem of adolescent girls as related to weight. *Perceptual and Motor Skills, 67,* 879–884.

Media Literacy Clearinghouse. (2006). Body image. Retrieved November 29, 2006, from *www.frankwbaker.com/body_image.htm*

Mellin, A. E., Neumark-Sztainer, D., Story, M., Ireland, M., & Resnick, M. D. (2002). Unhealthy behaviors and psychosocial difficulties among overweight adolescents: The potential impact of familial factors. *Journal of Adolescent Health, 31,* 145–153.

Mendelson, B. K., & White, D. R. (1982). Relation between body esteem and self-esteem of obese and normal children. *Perceptual and Motor Skills, 54,* 899–905.

Mendelson, B. K., & White, D. R. (1985). Development of self-body-esteem in overweight youngsters. *Developmental Psychology, 21,* 90–96.

Mendelson, B. K., White, D. R., & Mendelson, M. J. (1996). Self-esteem and body esteem: Effects of gender, age, and weight. *Journal of Applied Developmental Psychology, 17,* 321–346.

National Eating Disorders Association. (1999). *Go Girls!* curriculum.

National Eating Disorders Association. (1999). *Go Girls! Giving our girls inspiration and* resources for lasting self esteem: A curriculum for high school girls. Seattle, WA: Eating Disorders Awareness and Prevention.

Nestle M. (2002). Food politics: How the food industry influences nutrition and health. Berkeley: University of California Press.

Neumark-Sztainer, D., Falkner, N., Story, M., Perry, C., Hannan, P. J., & Mulert, S. (2002). Weight-teasing among adolescents: Correlations with weight status and disordered eating behaviors. International Journal of Obesity, 26, 123–131.

Neumark-Sztainer, D., Story, M., & Faibisch, L. (1998). Perceived stigmatization among overweight African-American and Caucasian adolescent girls. Journal of Adolescent Health, 23, 264–270.

Painter, J. E., Wansink, B., & Hieggelke, J. B. (2002). How visibility and convenience influence candy consumption. Appetite, 38, 237–258.

Pierce, J. W., & Wardle, J. (1997). Cause and effect: Beliefs and self-esteem of overweight children. Journal of Child Psychology and Psychiatry, 38, 645–650.

Puhl, R., & Brownell, K. D. (2001). Bias, discrimination, and obesity. Obesity Research, 9, 788–805.

Puhl, R., & Schwartz, M. B. (2003). If you are good you can have a cookie: The link between childhood food rules and adult eating behaviors. Eating Behaviors, 4, 283–293.

Rampersaud, G. C., Pereira, M. A., Girard, B. L., Adams, J., & Metzl, J. D. (2005). Breakfast habits, nutritional status, body weight, and academic performance in children and adolescents. Journal of the American Dietetic Association, 105, 743–760.

Rippe, J. M., Ward, A., Porcari, J. P., & Freedson, P. S. (1998). Walking for health and fitness. Journal of the American Medical Association, 259, 2720–2724.

Rolls, B., & Barnett, R. A. (2003). The Volumetrics weight control plan: Feel full on fewer calories. New York: HarperCollins.

Rolls, B. J., Roe, L. S., Kral, T. V. E., Meengs, J. S., & Wall, D. E. (2004). Increasing the portion size of a packaged snack increases energy intake in men and women. Appetite, 42, 63–69.

Sallade, J. (1973). A comparison of the psychological adjustment of obese vs. non-obese children. Journal of Psychosomatic Research, 17, 89–96.

Samaha, F. F., Iqbal, N., Seshadri, P., Chicano, K. L., Daily, D. A., McGrory, J., et al. (2003). A low-carbohydrate as compared with a low-fat diet in severe obesity. New England Journal of Medicine, 348, 2074–2081.

Schlosser, E. (2001). Fast food nation: The dark side of the all-American meal. New York: Houghton Mifflin.

Schwartz, M. B., Chambliss, H. O., Brownell, K. D., Blair, S. N., & Billington, C. (2003). Weight bias among health professionals specializing in obesity. Obesity Research, 11, 1033–1039.

Sheslow, D., Hassink, S., Wallace, W., & DeLancey, E. (1993). The relationship between self-esteem and depression in obese children. Annals of the New York Academy of Sciences, 699, 289–291.

Simkin-Silverman, L. R., Wing, R. R., Boraz, M. A., & Kuller, L. H. (2003). Lifestyle intervention can prevent weight gain during menopause: Results from a 5-year randomized clinical trial. Annals of Behavioral Medicine, 26, 212–220.

Stafford, M. R., & Faber, R. J. (Eds.). (2004). Advertising, Promotion, and New Media. Armonk, NY: Sharpe.

Tsai, A. G., & Wadden, T. A. (2005). Systematic review: An evaluation of major commercial weight loss programs in the United States. Annals of Internal Medicine, 142, 56–66.

Vandewater, E. A., Shim, M., & Caplovitz, A. G. (2004). Linking obesity and activity level with children's television and video game use. Journal of Adolescence, 27, 71–85.

Vartanian, L., Schwartz, M. B., & Brownell, K. D. (in press) Soft drinks, nutrition, and health. American Journal of Public Health.

Wansink, B. (2004). Environmental factors that influence the food intake and consumption volume of unknowing consumers. *Annual Review of Nutrition, 24,* 455–479.

Willett, W. C. (2002). *Eat, drink, and be healthy: The Harvard Medical School guide to healthy eating.* New York: Free Press.

Yamamiya, Y., Cash, T. F., Melnyk, S. E., Posavac, H. D., & Posavac, S. S. (2005). Women's exposure to thin-and-beautiful media images: Body image effects of media-ideal internalization and impact-reduction interventions. *Body Image, 2,* 74–80.

15

Self-Help for Night
Eating Syndrome

KELLY C. ALLISON
and ALBERT J. STUNKARD

DEFINITION OF NIGHT EATING SYNDROME

The night eating syndrome (NES) was first described in 1955 as a disorder of morning anorexia, evening hyperphagia, and insomnia, usually accompanied by a depressed mood and stressful life circumstances (Stunkard, Grace, & Wolff, 1955). In 1999, Birketvedt and colleagues (1999) reported awakenings with ingestions (*nocturnal ingestions*), which were added to the diagnostic criteria. There have been several definitions of NES (for a review, see de Zwaan, Burgard, Schenck, & Mitchell, 2003), and they have varied in their requirements for the amount of food ingested in the evening and nighttime and in the frequency of nocturnal ingestions. NES can be conceptualized as a delay in the circadian pattern of food intake such that food intake begins later in the day, with overeating in the evening and/or awakenings during the night to eat. O'Reardon and colleagues (O'Reardon, Ringel et al., 2004) reported that, although food intake is clearly delayed among night eaters, sleep onset and offset are not. Evidently, the rhythms of eating and sleeping are dissociated. Although the circadian sleep rhythm is intact, sleep is disturbed by awakenings to eat.

Additional criteria for NES can be derived from the study by O'Reardon, Ringel, et al. (2004). Patients initially reported that they consumed at least half of their intake after the evening meal. However, 7-day food intake diaries revealed that their caloric intake after dinner averaged 35% (*SD* = 10) compared with 10% (*SD* = 7) by control participants. An intake of two standard deviations above the control group mean would be 24%, therefore the consumption of at least 25% of the total daily caloric intake after the evening meal would appear to be an unusually large amount. O'Reardon, Ringel, et al. (2004) also reported that NES participants awoke 1.5 times per night and ate on 74% of those occasions. Accordingly, we propose the following criteria for NES: (1) the consumption of at least 25% of the total daily intake after the evening meal and/ or (2) three or more nocturnal ingestions per week. Morning anorexia is an associated, but not necessary, feature of NES, as it was not predictive of NES diagnosis in an item response theory analysis (IRT; Engel, 2005). Work is currently continuing to construct a valid and useful set of diagnostic criteria.

PREVALENCE OF NES

Prevalence of NES ranges from 1.5% in the general population (Rand, Macgregor & Stunkard, 1997) to between 9 and 14% in obesity clinics (Gluck, Geleibter, & Satov, 2001; Stunkard et al., 1996), and from 9% (Allison et al., 2006) to 42% (Hsu, Betancourt, & Sullivan, 1996) among bariatric surgery patients. NES is associated with depressed mood (Allison, Grilo, Masheb, & Stunkard, 2005; Gluck et al., 2001) and elevated lifetime incidence of DSM-IV-TR (American Psychiatric Association, 2000) Axis I disorders, such as mood, anxiety, and substance use disorders (Stunkard & Allison, 2003; Lundgren et al., 2006). In psychiatric outpatient clinics, 12.3% met criteria for NES (Lundgren, et al., 2006). Normal-weight persons also suffer from NES, and their symptoms appear similar to those of obese night eaters (Marshall, Allison, O'Reardon, Birketvedt, & Stunkard, 2004). Normal-weight night eaters in this study were significantly younger than their obese counterparts, and half of the obese night eaters reported that their night eating preceded their obesity, suggesting that NES may contribute to excess weight.

Unlike anorexia nervosa and bulimia nervosa, NES occurs in approximately equal proportions of men and women and of white (non-Hispanic) and black persons. In three recent prevalence studies, the breakdown of NES among males and females and white and black participants did not differ from the distribution of these demographics in the general samples (Allison, Crow, et al., 2004; Allison et al., 2005; Lundgren et al., 2006). A study of night-eating behaviors among persons with binge-eating disorder was the only one to report that nocturnal ingestions were more common among men (Grilo & Masheb, 2004). Little is known about the occurrence of NES among other racial or ethnic groups.

TREATMENT OF NES

The appearance of this volume could not be timelier. Growing numbers of persons are realizing that they suffer from this disorder and are embarrassed and ashamed by their eating behaviors. During the past 3 years, for example, more than 2,000 persons have approached our website or e-mail address asking for help with night eating. Few health care providers know much about NES, and fewer still know how to treat it. As a result, only a small minority of patients receive adequate, if any, treatment. For these reasons, providing information about self-help for NES has the potential to help many silent sufferers. The time is ripe for a major self-help effort. This effort can be advanced by the recently published self-help manual *Overcoming Night Eating Syndrome: A Step-by-Step Guide to Breaking the Cycle* (Allison, Stunkard, & Thier, 2004).

We first discuss the development of cognitive-behavioral therapy (CBT) for NES, which is the basis for the self-help manual. We then describe the self-help approaches as detailed in the manual. Finally, we describe the significant advances in pharmacotherapy of NES, which may help persons who cannot benefit from psychological approaches.

Psychological Treatment

Case studies of psychological treatments of NES patients have shown mixed results. Only one placebo-controlled trial has been carried out (Pawlow, O'Neil, & Malcolm, 2003) which compared progressive muscle relaxation (PMR) with a control condition in which participants sat quietly for the same duration of time. Pawlow and colleagues (2003) showed that a 1-week period of PMR decreased evening appetite and increased morning appetite, with nonsignificant decreases in nighttime food intake.

CBT has effectively treated disorders associated with NES, such as insomnia (Morin, 2002) and depression (DeRubeis et al., 2005). Its effectiveness in the treatment of binge-eating disorder and bulimia nervosa is described in Chapters 4 and 5 of this volume, respectively. It has also been the foundation for the only self-help resource for NES (Allison, Stunkard, & Thier, 2004).

An initial step in developing a CBT treatment for NES involved asking patients to record thoughts in diaries before and after they ate at night (examples are shown in Figure 15.1). Based on these experiences, we identified four main themes associated with these nocturnal ingestions. The most common themes were: (1) experiencing a craving for a specific food, (2) feeling anxious or agitated, (3) needing to eat to fall back to sleep, and (4) feeling physically hungry or compelled to eat (without a craving for a specific food). Examples of these themes are found in Table 15.1. Other, less common themes were feeling stressed, depressed, or bored. Most partici-

Time	Thoughts Before Eating/ Emotion or Feeling	Food/Beverage Consumed	Amount/ Quantity	Calories	Thoughts after Eating
8:30 pm	Anxious—I'm worried about going to family picnic tomorrow.	Chocolate chip cookies	4	240	That tasted good, but was too many calories! Still anxious.
10:00 pm	I should eat something before I go to bed.	Brownies	2	440	I'm sleepy, but now I'm too full. I'll have indigestion.
1:10 am	I am not hungry—just sleepy. This food will put me back to sleep.	Peanut Butter & crackers	4 tbs. 10	420 80	I am too full again. I will end up gaining weight! This is ridiculous.
3:30 am	I can't believe I'm up again. This will put me back to sleep quickly.	Shredded Wheat & 2% milk	2 cups 3/4 cup	270 90	I feel sick from eating too much. I'll regret this tomorrow.

FIGURE 15.1. Sample thought and food record for night eating syndrome.

TABLE 15.1. Examples of Four Common Themes of Thoughts Recorded before and after Night Eating Episodes

Theme	Thoughts before eating	Thoughts after eating
Compelled evening hyperphagia	"Oh, no! Why do I need this?! The urge is strong to eat something filling."	"I feel bad and angry with myself for eating."
Anxious/agitated	"I woke up from a bad dream. I am feeling upset and uptight, and hungry, too."	"I am more calm and relaxed and not hungry, but angry at myself for not having control over my hunger and feeling a little depressed."
Cravings	"I bolted out of bed with a radar (that's what it feels like—I remembered where there was chocolate without having to travel far). This is gross. I knew I threw out a box of chocolate truffles because I don't like them. I rifled through the trash . . . found the box and ate two."	"I feel ridiculous—I just want to stop doing this."
Need to eat to sleep	"I just wish I could go to sleep like a normal person. It's either eat so I can go back to sleep or just get up for the day."	"God, let me go to sleep." (In the morning): "Feel sick to my stomach and frustrated. I feel like I have no control over what is happening."

pants reported that they were able to resume sleep quickly after eating, and the impression was validated by all-night *polysomnography*, or sleep study. The average time between awakening and returning to EEG-validated sleep averaged 22.5 (SD= 24.7) minutes (O'Reardon et al., 2003).

The themes were incorporated into an assessment tool, the Night Eating Assessment (Figure 15.2), that patients complete just before each late evening and nocturnal eating episode during the initial phase of treatment. These visual analog scales help sufferers to identify whether or not they are physically hungry; whether they are experiencing negative moods, such as sadness, anxiety, or physical agitation; and whether they are craving a specific food or are just feeling generally compelled to eat something. This exercise raises awareness about the nature of the night-eating episodes, and it helps to identify possible antecedents by linking these feelings with their thoughts or with negative situations during the day.

In addition to identifying the stressors and thoughts that precipitate unwanted eating, the circadian pattern of food intake is explored in detail

Please mark an **X** on the line where appropriate for how much
you are experiencing each feeling before you eat at night.

Day_____   Time_____

Hungry
not at all ———————————————— extremely
Craving food
not at all ———————————————— extremely
Anxious
not at all ———————————————— extremely
Agitated
not at all ———————————————— extremely
Sad
not at all ———————————————— extremely
Bored
not at all ———————————————— extremely
Tired
not at all ———————————————— extremely
Compelled to eat
not at all ———————————————— extremely

FIGURE 15.2. Nighttime eating assessment

during the initial stage (sessions 1–4) of treatment. Patients are encouraged to confine their eating to scheduled meals and snacks during the waking hours and to keep a detailed food diary. The rationale for this eating schedule is explained as an attempt to retrain the patient's body to expect food at regular intervals during the day and not to expect food during the night. Anxiety is often associated with increasing food intake earlier in the day for fear of causing more weight gain. It is explained that eating earlier in the day is not sufficient to eliminate the nighttime eating, but it is necessary to regulate eating patterns, which are often chaotic among night eaters. Furthermore, consuming an adequate amount of calories throughout the day can be a counterargument to automatic thoughts during the night that compel the night eater to engage in nocturnal ingestions (e.g., "I didn't eat very much today, so it is okay to eat that piece of chocolate cake that is calling my name. I won't be able to sleep knowing that cake is there. I just have to go eat it").

Experimentation with behavioral techniques begins with nocturnal awakenings and ingestions and includes paying attention to the energy and nutrient content of the snacks and an official time chosen for the kitchen to be "closed." A behavioral chain that describes their typical patterns of nighttime eating should be completed and given to the patients for reference at home (Figure 15.3). In addition to recording the content and timing of food intake, overweight and obese patients start to keep records of caloric intake in session 3, with the help of a calorie counter (e.g., *The Doctor's Pocket Calorie, Fat & Carbohydrate Counter*;

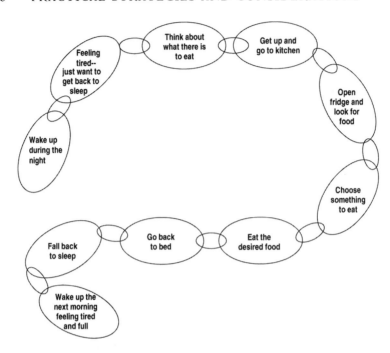

FIGURE 15.3. Behavioral chain for night eating syndrome.

Borushek, 2004). If patients have a weight-loss goal, they are encouraged to limit calories to 1,200 to 1,500 calories for women and 1,500 to 1,800 calories for men. No specific diet or macronutrient content is recommended. Clinical experience suggests that implementing a calorie goal improves motivation for change and compliance with therapy among overweight and obese night eaters.

Treatment for BED formerly had not restricted food intake based on the theory that such restriction encouraged binge eating. Both the National Task Force on the Prevention and Treatment of Obesity (2000) and Wadden et al. (2004) have reported that there is sufficient evidence to indicate that dieting does not cause binge-eating problems among overweight adults. Likewise, there is no evidence that would link caloric restriction to the occurrence of evening hyperphagia or nocturnal eating episodes. Accordingly, caloric restriction is included in our treatment of overweight and obese night eaters.

The middle stage of therapy (sessions 4–8) builds on the awareness the patients have gained about their night eating and the improved regulation of their daily eating schedule and seeks to build on coping skills and interventions for eliminating night eating behaviors. In this stage, deep breathing and relaxation scripts are introduced and practiced by the patients as a means of reducing their anxiety and distracting themselves from their compulsion to eat. Sleep hygiene, including establishing a regular bedtime and turning off the television before falling asleep, and physical activity are also addressed. Overall reinforcement of stimulus control of food and recording automatic thoughts continue to be important themes.

The final stage of therapy includes sessions 9 and 10, which occur biweekly, and addresses the typical concepts of "lapse" versus "relapse" and provides a general review of skills that have proven most helpful for the patients. Booster sessions at 4, 8 and 12 months are also encouraged.

This 10-session individual treatment was tested in a pilot study of 16 persons with NES (Allison, Martino, O'Reardon, & Stunkard, 2005). Last-observation-carried-forward analyses revealed significant reductions in the four major outcome measures at treatment end, including the Night Eating Symptom Scale (NESS; O'Reardon, Stunkard, & Allison, 2004;30.1 to 19.8, $p < .001$), percent of caloric intake after dinner (32.4 to 24.4%, $p < .01$), number of awakenings (11.7 to 8.3, $p < .01$), and number of nocturnal ingestions (8.6 to 3.9, $p < .001$). Completers ($n = 9$) showed more dramatic improvements, decreasing their nocturnal ingestions from 6.4 to 0.3 per week ($p < .01$) and reducing the percentage of calories consumed after dinner from 33.7 to 18.7% ($p < .05$). Completers also lost a significant amount of weight, from 84.4 ($SD = 23.5$) kg at baseline to 81.5 ($SD = 22.0$) kg at session 10 ($p < .01$). Dropouts ($n = 7$) did not differ significantly from completers on baseline night eating and demographic measures, but they were 10 years younger, on average, and closer to normal weight. A controlled trial of CBT for NES is needed with longer term follow-up to investigate its efficacy further.

Self-Help for Night Eating Syndrome

The self-help strategies presented here are based on the CBT treatment explained here and in the self-help book (Allison, Stunkard, & Thier, 2004). The two main goals are to reduce excessive snacking after the evening meal and to eliminate nocturnal ingestions, on the theory that this would, in turn, decrease nocturnal awakenings. The impact on those who have met these goals is notable. One night eater said:

> I can't even begin to tell you the difference just three nights of good sleep has made on me! I'm 24 and already feel like a 24-year-old should! Clear thoughts . . . no morning anxiety, and even a somewhat more centered mind! My workout at the gym has improved because I am not fatigued the entire time. This answers so much for me. Forever this has been a vicious cycle—not knowing if anxiety was causing me to wake or the lack of sleep was causing the anxiety! (Personal communication, Robert Nolan, June 1, 2004).

Regulating Daytime Eating Patterns and Preventing Nighttime Eating

Persons with NES often do not eat meals and snacks at regular intervals during the day. This usually occurs for two reasons: first, many night eaters have little appetite during the first half of the day; and second, some actively try to restrict their daytime intake to conserve their calories for their inevitable nighttime snacks. The theory that there is a delay in the circadian, or daily, pattern of eating suggests the need for a concerted effort to retrain the body to expect regular food intake during the day and to teach it *not* to expect food during the night.

The first attempt at regulating food intake is to keep a comprehensive food and sleep diary, which includes all eating episodes, day and night, and notation of bedtimes, nocturnal awakenings, and morning rising times. Once a baseline is established, a goal should be set to eat breakfast, lunch, an afternoon snack, dinner, and a modest evening snack. A reasonable time should be set to declare the kitchen closed, considering dinner time and cleanup time after the evening meal. This declaration may be symbolic, but it is often useful. Additional behavioral techniques are often helpful, such as putting up a physical barrier to the kitchen (e.g., painter's tape, which can be removed easily from walls and doors in the morning) or locks on cabinets and the refrigerator. Extra barriers such as these are often needed initially to help the night eater to resist eating and to ask the following questions during the night: (1) "What is the worst thing that will happen to me if I do not eat something right now?" and (2) "How great do I feel when I awake and have not eaten, and how awful do I feel when I do eat?"

Stimulus control, a basic tenet in behavioral weight-loss programs, plays an important part in this treatment. For example, seeing a bag of cookies (the stimulus) before bedtime may make a nighttime snack more probable. By not buying those cookies or by putting them out of sight and out of reach, this snack becomes less probable. Completing a night eating behavioral chain (Figure 15.3) helps to identify the best targets for intervention. Food in the kitchen must be made less accessible, and it must be cleared from bedrooms and the family room or other rooms where night eaters spend their late evening time. Some night eaters keep a small refrigerator in their bedrooms to shorten the amount of time they are awake and minimize the effort expended during nocturnal ingestions. Although this may help to increase total sleep time, it reinforces the drive to awaken and eat. For some night eaters, just knowing there is food in the room increases the number of times they awaken during the night. This makes it harder to resist temptation than if they were forced to get up and eat in a more remote location. After banishing all food from the bedroom, patients have reported that their compulsion to eat lessens and that they awaken less frequently. As reported in the aforementioned CBT study, nocturnal ingestions were particularly well managed with this method, decreasing them from once a night to less than once a week in the group that completed treatment.

We ask night eaters to experiment with their usual chain of behaviors. For example, if they usually get out of bed as soon as they wake up, we ask that they make themselves wait at least 5 minutes. At the end of those 5 minutes, they should reassess that craving. If it has lessened, they should ask themselves if they can wait another 5 minutes. We tell them that only they will know if the cravings are so intolerable that they absolutely must get up to eat. If their cravings overwhelm them, we focus their attention on another part of the chain by trying to limit the size of their snacks.

Eliminating all nocturnal ingestions abruptly is very difficult. Accordingly, cutting portion sizes and choosing low-calorie options are ways to begin to reduce this behavior. This strategy may include preplanning a healthy, calorie-controlled nocturnal snack. Tempting, high-calorie foods should not be left near this preplanned snack so as to help the individual resist eating more than the predetermined amount. Efforts should be made to slowly decrease the amount of food eaten. Successfully eating a smaller amount has the potential to increase feelings of self-efficacy and accomplishment. Keeping water at the bedside is also helpful. It may reduce the drive for some people sufficiently to help them stay in bed and resume sleep.

Raising Awareness of Automatic Thoughts and Feelings

To complement these behavioral measures, it is important to raise awareness of the feelings and the content of the automatic thoughts. The Night Eating Assessment (Figure 15.2) is a quick way to assess what the person is experiencing internally. This is especially helpful in determining whether someone is feeling physically hungry or is eating to decrease anxiety or negative affect.

Recording automatic thoughts before and after eating during the night is another helpful measure. When we asked our patients to write down what they were thinking, many responded that they did not think much about their nighttime eating. They reported that they ate in an automatic manner with very little control. We believe that they were probably not completely aware of their decision processes at that time of night. This belief, that their thoughts are automatic, can be challenged by having them consider the following: If their food choices during their night eating episodes were so automatic, why did they not reach for carrots or apples as often as they reached for cookies or peanut butter? Furthermore, when they began to stop and actually monitor their thoughts, they often remembered many different statements that they were telling themselves, and many of them were personally demeaning (see Table 15.1). Once awareness is raised about the circumstances of night eating episodes (including the environmental, psychological, and physiological cues), then it is important to address alternatives to eating.

Alternatives to Eating

Once night eaters have decided to stay in bed or have eaten a reduced portion and are unable to fall asleep as quickly as usual, what should they do? Activities that cause physiological arousal, such as cleaning the house, paying bills, or other household tasks, should be avoided. They must find an alternative to eating that would encourage sleep onset.

The stress-related component of NES often causes anxiety and tension in the evening when night eaters are trying to fall asleep initially or in the middle of the night. People have many different ways to unwind after a stressful day. However, most do not have the time or make the time to do what works best for them. This may include taking a bubble bath, reading a book, talking with a friend who makes them laugh, or spending some romantic time with a partner or spouse.

Deep breathing and PMR exercises are particularly effective for a few reasons. First, implementing them is not dependent on anyone else's schedule or help. Second, they do not require elaborate equipment or much space. Third, they do not disturb other people in the household, even at night. Many scripts are available to teach deep breathing and PMR. It is important to practice them consistently. Night eaters must remember to use these approaches so that they can be easily implemented, even in the middle of the night.

Sleep Hygiene and Physical Activity

Because persons with NES often have some form of insomnia and problems with weight gain, it is important to implement good sleep hygiene and adequate physical activity. Sleep hygiene is important in the treatment of insomnia. Some of the salient factors include limiting caffeine, cigarettes, and alcohol. Night eaters may be relying on caffeinated drinks and the nicotine in cigarettes to help overcome the sleep debt they have acquired from waking to eat. However, using these substances may perpetuate the cycle of difficulty in falling asleep initially or waking in the middle of the night. For this reason, caffeine and cigarettes should be avoided, particularly during the afternoon, evening, and nighttime hours. Alcohol consumption also influences sleep. Falling asleep initially may be facilitated by having a few drinks in the late evening, but the quality of sleep suffers, and awakenings during the night occur more frequently. Therefore, drinking before bedtime should be discouraged.

Another aspect of sleep hygiene is having regular bedtime and waking hours. This way the body adjusts to a routine set of times. Television should not be kept on during sleep, as its brightness and volume vary, potentially awakening the person. These awakenings may be brief for persons without NES, but night eaters should avoid any stimuli for waking. A white-noise machine or fan may be a good substitute for those who prefer a constant noise in the background while falling asleep.

Engaging in physical activity is important for two reasons. First, most night eaters are concerned about the weight gain associated with the extra calories they consume at night. Exercising, including increasing lifestyle activities such as walking, climbing stairs, and heavy housework, can aid in weight loss or weight maintenance. Second, an adequate level of physical activity during the day helps to promote sleepiness at night. Being physically tired at the end of the day can improve the quality and duration of sleep.

Social Support

Finally, it is often helpful to have social support from family, friends, or housemates. They may help to make food less accessible during the night, keep the combination or keys to locks on food, and remind the night eaters of their goals. Aside from these instrumental roles, listening and supporting the sufferers as they attempt to regulate their eating is also important in helping them to overcome their NES.

Pharmacotherapy

Self-help and individual psychotherapy may leave individuals still suffering from some elements of NES. For these persons, pharmacotherapy may be useful. In fact, more is known about pharmacotherapy approaches to NES than about self-help approaches.

Most NES treatment studies have relied heavily on selective serotonin reuptake inhibitors (SSRIs). A case series reported that all four NES patients responded to the SSRI paroxetine (Miyaoka, Yasukawa, Tsubouchi, et al., 2003). Additionally, an open-label treatment study used sertraline with 17 patients (O'Reardon, Stunkard, & Allison, 2004). This 12-week trial was also successful, showing significant decreases in the NESS, percentage of calories consumed after dinner, and the number of awakenings and nocturnal ingestions (O'Reardon, Stunkard, & Allison, 2004).

A double-blind placebo-controlled trial of sertraline with 34 patients was also successful (O'Reardon et al., 2006). Seventy-one percent of all participants were classified as "responders," according to the Clinical Global Impression of Improvement Scale (CGI-I ≤ 2), and 41% as "remitters" (CGI-I = 1) (also included in the responder category). Only 18% in the placebo group reached responder status. Overall, significant reductions were achieved in the sertraline group versus the placebo group. Scores on the NESS fell by 57% (31.7 to 13.6) in the sertraline group versus a 16% reduction (30.5 to 20.5) in the placebo group ($p < .0001$); awakenings fell by 74% (8.8 to 2.3 per week) in the sertraline group versus only 14% (6.8 to 5.6; $p < .01$) in the placebo group; and nocturnal ingestions were reduced by 81% (8.3 to 1.6 per week) in the sertraline group versus only 14% (6.4 to 5.5, $p = .03$) in the placebo group. Percentage of caloric intake after the evening meal was reduced by 68% in the sertraline group versus 29% in the placebo group. Participants with a body mass index (BMI) over 25 kg/m² lost –2.9 ($SD = 3.8$) kg on sertraline versus –0.3 ($SD = 2.7$) kg on placebo ($p = .013$).

Long-Distance Community Study of Sertraline

Many sufferers of NES have contacted our program to ask for advice about their NES. Persons interested in treatment for NES who had contacted us through our website or by e-mail or telephone underwent a semistructured interview, the Night Eating Syndrome History and Inventory (Allison, O'Reardon, & Stunkard, 2001), by phone to confirm a diagnosis of NES. After giving informed consent, patients approached their personal physicians regarding treatment, and we offered the physicians consultation. Participants' doctors were then sent information regarding treatment of NES with sertraline. Fifty participants were treated by their own physicians and completed the questionnaires to assess their progress every 2 weeks for an 8-week trial. Dosage averaged 122 mg per day at the end of 8 weeks (Stunkard, Allison, Lundgren, Martino, Heo, et al,, 2006).

Results of this long-distance study were comparable to those of our face-to-face studies (O'Reardon et al., 2006; O'Reardon, Stunkard, & Allison, 2004). Significant improvement was shown on the NESS (60%), in percentage of caloric intake after dinner (67%), in number of awakenings (64%), and in number of nocturnal ingestions (70%; all $p < .001$). Weight of the 41 overweight and obese participants decreased by 2.9 kg ($p < .01$). Depressed mood decreased and quality of life increased significantly. These findings suggest that NES sufferers in the community may be able to receive successful treatment for their NES with sertraline. Combining pharmacotherapy with the psychotherapeutic and self-help approaches discussed here may improve the results over those obtained by each method alone, although more research is needed to address the additive effects of these approaches.

CONCLUSIONS AND FUTURE DIRECTIONS

More research is needed to develop the psychotherapeutic approaches described in this chapter and to compare them with treatments such as supportive therapy, interpersonal therapy, and behavioral weight-loss programs. These developments should lead to more effective self-help programs, and these programs should be widely disseminated. Self-help efforts using the Internet would be ideal for such dissemination and for assessment of their effectiveness and cost-effectiveness. There appears to be an opportunity to combine self-help behavioral measures with the medications of established effectiveness, much as is being undertaken in the treatment of obesity.

REFERENCES

Allison, K., Crow, S., Stunkard, A., & Eating Disorders Look AHEAD Study Group. (2004). The prevalence of binge eating disorder and night eating syndrome in adults with type 2 diabetes mellitus. *Obesity Research, 12,* A89.

Allison, K., Martino, N., O'Reardon, J., & Stunkard, A. (2005). CBT treatment for night eating syndrome: A pilot study. *Obesity Research, 13,* A83.

Allison, K. C., Grilo, C. M., Masheb, R. M., & Stunkard, A. J. (2005). Binge eating disorder and night eating syndrome: A comparative study of disordered eating. *Journal of Consulting and Clinical Psychology, 73,* 1107–1115.

Allison, K. C., O'Reardon, J. P., & Stunkard, A. J. (2001). *Night Eating Syndrome History and Inventory.* Unpublished interview.

Allison, K. C., Stunkard, A. J., & Thier, S. L. (2004). *Overcoming night eating syndrome: A step-by-step guide to breaking the cycle.* Oakland, CA: New Harbinger.

Allison, K. C., Wadden, T. A., Sarwer, D. B., Fabricatore, A. N., Crerand, C. E., Gibbons, L. M., et al. (2006). Night eating syndrome and binge eating disorder among persons seeking bariatric surgery: Prevalence and related features. *Obesity Research, 14*(Suppl. 2), 77S–82S.

American Psychiatric Association. (2000). *Diagnostic and statistical manual of mental disorders* (4th ed., text rev.). Washington, DC: Author.

Birketvedt, G., Florholmen, J., Sundsfjord, J., Osterud, B., Dinges, D., Bilker, W., et al. (1999). Behavioral and neuroendocrine characteristics of the night-eating syndrome. *Journal of the American Medical Association, 282,* 657–663.

Borushek, A. (2004). *The doctor's pocket calorie, fat & carbohydrate counter.* Costa Mesa, CA: Family Health Publications.

DeRubeis, R. J., Hollon, S. D., Amsterdam, J. D., Shelton, R. C., Young, P. R., Salomon, R. M., et al. (2005). Cognitive therapy vs. medications in the treatment of moderate to severe depression. *Archives of General Psychiatry, 62,* 409–416.

de Zwaan, M., Burgard, M. A., Schenck, C. H., & Mitchell, J. E. (2003). Night time eating: A review of the literature. *European Eating Disorders Review, 11,* 7–24.

Engel, S. (2005, September 30). *Night Eating Syndrome.* Symposium conducted at the annual meeting of the Eating Disorders Research Society, Toronto, Ontario, Canada.

Gluck, M. E., Geliebter, A., & Satov, T. (2001). Night eating syndrome is associated with depression, low self-esteem, reduced daytime hunger and less weight loss in obese outpatients. *Obesity Research, 9,* 264–267.

Grilo, C. M., & Masheb, R. M. (2004). Night-time eating in men and women with binge eating disorder. *Behaviour Research and Therapy, 42*, 397–407.

Hsu, L. K. G., Betancourt, S., & Sullivan, S. P. (1996). Eating disturbances before and after vertical banded gastroplasty: A pilot study. *International Journal of Eating Disorders, 19*, 23–34.

Lundgren, J. D., Allison, K. C., Crow, S., O'Reardon, J. P., Berg, K. C., Galbraith, J., et al. (2006). Prevalence of the night eating syndrome in a psychiatric population. *American Journal of Psychiatry, 163*, 156–158.

Marshall, H. M., Allison, K. C., O'Reardon, J. P., Birketvedt, G. S., & Stunkard, A. J. (2004). Night eating syndrome among nonobese persons. *International Journal of Eating Disorders, 35*, 217–222.

Miyaoka, T., Yasukawa, R., Tsubouchi, K., Miura, S., Shimizu, Y., Sukegawa, T., et al. (2003). Successful treatment of nocturnal eating/drinking syndrome with selective serotonin reuptake inhibitors. *International Clinical Psychopharmacology, 18*, 175–177.

Morin, C. (2002). Contributions of Cognitive-behavioral approaches to the clinical managment of insomnia. *Primary Care Companion Journal of Clinical Psychiatry, 4*(1), 21–26.

National Task Force on the Prevention and Treatment of Obesity. (2000). Dieting and the development of eating disorders in overweight and obese adults. *Archives of Internal Medicine, 160*, 2581–2589.

O'Reardon, J. P., Allison, K. C., Fox, C. G., Martino, N. S., Dinges, D. F., & Stunkard, A. J. (2003). Comparison of in-lab polysomnography in night eating syndrome and overweight controls. *Sleep, 26*(Suppl.), A378.

O'Reardon, J. P., Allison, K. C., Martino, N. S., Lundgren, J. D., Heo, M., & Stunkard, A. J. (2006). A randomized placebo-controlled trial of sertraline in the treatment of the night eating syndrome. *American Journal of Psychiatry, 163*, 893–898.

O'Reardon, J. P., Ringel, B. L., Dinges, D. F., Allison, K. C., Rogers, N. S., Martino, N. S., et al. (2004). Circadian eating and sleeping patterns in the night eating syndrome. *Obesity Research, 12*, 1789–1796.

O'Reardon, J. P., Stunkard, A. J., & Allison, K. C. (2004). A clinical trial of sertraline in the treatment of the night eating syndrome. *International Journal of Eating Disorders, 35*, 16–26.

Pawlow, L. A., O'Neil, P. M., & Malcolm, R. J. (2003). Night eating syndrome: Effects of brief relaxation training on stress, mood, hunger, and eating patterns. *International Journal of Obesity, 27*, 970–978.

Rand, C. S. W., Macgregor, M. D., & Stunkard, A. J. (1997). The night eating syndrome in the general population and among post-operative obesity surgery patients. *International Journal of Eating Disorders, 22*, 65–69.

Stunkard, A. J., & Allison, K. C. (2003). Two forms of disordered eating in obesity: Binge eating and night eating. *International Journal of Obesity, 27*, 1–12.

Stunkard, A. J., Allison, K. C., Lundgren, J. D., Martino, N. S., Heo, M., Etemad, B., et al. (2006). A paradigm for facilitating pharmacotherapy at a distance: Sertraline treatment of the night eating syndrome. *Journal of Clinical Psychiatry, 67*, 1568–1572.

Stunkard, A. J., Berkowitz, R., Wadden, T., Tanrikut, C., Reiss, E., & Young, L. (1996). Binge eating disorder and the night eating syndrome. *International Journal of Obesity and Related Metabolic Disorders, 20*, 1–6.

Stunkard, A. J., Grace, W. J., & Wolff, H. G. (1955). The night-eating syndrome: A pattern of food intake among certain obese patients. *American Journal of Medicine, 19*, 78–86.

Wadden, T. A., Foster, G. D., Sarwer, D. B., Anderson, D. A., Gladis, M., Sanderson, R. S., et al. (2004). Dieting and the development of eating disorders in obese women: Results of a randomized controlled trial. *American Journal of Clinical Nutrition, 80*, 560–568.

16

Appetite-Focused Cognitive-Behavioral Therapy for Binge Eating

VIRGINIA V. W. MCINTOSH, JENNIFER JORDAN,
JANET D. CARTER, JANET D. LATNER,
and ALISON WALLACE

Bulimia nervosa and binge-eating disorder are characterized by recurrent binge-eating episodes during which the individual feels out of control while consuming abnormally large quantities of food. Cognitive-behavioral therapy (CBT) is well established as an effective treatment for binge eating in bulimia nervosa and binge-eating disorder (National Institute for Health and Clinical Excellence, 2004). However, for some individuals, binge eating continues despite treatment with CBT; other individuals cease binge eating with treatment but relapse at some later time (Quadflieg & Fichter, 2003; Wonderlich, de Zwaan, Mitchell, Peterson, & Crow, 2003). Appetite-focused CBT (CBT-A) is a modification of standard CBT for bulimia nervosa and binge eating that aims to improve the efficacy of standard CBT. CBT-A has a primary focus on the role of appetite in problems with binge eating. Appetite comprises both hunger and fullness. In normal eating, hunger prompts the initiation of eating, and fullness is the signal for stopping eating. For individuals who binge, one or both of the normal appetite mechanisms may be disturbed.

Many individuals who binge alternate between dietary restraint and overeating. These individuals have been well represented in models of binge eating, in which dieting is viewed as central to the development and maintenance of binge eating. Strict dieting leads to intense hunger, which, because dieting frequently involves overriding normal appetite cues, may go unnoticed. Alternatively, hunger may be recognized but ignored. Such individuals are at risk for binge eating once eating begins, partly because of the intensity of hunger cues. For other individuals who have less current dietary restraint and may have a general pattern of overeating, in addition to frank binge-eating episodes, hunger may make a smaller contribution to the maintenance of binge eating. For these individuals, past dieting and regular overeating contribute to impaired recognition of fullness. Reduced awareness of satiety results in continuing to eat beyond moderate levels of fullness.

Although it is not known whether the disturbances in appetite and satiety among individuals with frequent binge eating are a cause or a consequence of dysfunctional eating behavior (Walsh & Devlin, 1998), there is some evidence that addressing these appetitive disturbances can be therapeutic. Ventura and Bauer (1999) implemented an expanded version of CBT that focused on resynchronizing the appetite system. Participants were taught about the psychobiological mechanisms controlling appetite and were encouraged to recognize hunger and satiety and to experiment with different foods in order to maximize satiation. The expanded treatment led to lower rates of binge eating and purging than standard CBT at treatment termination and at 9- and 12-month follow-up. Another treatment designed to help the self-regulation of eating through heightened responsiveness to hunger and satiety cues has shown preliminary efficacy in reducing binge eating among women with binge-eating disorder and bulimia nervosa (Craighead & Allen, 1995; Dicker & Craighead, 2004). This treatment modified CBT by teaching participants to self-monitor hunger and fullness (rather than monitoring food and fluid intake) and to initiate eating in response to moderate hunger and stop eating in response to moderate fullness.

CBT-A aims to eliminate binge eating by retraining the individual to respond to internal appetite cues. This intervention includes responding to internal cues of hunger (to cue the initiation of eating) and fullness (to cue the cessation of eating). Learning to recognize and respond to *moderate* hunger and *moderate* fullness levels is a key goal of treatment.

The distinction between standard CBT for binge eating and CBT-A is that the primary emphasis of CBT-A is on the role of appetite and satiety in the onset and maintenance of binge eating and also its treatment. This includes a major and systematic focus on appetite in self-monitoring, education about satiety, and emphasis on selecting foods that promote satiety. All other aspects of standard CBT for binge eating and bulimia nervosa are included in CBT-A.

This chapter is an overview of CBT-A for binge eating and bulimia nervosa. The chapter first introduces the rationale for focusing on appetite in the treatment of binge eating. The experimental and applied research on the role of appetite in binge eating is reviewed. As CBT-A augments standard CBT, an overview of the components of standard CBT for bulimia nervosa and binge eating are briefly described. Specific appetite-focused strategies are also outlined. First, an appetite-focused model of the development and maintenance of binge eating is presented. Second, the self-monitoring of appetite—both hunger and fullness—is described. Third, the principles of choosing foods that promote satiety are reported—increasing food volume, increasing the proportion of protein, and choosing longer lasting carbohydrates. The adaptation of CBT-A to a self-help format is then discussed.

THE ROLE OF APPETITE IN BINGE EATING

Individuals who frequently binge have impaired satiety and hunger responses. The deficits may be partly due to physiological abnormalities in appetite functioning and partly due to a psychological or learned insensitivity to satiety signals. By definition, individuals with bulimia nervosa and binge-eating disorder consume abnormally large amounts of food, both during binge episodes and over a 24-hour period (Weltzin, Hsu, Pollice, & Kaye, 1991; Yanovski et al., 1992). This appears, at least in part, to be caused by disturbances in appetite signals. For example, compared with those without eating disorders, individuals with bulimia nervosa report little increase in fullness over the course of a meal (Halmi, Sunday, Puglisi, & Marchi, 1989), lower than normal fullness at the end of a meal (Geracioti & Liddle, 1988; Hadigan, Walsh, Devlin, LaChaussee, & Kissileff, 1992), and lower than normal decrease in the desire for a recently eaten food (Hetherington & Rolls, 1989). Individuals with bulimia nervosa and binge-eating disorder may also consume a lower than normal proportion of foods that are known to be satiating—binge episodes commonly consist of eating energy-dense dessert or snack foods (Rosen, Lietenberg, Fischer, & Khazam, 1986). Relative to those of control participants, the binge episodes (Walsh, Hadigan, Kissileff, & LaChaussee, 1992) and daily intake (Hetherington, Altemus, Nelson, Bernat, & Gold, 1994) of those with bulimia nervosa are lower in dietary protein. During binge episodes, individuals with binge-eating disorder consume more of their energy from fat and less from protein than weight-matched controls (Yanovski et al., 1992).

These disturbances may be linked to physiological abnormalities in neuropeptides that govern eating behavior (Jimerson & Wolfe, 2004). In individuals with bulimia nervosa, the postmeal release of the satiety-inducing gut peptide cholecystokynin is significantly blunted (Devlin et al., 1997; Geracioti & Liddle, 1988). Ghrelin, a peptide hormone that stimulates hunger and food intake, normally decreases drastically after eating; however, it remains abnormally high after meals in individuals with bulimia nervosa. On the other hand, the release of the satiety agent peptide YY is blunted after meals (Monteleone et al., 2005). In addition, those with bulimia nervosa have abnormally large gastric capacity (Geliebter et al., 1992). Obese individuals with concurrent binge-eating disorder have increased gastric capacity relative to obese individuals without binge-eating disorder (Geliebter & Hashim, 2001). A larger stomach capacity necessitates a larger volume of food in the stomach to suppress food intake (Geliebter, 1988). This abnormality may severely inhibit gastric distension, which is usually involved in the development of satiety following food intake.

There is also evidence that satiety-related abnormalities in binge eaters may be related to psychological phenomena. An investigation of *interoceptive awareness*, a subscale of the Eating Disorders Inventory (EDI; Garner, Olmsted, & Polivy, 1983) that measures the self-perceived ability to recognize and accurately identify emotions and sensations of hunger and satiety, showed disturbances in interoceptive awareness among individuals with bulimia nervosa compared with obese individuals without eating disorders (Fassino, Piero, Gramaglia, & Abbate-Daga, 2004). Impaired interoceptive awareness was related to low mood and to the personality dimensions of low self-directedness and high persistence on the Temperament and Character Inventory (Cloninger, Svrakic, & Przybeck, 1993), suggesting that both psychopathological and personality factors may influence the way that individuals with eating disorders perceive their emotions and sensations related to food (Fassino et al., 2004). In another study, individuals who scored high on the EDI Bulimia and Body Dissatisfaction subscales reported being less aware and less responsive to satiety cues, especially when they were also low on the ability to narrow their attentional focus (Heilbrun & Worobow, 1991).

The lack of awareness or neglect of internal cues of hunger and satiety may put people at risk for binge eating. Eating behavior and binge eating may instead come to be driven by external cues, such as the presence of highly palatable food (Lowe & Levine, 2005; McManus & Waller, 1995), or by internal cues not related to appetite, such as emotional and cognitive cues. Individuals with binge-eating disorder may be motivated by the sensory pleasures of the taste, smell, and texture of food during binges (Mitchell et al., 1999); those with bulimia nervosa may be more responsive to sweetness than are control participants (Drewnowski, Bellisle, Aimez, & Remy, 1987; Drewnowski, Halmi, Pierce, Gibbs, & Smith, 1987). Internal antecedents to binge eating include negative emotional states (Stickney, Miltenberger, & Wolff, 1999) that precede binge episodes in individuals with binge-eating disorder but not in weight-matched participants without binge-eating disorder (Greeno, Wing, & Shiffman, 2000). People with frequent binge eating may notice and respond to their hunger and fullness signals only once they have reached extreme states—either ravenous or overfull (Craighead & Allen, 1995).

COMPONENTS OF CBT-A FOR BINGE EATING

The appetite component of CBT-A is integrated into the standard cognitive-behavioral approach to facilitate normalization of eating. For further reading about standard CBT for bulimia nervosa and binge eating, refer to Fairburn and colleagues (Fairburn, Marcus, & Wilson, 1993; Fairburn, Cooper, & Shafran, 2003). This section reviews standard CBT strategies, which remain part of CBT-A.

A comprehensive assessment is conducted prior to the beginning of treatment, and the case formulation and intervention strategies utilized stem directly from cognitive and behavioral conceptualizations of binge eating. Therapy commences by introducing the cognitive-behavioral model of binge eating. Initially, a psychoeducational focus is taken, with information provided about the influence of sociocultural factors in the development and maintenance of eating disorders; the biological and genetic contributions to weight and body shape; the cycle and consequences of disordered eating, such as dieting and binge eating; and the role of compensatory behaviors, including purging and engaging in excessive exercise for the purpose of weight and shape control.

Information and advice are given about good nutrition and the principles of normal eating—eating *regularly*, eating from a *variety* of food groups, and eating *sufficient* amounts of food (Beumont & Touyz, 1995). Self-monitoring involves prospectively recording information about the amount and type of food eaten, episodes of overeating, subjective or objective binge eating, and the context or situation in which the eating occurs, along with the thoughts and feelings associated with binge eating. Self-monitoring food and fluid intake enables the identification of problem eating, examination of dietary intake, identification of cues for binge eating (including unhelpful cognitions and particular emotions), and tracking progress and changes in behavior. Based on the principles of *regularity*, *variety*, and eating *a sufficient quantity*, manageable goals are agreed on for normalizing eating.

Cognitive strategies focus on the dysfunctional thoughts the individual has about food, weight, shape, binging, purging, and other behaviors related to the eating disorder. Unhelpful automatic thoughts are monitored between sessions in order to identify, evaluate, and restructure these cognitions. Behavioral strategies, such as the use of behavioral experiments and graded exposure, are used along with cognitive strategies to facilitate change. Behavioral principles are used to understand the cues for and consequences of eating-disordered behaviors. Consideration is given to social, food-related, situational, physiological/nutritional, emotional, and thought cues and to the negative and positive consequences of problem eating-related behaviors. Individuals are encouraged to increase their repertoire of alternative activities that are incompatible with binge eating, to develop behaviors that help manage urges to binge between episodes of normal eating, and to increase their range of self-care activities, such as meeting emotional needs (affect regulation) in more appropriate ways than through binge eating. The therapist assists in identifying, understanding, and finally breaking the links between these cues and binge eating.

Practicing newly acquired techniques between therapy sessions and continuing with these after the completion of therapy is encouraged. Homework, maintenance, and relapse prevention are central to CBT. During the final sessions of CBT, discussions occur about managing eating and other issues that have been a focus of therapy once treatment has ended, identifying potential problems and generating possible solutions. Expectations about future eating and weight- and shape-related issues are explored, and unrealistic or unhelpful cognitions are challenged. Occasional setbacks are conceptualized as a normal part of recovery and to be expected. A written maintenance and relapse prevention plan is developed that incorporates important ongoing maintenance strategies, plans for coping with future problems, and ideas to prevent setbacks while also documenting strategies for lapses or relapses.

SPECIFIC APPETITE FOCUS WITHIN CBT

An Appetite-Focused Model

An appetite-focused model of bulimia nervosa and binge eating differs from other models of binge eating with appetite conceptualized as central to the diet–binge–purge cycle. The model in Figure 16.1 is based on Bulik's (1994) model but emphasizes the pivotal role of appetite in the development and maintenance of binge eating. This model can be helpful when used with patients, who can adapt the generic model to their own situation, adding their own personal experiences.

The model highlights risk factors that contribute to the onset of the eating problems. For any individual, a unique combination of family, sociocultural, and personal risk factors combine to begin the cycle. For most individuals with these eating disorders, dieting to lose weight is the entry to the diet–binge–purge cycle. Dieting inevitably requires that the individual ignore her or his body's messages to eat (hunger). Increased hunger or symptoms of starvation become cues for binge eating. Because binge eating involves consuming large quantities of food beyond the amount that feels comfortable, the body's normal mechanisms for signaling the cessation of eating are overridden. This has the effect of "turning down the volume" on appetite, which in turn further disinhibits eating. During vomiting, normal physiological deterrents are overridden. Vomiting is the body's "emergency" response to the presence of dangerous substances. Repeated or regular vomiting overrides the body's natural processes and in-

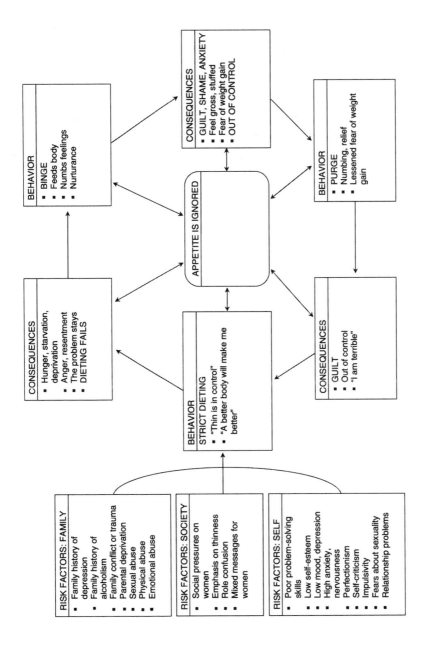

FIGURE 16.1. Appetite-focused CBT model of binge eating.

terferes with normal digestion and normal satiety signals. In turn, ignoring appetite has the effect of making dieting, binging, and purging less difficult. Appetite is like the hub of a wheel around which the diet–binge–purge cycle spins.

Self-Monitoring of Appetite

A major innovation in self-monitoring in CBT-A is the routine focus on monitoring appetite—both hunger and satiety—in addition to monitoring food and fluid intake, cues, thoughts, and feelings. One model of therapy for binge eating advocates self-monitoring appetite rather than daily food and fluid intake (Craighead & Allen, 1995). However, in CBT-A, both appetite and food and fluid intake are monitored. This enables discussion about quantities of food eaten so that the therapist can gradually retrain the awareness of hunger and fullness. The self-monitoring form (see Figure 16.2) includes a column for monitoring aspects of appetite, both hunger and satiety, alongside details of food and fluid intake. When first approaching the task of monitoring appetite, the individual may be unable to accurately read her or his body's appetite signals. By referring to the quantity of food eaten and time since previous eating, the therapist gradually retrains awareness of hunger and fullness.

The goal of monitoring appetite is to gradually resensitize the individual to feelings of hunger and fullness and to encourage eating in response to these appetite cues. Recognizing and responding to appetite cues involves retraining to start and stop eating in response to feelings of hunger and fullness rather than in response to other cues—environmental, cognitive, or affective. In particular, the focus is on learning to respond to *moderate* hunger cues and *moderate* satiety cues while relearning to eat regularly.

An assumption of CBT-A is that the individual has, at some time in the past, responded appropriately to appetite cues. A variety of factors may contribute to ignoring appetite cues. When an individual has attempted to restrict her or his food intake over a period of time, she or he is likely to have worked hard to ignore and override hunger cues and in so doing has trained her- or himself to ignore the body's messages of hunger. A useful metaphor is that, like the volume control on a radio or television, the individual has turned down the volume on hunger signals. CBT-A aims to retrain the individual to "turn up the volume" on hunger messages. For some individuals, binge eating has the effect of providing comfort, filling in time when they are at loose ends, or allowing them to avoid unpleasant tasks or activities. In these situations binging may have allowed the individual to temporarily ignore or disregard negative emotions. If binges have served the function of dulling negative affect, this may have worked like a "mute button" on a radio or television.

The person's first attempts at monitoring appetite are likely to be by

Self-Monitoring Record Form

Name: Joanna   Date: 22 December   Day: Thursday

Date/Time	Food & Fluid	B/P	Situation	Hunger/Fullness (before & after)	Thoughts	Feelings
7.30 am	1 cup black coffee		making lunches	H 6 F 0,2	I must not overeat today. I am so fat. I need to lose weight	strong
12.00	2 rice wafers, 2 t weight watchers cottage cheese		In lunchroom at work	2, 6 0, 3	I want to eat the chocolate muesli bars from the snack machine. I must be strong.	determined
4.00 pm	1 espresso coffee		At home with children doing homework	10 3 0, 2	The children's oatmeal cookies look delicious but I must not eat them.	stressed
5.00 pm	1 espresso coffee, 2 cherries		Cooking dinner. Answering phone. My mother asking about Xmas plans.	10 9 0, 1	I can't resist these.	weak, hassled
5.45	3 T satay sauce		Hearing children's reading	10 9 5, 3	I shouldn't eat this. It is so fattening.	weak, worn out
7.00pm	2 cherries, 1 litre water			10 9 5		
7.30 pm	2 pieces toast, 2 T butter, 3 T peanut butter	B	standing in kitchen	10 0	I am disgusting. This is gross. No wonder I am so fat. I am a pig	disgusted, guilty
7.45 pm	large pizza hut seafood pizza, 2 c french fries, 1 litre icecream			0 10		
8.00 pm		V		0, 0 10, 8		disgusted, weak, relief.

FIGURE 16.2. Self-monitoring record form.

333

retrospective recall with the therapist while reviewing self-monitoring during a therapy session: "How full is your body likely to have been after eating the pizza?" Hunger is rated at salient points throughout the day using a simple 0–10 scale, with 0 being "not at all hungry" and 10 being "the most hungry imaginable." This may include rating hunger before eating or drinking, at times when others are eating even if the individual is not, or at particular times that have been agreed on. An individual who tries very hard not to eat during the early part of the day may be encouraged to monitor her or his hunger at usual mealtimes, when others are eating, or when feeding her or his children.

Initially, the monitoring of hunger and fullness is likely to be hypothetical or cognitive. When reviewing self-monitoring, the therapist guides discussion about how hungry or full the body is *likely* to have been at the time of self-monitoring. This will include a consideration of how long it has been since last eating, how much was eaten at the last meal or snack, and how much has been eaten through the day. Using language that promotes the externalization of appetite can be useful at this first hypothetical or cognitive appraisal of likely hunger. Many individuals with bulimia nervosa and binge-eating disorder do not think of food as nourishing the body. Rather, not eating is viewed as a means of achieving a desired body shape or weight and, as such, is appraised positively. Speaking of "the body's hunger" rather than "how hungry you are feeling" or "how hungry you are" can circumvent the denial of hunger.

If speculating about one's own body's likely hunger level is very difficult, it may be useful for the person to think about how hungry a third person might be in this situation. Choosing someone whom the patient would want to adequately nourish will assist with the realistic appraisal of the other's hunger. Choosing someone as similar to the individual as possible helps this appraisal to be generalized to her or his own likely appetite. The therapist may also use him- or herself as the model if it is difficult to identify a known third person: "How hungry do you think my body would be if I had been up since 6.30 A.M., had gone for a long run, and had had a busy morning at work?" If speculating about others' hunger is very difficult, the therapist may make accurate and honest self-disclosures about his or her own appetite: "By midday, if I had skipped breakfast and had only sipped a cup of black coffee through the morning, I would have been extremely hungry. I would probably rate my hunger at 9 by lunch time."

For some individuals who have a pattern of undereating with infrequent binge-eating episodes, monitoring of appetite may begin with increasing awareness of hunger. For other individuals who binge or eat constantly and have little dietary restraint or restriction, more emphasis may need to be placed on awareness of fullness and the absence of hunger. Becoming aware of signs of fullness is also part of CBT-A. Fullness is rated using another 0–10 scale, with 0 being "not at all full" and 10 being "the most full imaginable."

It is important to note that "0" hunger gives no indication of fullness. A "0" hunger rating would be appropriate when one is either comfortably satisfied or uncomfortably overfull at the end of a binge. In both situations, hunger is not present and would be rated as "0"; however, ratings of fullness would be quite different. In the first situation, after eating a normal meal or snack, hunger is at 0, and fullness may be around 6. After a large binge, hunger is 0, but fullness may be 10.

Education and discussion about the various signs of hunger and fullness will also help facilitate awareness of appetite. As well as physical sensations, such as stomach emptiness and rumbling, noticing other signs of hunger is encouraged. These may include physical signs (increased salivation; cravings for particular foods; urges to binge; feeling tired, weak, dizzy, listless, apathetic, sleepy, unenergetic, slowed up, lightheaded, nauseated, cold, shaky, sped up; tingling extremities; headaches; visual disturbances; hypersensitivity to noise or light; poor motor control), emotional signs (feeling irritable, unmotivated, short-tempered, grumpy, anxious, argumentative, tearful, exhilarated, low, or down; mood swings), cognitive signs (preoccupation with thoughts of food or eating, increased negative thoughts) and behavioral signs (reading recipe books, looking at pictures of food in magazines, binging, drinking alcohol, drinking fluid, chewing gum, smoking).

Appetite-Focused Food Choices

So far we have considered the key CBT-A concept of retraining individuals to eat in response to internal appetite cues of hunger and satiety. A second major focus of CBT-A is education about satiety mechanisms and the choice of foods that promote satiety—foods that are more satisfying or last longer, supplying energy over a longer time.

Powerful triggers for binge eating are physiological cues of hunger, the depletion of particular nutrients, and the elimination of enjoyed foods from the daily diet. Many individuals who binge restrict their food intake. This is particularly so early in the day, in an attempt to limit the intake of calories in order to lose weight or to compensate for binge eating the previous day. Although this is not difficult early in the day, as the day progresses, the body's drive for food increases, and this may become a strong cue for binge eating later in the day.

Many forbidden or binge foods are not highly satiating and provide a rapidly available burst of energy that is soon used up. In order to keep food available to the body for longer periods of time, both to increase satiation after eating and also to reduce the presence of hunger as a cue for bingeing, individuals are encouraged to increase their consumption of more highly satiating foods. Three principles of choosing foods to promote satiety are: (1) choosing foods with greater volume, (2) eating a higher proportion of protein, and (3) choosing carbohydrates that have a more sustained release of energy and therefore last longer (i.e., have a lower glycemic index and glycemic load).

As well as incorporating more highly satiating foods in the daily diet in order to decrease the general risk of binge eating, it is also important to eat more satiating foods prior to specific high-risk times, such as before a long meeting without a meal or snack break or when a meal or snack will be later than usual in order to reduce hunger-related cues for binge eating.

Food Volume

Overall, people eat a relatively constant weight or volume of food over a day. Because of this, the energy density of foods (i.e., the amount of available energy—calories or kilojoules for the portion size) is a critical determinant of energy intake. The energy density of food can have a marked effect on both satiation (the amount eaten in a meal) and satiety (the effect on subsequent intake), independently of palatability and macronutrient content (Rolls, 2000). In general, the water content of foods is a critical determinant of energy density. Whole foods generally have a lower energy density, with less processed foods being less energy dense. Fruits and vegetables typically have a low energy density, and whole fruits or vegetables have a lower energy density than the same foods juiced. Adding water to a food (such as adding water to a casserole so that it becomes a soup) also lowers the food's energy density and consequently increases satiety (Rolls, Bell, & Thorwart, 1999).

Eating normal portions of food is central to this approach. Being aware of food volume makes eating meals and snacks more satiating. This includes paying attention to portion size, eating normal portions of food, but increasing the proportion of higher volume, lower energy density foods (including wet or soupy foods, fruits, vegetables, whole foods, and higher fiber foods).

Strategies for increasing food volume include:

- Eating normal portions
- Increasing the proportion of higher volume foods.

EDUCATION ABOUT SATIETY-SIGNALING MECHANISMS

Information is given to the individual about the body's many "satiety" systems that signal that the individual has eaten enough. Higher volume food choices indicate via numerous sensory signals that a satisfying portion of food is being eaten. These include the individual's overall evaluation that the serving will be satisfying, indicated via specific visual, olfactory, and gustatory senses; stomach "stretch" receptors; the time taken for chewing and swallowing; intestinal contractions; and the time taken and physical sensations of the passage of food through the digestive system. Other satiety markers include hormones such as cholecystokinin (CCK, dubbed the "satiety hormone"). A larger volume of food stimulates more of the body's satiety signals as it moves through the digestive system.

Protein

Individuals who binge have a lower protein intake throughout the day (Hetherington et al., 1994). Consuming protein decreases subsequent food intake, both in the short (Latner, 2003; Latner & Schwartz, 1999) and long term (de Castro, 1987), and reduces subsequent binge eating in individuals with bulimia nervosa and binge-eating disorder (Latner & Wilson, 2004). There is some evidence that a moderate-to-high-protein diet may be effective for weight loss in an overweight sample (Foster et al., 2003). One possible mechanism for this may be a reduction in binge eating. Increased protein consumption may reduce the likelihood of subsequent binging or overeating by increasing satiety.

Sources of protein include meat, poultry, and fish, eggs, dairy products, seeds and nuts, beans and lentils, soy products, and grains, especially wheat, but less so barley and corn. As the human body cannot store protein, it must be supplied on a daily basis from the foods eaten. The nutritional value of a protein is judged by how many of the essential amino acids it provides and in what quantity. Generally speaking, animal proteins (such as chicken, beef, or fish) contain all of the essential amino acids. Plant proteins usually lack at least one amino acid, except for soy and the seed of the leafy green amaranth (consumed in Asia and the Mediterranean). Strict vegetarians can solve this dietary problem by eating a combination of plant foods. For example, a single meal containing cereals and legumes provides all the essential amino acids found in a typical meat dish.

Health professionals recommend that protein make up 10 to 35% of the daily diet for the general population. In general terms, eating a moderate amount of protein—in one or two meals every day—will be sufficient. For individuals who binge, however, increasing the daily percentage of food intake from protein toward the upper end of this range (i.e., 20–35%) is likely to aid in the reduction of binge eating by increasing satiety.

Individuals who binge are likely to benefit from eating protein-rich foods regularly throughout the day and at most meals and snacks rather than having one or two meals each day that contain moderate amounts of protein. It is important to note, however, that although higher levels of protein may be helpful, there is evidence that a *very*-high-protein–low-carbohydrate diet increases calcium excretion and therefore increases the risk of osteoporosis and of developing kidney stones (Mann & Truswell, 2002).

Strategies for increasing protein include:

- Increasing the overall daily intake of protein foods (meat, poultry, fish, eggs, dairy products, seeds and nuts, beans and lentils, soy products, and grains) to 20–35% of the daily diet.
- Including a protein food at most or all meals and snacks.

Choosing Carbohydrates That Last Longer

Food provides fuel for the body in the form of fat, protein, and carbohydrates, but carbohydrates are the body's preferred fuel source. Carbohydrate-containing foods include bread, cereals, rice, pasta, legumes, corn, potato, fruit, milk, yogurt, sugar, biscuits, cakes and sweets, and chocolate or candy.

DIGESTING AND ABSORBING CARBOHYDRATES

The digestive system breaks down carbohydrate-containing foods into simple sugars, mainly glucose. This simple sugar is then carried to each cell via the bloodstream. Once inside a cell, the glucose is "burned" along with oxygen to produce energy. The body converts any excess glucose from food into another form, called glycogen. Glycogen is stored inside muscle tissue and the liver, ready to supplement blood sugar levels should they drop between meals or during physical activity (Mann & Truswell, 2002).

Many researchers have begun to pay more attention to the ways carbohydrates in foods break down into and affect blood sugar or blood glucose levels. In certain situations a rapid burst of energy is necessary (e.g., elite athletes often eat foods of this type in order to have energy available quickly). However, this energy spike is followed by a dramatic drop in energy (a hypoglycemic state, often referred to as a "hypo"). This results in dramatically increased hunger and is often accompanied by feeling weak, light-headed, and irritable. For individuals who are prone to binge eating, this drop in energy can lead to overeating or binge eating.

MEASURING THE EFFECTS OF CARBOHYDRATE ON BLOOD GLUCOSE

Carbohydrate-containing foods can be rated according to their immediate effect on blood sugar levels. Various rating systems have been devised, including the glycemic index and glycemic load.

Glycemic Index. The glycemic index (or GI) is a ranking of how rapidly a given food triggers a rise in the blood sugar level. The developers of GI used pure glucose as the standard, giving it a rating of 100. Therefore, the closer a particular food is to 100, the higher its GI and the more rapidly it raises blood sugar levels (see Table 16.1). All foods with a GI rating are based on 50 grams of carbohydrates, regardless of the size of the serving that constitutes 50 grams. Publications are available that contain GI rankings of particular food types (Foster-Powell, Holt, & Brand-Miller, 2002).

Glycemic Load. The GI ranks how rapidly a particular food turns into sugar but does not take into account the amount of the food that a person eats. For example, pasta is a slower releasing carbohydrate (with a lower GI) than a cookie, but people with diabetes or impaired glucose tolerance are not advised to eat a large serving of pasta because the total amount of carbohydrate, and therefore the total blood glucose response, will be too high. To overcome these problems, the glycemic load (GL) has been developed to rank how much a standard serving of a particular food raises blood sugar. Therefore, GL takes into account both the type and the amount of carbohydrate eaten. The lower the GL, the less likely it will be that a serving of that food will cause blood sugar to spike (see Table 16.1).

Physiological Responses to High- versus Low-Glycemic-Load Foods. The consumption of high-GL foods results in higher and more rapid increases in blood glucose levels than the consumption of low-GL foods. Rapid increases in blood glucose are potent signals to the beta cells of the pancreas to increase insulin secretion (Ludwig, 2002), which creates a sharp decrease in blood glucose levels (hypoglycemia). In contrast, the consumption of low-GL foods results in lower but more sustained increases in blood glucose and lower insulin demands on pancreatic beta cells (Willett, 2001). A majority of published studies have found that the consumption of low-GL foods delays the return of hunger, decreases subsequent food intake, and increases satiety compared with high-GL foods (Ludwig, 2003). Some examples of the glycemic load of various carbohydrates include:

TABLE 16.1. Glycemic Index and Glycemic Load Ratings

	Glycemic index	Glycemic load
High	70+	20+
Moderate	56–69	GL of 11-19
Low	55 or less	GL of 10 or less

- Low GL (slow release): soy products, beans, fruit, milk, whole-grain bread
- Medium GL (medium release): sugar, orange juice, oats
- High GL (fast release): potatoes, whole-meal and white bread, rice.

For a more comprehensive list of the glycemic load of foods, refer to Foster-Powell, Holt, and Brand-Miller (2002).

Some strategies for lowering dietary GL include:

- Increasing the consumption of fruits, vegetables, legumes (peas and beans), nuts, and whole grains
- Decreasing the consumption of starchy high-GL foods such as potatoes, white rice, and white bread
- Decreasing the consumption of sugary foods such as cookies, cakes, sweets or candy, and soft drinks or sodas.

In summary, appetite-focused food choices are those that promote satiety, including foods with a lower energy density and a higher proportion of protein, and choosing carbohydrates with a longer lasting, slower, and more sustained release of energy. CBT-A also promotes the awareness of appetite by retraining the individual to recognize and respond to hunger and fullness signals.

ADAPTING CBT-A TO SELF-HELP

Adapting CBT-A to a self-help format is potentially important because of the large number of individuals with bulimia nervosa or binge-eating disorder who do not present to clinics for treatment (Fairburn & Carter, 1997; Wilson & Agras, 2001) and the shortage of therapists in general, particularly those trained in manualized CBT (Mussell et al., 2000; see Chapters 4 and 5, this volume). Self-help formats have the potential for increased self-efficacy and acceptability of the therapy, as well as greater accessibility and lower treatment cost.

A number of commercially available self-help formats that use standard CBT principles for bulimia nervosa and binge-eating disorder are available, including self-help books (Fairburn, 1995), CD-ROMs for personal computers (Williams, Aubin, Cottrell, Harkin, & Schmidt, 2005), and Internet-based programs. The use of innovative technologies and alternative delivery formats for eating disorders has been favorably reviewed (Myers, Swan-Kremeier, Wonderlich, Lancaster, & Mitchell, 2004).

Self-help has been delivered in pure form (Carter & Fairburn, 1998; Carter et al., 2003) and with varying levels and types of guidance (Bailer et al., 2004; Cooper, Coker, & Fleming, 1996; Pritchard, Bergin, & Wade,

2004; Wells, Garvin, Dohm, & Striegel-Moore, 1997). It has been used alone or as an adjunct to usual treatment, such as while on a waiting list (Schmidt, Tiller, & Treasure, 1993). Initial open-trial pilot studies have reported promising results (Cooper, Coker, & Fleming, 1994; Schmidt et al., 1993), and several randomized clinical trials have found that both pure self-help and guided self-help are more effective than a no-treatment waiting list for binge-eating disorder (Carter & Fairburn, 1998) or a comparison group controlling for amount of professional contact (Grilo & Masheb, 2005; see also Chapters 4, 5, and 8, this volume).

CBT-A would be readily adaptable to a self-help format by incorporating an appetite focus that would be introduced at the beginning of the program and then interwoven throughout the other standard CBT components. This could be achieved by systematic psychoeducation regarding core CBT-A components, including attention to and monitoring of hunger and satiety, and enhancing satiation by increasing food volume, increasing protein, and choosing carbohydrates that have a slower and more sustained glycemic response. These appetite-focused principles would be added to the usual goals of normalizing eating: eating *regularly* from a *variety* of food groups and eating a *sufficient* quantity of food.

Certain components of a CBT-A approach, particularly advice about appetite-focused food choices, have for some time been reported in popular literature as weight-reduction strategies. These include advice about choosing carbohydrates with a low glycemic index, increasing the proportion of protein in the daily food intake, and choosing foods with lower energy density (or higher volume). Although education about appetite-focused food choices is part of CBT-A, these strategies, in isolation, are unlikely to bring about the cessation of binge eating. The cornerstone of CBT-A is relearning to recognize and respond to hunger and satiety cues. This may be the most difficult skill to learn through self-help, as many individuals with eating disorders have trained themselves to minimize and ignore signs of hunger and have come to routinely override physical sensations of fullness during binge-eating episodes. Retraining awareness of hunger and fullness often takes considerable therapist skill in the use of successive approximation and careful questioning. A series of questions could be used to help increase the individual's awareness in this area. Questions could include the following: "How hungry would your body have been when you had your first cup of coffee?" "How hungry would your sister (or close friend) be by dinner time if she had eaten what you have eaten today?" "If your sister were visiting from out of town and you were responsible for taking care of her, how would the meals and snacks you would provide for her differ from your day's eating?" "At what point in the binge would you have been comfortably full?"

CBT-A in a self-help format may be useful as a first-line treatment for those with less severe difficulties. As with other self-help programs, those with more severe eating disorders and who have potential health concerns require assessment and monitoring by health professionals experienced in the treatment of eating disorders (Wilson, Vitousek, & Loeb, 2000). Of particular relevance to CBT-A are concerns about the potential negative health consequences of high-protein diets (Bravata et al., 2003). It is also possible that without therapist supervision, some individuals with eating disorders may use the principles of increasing satiety as an aid to "better dieting" and may risk developing problems related to weight loss or low weight, including anorexia nervosa. Indeed, one study has reported that those with a history of anorexia nervosa and/or personality disorder were more likely to drop out or have poor outcomes from self-help treatment (Cooper, Coker, & Fleming, 1996).

Adding appetite-focused principles to standard CBT in a self-help format, with or without professional guidance, needs to be studied systematically. Incorporating established laboratory research on appetite and satiety with psychoeducation promoting appetite-focused food choices offers the promise of further enhancing the effectiveness of existing CBT self-help approaches.

SUMMARY

CBT has the best evidence of effectiveness in treating binge eating, being equal to or better than other psychological therapies for binge eating. However, the proportion of those participants who do poorly or who only partially respond to treatment is still unacceptably high. Continued effort is needed to improve treatment efficacy by developing new treatments or enhancing the outcome of existing treatments. Traditional CBT has paid relatively little attention to the role of appetite and satiety, instead attending to the pattern of eating and dismantling the binge–purge cycle. Although there is much to learn about the biological underpinnings of binge-eating behaviors, there is now good evidence from laboratory and feeding studies of the role of dysregulation of hunger and satiety in those with binge-eating disorders. There have also been several promising studies adapting CBT to include greater attention to appetite. CBT-A builds on this research by promoting the role of appetite and satiety within the treatment model and by introducing a major focus on food choices that maximize satiety. Although CBT-A builds on existing elements of effective treatments, this combination of CBT components has yet to be systematically evaluated.

REFERENCES

Bailer, U., de Zwaan, M., Leisch, F., Strnad, A., Lennkh-Wolfsberg, C., El-Giamal, N., et al. (2004). Guided self-help versus cognitive-behavioral group therapy in the treatment of bulimia nervosa. *International Journal of Eating Disorders, 35*(4), 522–537.
Beumont, P. J. V., & Touyz, S. W. (1995). The nutritional management of anorexia and

bulimia nervosa. In K. D. Brownell & C. G. Fairburn (Eds.), *Eating disorders and obesity: A comprehensive handbook* (pp. 306–312). New York: Guilford Press.

Bravata, D. M., Sanders, L., Huang, J., Krumholz, H. M., Olkin, I., Gardner, C. D., et al. (2003). Efficacy and safety of low-carbohydrate diets. *Journal of the American Medical Association, 289*(14), 1837–1850.

Bulik, C. (1994). *Eating disorders: Detection and treatment.* Palmerston North, New Zealand: Dunmore Press.

Carter, J. C., & Fairburn, C. G. (1998). Cognitive-behavioral self-help for binge-eating disorder: A controlled effectiveness study. *Journal of Consulting and Clinical Psychology, 66*(4), 616–623.

Carter, J. C., Olmsted, M. P., Kaplan, A. S., McCabe, R. E., Mills, J. S., & Aime, A. (2003). Self-help for bulimia nervosa: A randomized controlled trial. *American Journal of Psychiatry, 160*(5), 973–978.

Cloninger, C. R., Svrakic, D. M., & Przybeck, T. R. (1993). A psychobiological model of temperament and character. *Archives of General Psychiatry, 50*, 975–990.

Cooper, P. J., Coker, S., & Fleming, C. (1994). Self-help for bulimia nervosa: A preliminary report. *International Journal of Eating Disorders, 16*(4), 401–404.

Cooper, P. J., Coker, S., & Fleming, C. (1996). An evaluation of the efficacy of supervised cognitive behavioral self-help for bulimia nervosa. *Journal of Psychosomatic Research, 40*(3), 281–287.

Craighead, L. W., & Allen, H. N. (1995). Appetite awareness training: A cognitive behavioral intervention for binge eating. *Cognitive and Behavioral Practice, 2*(2), 249–270.

de Castro, J. M. (1987). Macronutrient relationships with meal patterns and mood in the spontaneous feeding behavior of humans. *Physiology and Behavior, 39*(5), 561–569.

Devlin, M. J., Walsh, B. T., Guss, J. L., Kissileff, H. R., Liddle, R. A., & Petkova, E. (1997). Postprandial cholecystokinin release and gastric emptying in patients with bulimia nervosa. *American Journal of Clinical Nutrition, 65*(1), 114–120.

Dicker, S. L., & Craighead, L. W. (2004). Appetite-focused cognitive-behavioral therapy in the treatment of binge eating with purging. *Cognitive and Behavioral Practice, 11*, 213–221.

Drewnowski, A., Bellisle, F., Aimez, P., & Remy, B. (1987). Taste and bulimia. *Physiology and Behavior, 41*, 621–626.

Drewnowski, A., Halmi, K. A., Pierce, B., Gibbs, J., & Smith, G. P. (1987). Taste and eating disorders. *American Journal of Clinical Nutrition, 46*(3), 442–450.

Fairburn, C. G. (1995). *Overcoming binge eating.* New York: Guilford Press.

Fairburn, C. G., & Carter, J. C. (1997). Self-help and guided self-help for binge-eating problems. In D. M. Garner (Ed.), *Handbook of treatment for eating disorders* (2nd ed., pp. 494–499). New York: Guilford Press.

Fairburn, C. G., Cooper, Z., & Shafran, R. (2003). Cognitive behaviour therapy for eating disorders: A "transdiagnostic" theory and treatment. *Behaviour Research and Therapy, 41*(5), 509–528.

Fairburn, C. G., Marcus, M. D., & Wilson, G. T. (1993). Cognitive-behavioural therapy for binge eating and bulimia nervosa: A comprehensive treatment manual. In C. G. Fairburn & G. T. Wilson (Eds.), *Binge eating: Nature, assessment and treatment* (pp. 361–404). New York: Guilford Press.

Fassino, S., Piero, A., Gramaglia, C., & Abbate-Daga, G. (2004). Clinical, psychopathological and personality correlates of interoceptive awareness in anorexia nervosa, bulimia nervosa and obesity. *Psychopathology, 37*(4), 168–174.

Foster, G. D., Wyatt, H. R., Hill, J. O., McGuckin, B. G., Brill, C., Mohammed, B. S., et al. (2003). A randomized trial of a low-carbohydrate diet for obesity. *New England Journal of Medicine, 348*(21), 2082–2090.

Foster-Powell, K., Holt, S. H., & Brand-Miller, J. C. (2002). International table of glycemic index and glycemic load values: 2002. *American Journal of Clinical Nutrition, 76*(1), 5–56.

Garner, D. M., Olmsted, M. P., & Polivy, J. (1983). The Eating Disorder Inventory: a measure of cognitive-behavioral dimensions of anorexia nervosa and bulimia. In P. L. Darby, P. E. Garfinkel, D. M. Garner, & D. V. Coscina (Eds.), *Anorexia nervosa: Recent developments in research* (pp. 173–184). New York: Liss.

Geliebter, A. (1988). Gastric distension and gastric capacity in relation to food-intake in humans. *Physiology and Behavior, 44*(4–5), 665–668.

Geliebter, A., & Hashim, S. A. (2001). Gastric capacity in normal, obese, and bulimic women. *Physiology and Behavior, 74*, 743–746.

Geliebter, A., Melton, P. M., McCray, R. S., Gallagher, D. R., Gage, D., & Hashim, S. A. (1992). Gastric capacity, gastric emptying, and test-meal intake in normal and bulimic women. *American Journal of Clinical Nutrition, 56*(4), 656–661.

Geracioti, T. D. J., & Liddle, R. A. (1988). Impaired cholecystokinin secretion in bulimia nervosa. *New England Journal of Medicine, 319*(11), 683–688.

Greeno, C. G., Wing, R. R., & Shiffman, S. (2000). Binge antecedents in obese women with and without binge-eating disorder. *Journal of Consulting and Clinical Psychology, 68*(1), 95–102.

Grilo, C. M., & Masheb, R. M. (2005). A randomized controlled comparison of guided self-help cognitive behavioral therapy and behavioral weight loss for binge-eating disorder. *Behaviour Research and Therapy, 43*(11), 1509–1525.

Hadigan, C. M., Walsh, B. T., Devlin, M. J., LaChaussee, J. L., & Kissileff, H. R. (1992). Behavioral assessment of satiety in bulimia nervosa. *Appetite, 18*(3), 233–241.

Halmi, K. A., Sunday, S., Puglisi, A., & Marchi, P. (1989). Hunger and satiety in anorexia and bulimia nervosa. *Annals of the New York Academy of Sciences, 575*, 431–444.

Heilbrun, A. B., & Worobow, A. L. (1991). Attention and disordered eating behavior: 1. Disattention to satiety cues as a risk factor in the development of bulimia. *Journal of Clinical Psychology, 47*(1), 3–9.

Hetherington, M., & Rolls, B. J. (1989). Sensory-specific satiety in anorexia and bulimia nervosa. *Annals of the New York Academy of Sciences, 575*, 387–398.

Hetherington, M. M., Altemus, M., Nelson, M. L., Bernat, A. S., & Gold, P. W. (1994). Eating behavior in bulimia nervosa: Multiple meal analyses. *American Journal of Clinical Nutrition, 60*, 864–873.

Jimerson, D. C., & Wolfe, B. E. (2004). Neuropeptides in eating disorders. *CNS Spectrums, 9*(7), 516–522.

Latner, J. D. (2003). Macronutrient effects on satiety and binge eating in bulimia nervosa and binge-eating disorder. *Appetite, 40*(3), 309–311.

Latner, J. D., & Schwartz, M. (1999). The effects of a high-carbohydrate, high-protein or balanced lunch upon later food intake and hunger ratings. *Appetite, 33*(1), 119–128.

Latner, J. D., & Wilson, G. T. (2004). Binge eating and satiety in bulimia nervosa and binge-eating disorder: Effects of macronutrient intake. *International Journal of Eating Disorders, 36*, 402–415.

Lowe, M. R., & Levine, A. S. (2005). Eating motives and the controversy over dieting: Eating less than needed versus less than wanted. *Obesity Research, 13*(5), 797–806.

Ludwig, D. S. (2002). The glycemic index: Physiological mechanisms relating to obesity, diabetes, and cardiovascular disease. *Journal of the American Medical Association, 287*(18), 2414–2423.

Ludwig, D. S. (2003). Dietary glycemic index and the regulation of body weight. *Lipids, 38*(2), 117–121.

Mann, J., & Truswell, A. S. (Eds.). (2002). *Essentials of human nutrition.* New York: Oxford University Press.

McManus, F., & Waller, G. (1995). A functional analysis of binge-eating. *Clinical Psychology Review, 15*(8), 845–863.

Mitchell, J. E., Mussell, M. P., Peterson, C. B., Crown, S., Wonderlich, S. A., Crosby, R. D., et al. (1999). Hedonics of binge eating in women with bulimia nervosa and binge-eating disorder. *International Journal of Eating Disorders, 26,* 165–170.

Monteleone, P., Martiadis, V., Rigamonti, A. E., Fabrazzo, M., Giordani, C., Muller, E. E., et al. (2005). Investigation of peptide YY and ghrelin responses to a test meal in bulimia nervosa. *Biological Psychiatry, 57*(8), 926–931.

Mussell, M. P., Crosby, R. D., Crow, S. J., Knopke, A. J., Peterson, C. B., Wonderlich, S. A., et al. (2000). Utilization of empirically supported psychotherapy treatments for individuals with eating disorders: A survey of psychologists. *International Journal of Eating Disorders, 27*(2), 230–237.

Myers, T. C., Swan-Kremeier, L., Wonderlich, S., Lancaster, K., & Mitchell, J. E. (2004). The use of alternative delivery systems and new technologies in the treatment of patients with eating disorders. *International Journal of Eating Disorders, 36*(2), 123–143.

National Institute for Health and Clinical Excellence. (2004). *Eating disorders: Core interventions in the treatment and management of anorexia nervosa, bulimia nervosa and related eating disorders.* London: National Institute for Health and Clinical Excellence.

Pritchard, B. J., Bergin, J. L., & Wade, T. D. (2004). A case series evaluation of guided self-help for bulimia nervosa using a cognitive manual. *International Journal of Eating Disorders, 36*(2), 144–156.

Quadflieg, N., & Fichter, M. M. (2003). The course and outcome of bulimia nervosa. *European Child and Adolescent Psychiatry, 12*(Suppl. 1), i99–i109.

Rolls, B. J. (2000). The role of energy density in the overconsumption of fat. *Journal of Nutrition, 130*(2), 268s–271s.

Rolls, B. J., Bell, E. A., & Thorwart, M. L. (1999). Water incorporated into a food but not served with a food decreases energy intake in lean women. *American Journal of Clinical Nutrition, 70*(4), 448–455.

Rosen, J. C., Lietenberg, H., Fischer, C., & Khazam, C. (1986). Binge-eating episodes in bulimia nervosa: The amount and type of food consumed. *International Journal of Eating Disorders, 5,* 255–267.

Schmidt, U., Tiller, J., & Treasure, J. (1993). Self-treatment of bulimia nervosa: A pilot study. *International Journal of Eating Disorders, 13*(3), 273–277.

Stickney, M. I., Miltenberger, R. G., & Wolff, G. (1999). A descriptive analysis of factors contributing to binge eating. *Journal of Behavior Therapy and Experimental Psychiatry, 30*(3), 177–189.

Ventura, M., & Bauer, B. (1999). Empowerment of women with purging-type bulimia nervosa through nutritional rehabilitation. *Eating and Weight Disorders, 4,* 55–62.

Walsh, B. T., & Devlin, M. J. (1998). Eating disorders: Progress and problems. *Science, 280*(5368), 1387–1390.

Walsh, B. T., Hadigan, C. M., Kissileff, H. R., & LaChaussee, J. L. (1992). Bulimia nervosa: A syndrome of feast and famine. In G. H. Anderson & S. H. Kennedy (Eds.), *The biology of feast and famine* (pp. 3–20). New York: Academic Press.

Wells, A. M., Garvin, V., Dohm, F. A., & Striegel-Moore, R. H. (1997). Telephone-based guided self-help for binge-eating disorder: A feasibility study. *International Journal of Eating Disorders, 21*(4), 341–346.

Weltzin, T. E., Hsu, L. K., Pollice, C., & Kaye, W. H. (1991). Feeding patterns in bulimia nervosa. *Biological Psychiatry, 30*(11), 1093–1110.

Willett, W. C. (2001). *Eat, drink, and be healthy: The Harvard Medical School guide to healthy eating.* New York: Simon & Schuster.

Williams, C., Aubin, S., Cottrell, D., Harkin, P., & Schmidt, U. (2005). *Overcoming bulimia* [CD-ROM]. Leeds, UK: Leeds Innovations Multimedia Division.

Wilson, G. T., & Agras, W. S. (2001). Practice guidelines for eating disorders. *Behavior Therapy, 32*(2), 219–234.

Wilson, G. T., Vitousek, K. M., & Loeb, K. L. (2000). Stepped care treatment for eating disorders. *Journal of Consulting and Clinical Psychology, 68*(4), 564–572.

Wonderlich, S. A., de Zwaan, M., Mitchell, J. E., Peterson, C., & Crow, S. (2003). Psychological and dietary treatments of binge-eating disorder: Conceptual implications. *International Journal of Eating Disorders, 34*(Suppl.), S58–S73.

Yanovski, S. Z., Leet, M., Yanovski, J. A., Flood, M., Gold, P. W., Kissileff, H. R., et al. (1992). Food intake and selection of obese women with and without binge-eating disorder. *American Journal of Clinical Nutrition, 56*(6), 975–980.

17

Strategies for Coping
with the Stigma of Obesity

REBECCA M. PUHL *and* KELLY D. BROWNELL

Combining the prevalence of obesity with its medical consequences makes obesity a major public health problem. Attention to obesity as a medical and public health problem has increased, but much less emphasis has been placed on the social consequences of being obese, which are serious, pervasive, and damaging. Obese individuals face multiple forms of stigmatization in our society, frequently resulting in bias and discrimination.

EXTENT AND IMPACT OF WEIGHT BIAS

Abundant research documents the social disadvantages of being overweight in employment, health care, education, interpersonal relationships, and overall quality of life (Puhl & Brownell, 2001; Puhl, Henderson, & Brownell, 2005). In employment settings, obese individuals are less likely to be hired than thinner persons, even when they have the same qualifications (Roehling, 1999); they are perceived to be less competent, lazy, and lacking in self-discipline (Paul & Townsend, 1995); and weight stigma negatively affects their wages, promotions, and stability of employment (Bordieri, Drehmer, & Taylor, 1997; Pagan & Davila, 1997; Register & Williams, 1990; Rothblum, Brand, Miller, & Oetjen, 1990).

In health care settings, obese patients face stigmatizing attitudes from physicians, psychologists, nurses, dietitians, and medical students (Davis-Coelho, Waltz, & Davis-Coelho, 2000; Maddox & Liederman, 1969;

Maroney & Golub, 1992; Price, Desmond, Krol, Snyder, & O'Connell, 1987; Teachman & Brownell, 2001; Wiese, Wilson, Jones, & Neises, 1992). Research has demonstrated questionable obesity management practices among physicians and reluctance of obese patients to seek needed health care services, both of which may further exacerbate health consequences associated with obesity (Fontaine, Faith, Allison, & Cheskin, 1998; Galuska, Will, Serdula, & Ford, 1999; Kristeller & Hoerr, 1997; Olson, Schumaker, & Yawn, 1994).

Obese students confront teasing, harassment, and rejection from peers at school, as well as obstacles in education due to negative teacher attitudes, lower college acceptances, and wrongful dismissals from college (Canning & Mayer, 1966; Neumark-Sztainer, Story, & Faibisch, 1998; Weiler & Helmes, 1993). Obese children, who may be especially vulnerable to the negative consequences of stigma, can expect to be victims of negative attitudes from peers as early as age 3 (Cramer & Steinwert, 1998). In addition, obese children may experience stigma from their own parents, both in terms of receiving less financial support for education (Crandall, 1995) and in subtle forms of stigma that occur in parent–child interactions at home (Adams, Hicken & Salehi, 1988).

As members of a media-saturated culture, we need to look no further than the television or a magazine to observe negative attitudes toward obese individuals. Research has documented substantial weight stigma in multiple media sources (Greenberg, Eastin, Hofshire, Lachlan, & Brownell, 2003). Overall, widespread social attitudes fuel negative assumptions that obese individuals are impulsive and that they lack willpower, motivation, and personal control (Puhl & Brownell, 2001; Teachman, Gapinski, & Brownell, 2001).

Given the multiple domains in which weight stigma is prevalent, obese individuals may have increased vulnerability to negative outcomes such as depression, suicidal thoughts, and suicide attempts (Carpenter, Hasin, Allison, & Faith, 2000; Eaton, Lowry, Brener, Galuska, & Crosby, 2005). Research has also documented negative physical health consequences among people who experience stigma (Guyll, Matthews, & Bromberger, 2001), and it is plausible to predict that this may hold true for obese people who are stigmatized, which is a concern given the health risks that obese people already face.

The prevalence and acceptability of weight stigma make it necessary for obese individuals to cope with bias, stigma, and discrimination. The limited long-term success of existing weight-loss approaches also implies that people who remain overweight are exposed to stigma and must cope with it for years. Understanding how obese persons cope with these experiences is important in documenting the overall impact of obesity on health and well-being and in developing strategies that can improve daily functioning given the stigmatizing environment. Such an understanding may help temper the impact of prejudiced encounters. Identification of effective coping strategies is also important for health-care professionals, who could use these tools as an adjunct to treatment in efforts to improve emotional well-being in their obese clientsted to seminar ion will still count following the midterm!, and if you have any ideas aboutthey are . Self-help strategies may additionally provide an appropriate and empowering venue for learning ways to cope with stigma, both for obese individuals themselves and for parents and teachers who wish to help obese children.

Despite the vast numbers of people potentially affected by weight bias, there has been little discussion about reactions to weight prejudice among obese people. There is some indication that coping methods in general are used more frequently to deal with stigma as individuals become more obese (Myers & Rosen, 1999). Coping with stigma is rarely discussed as a component of treatments for obesity (but refer to Chapter 14, this volume, for additional discussion of this topic). Further, there is insufficient research to determine which coping strategies are most frequently used by obese people and which methods are most beneficial. This chapter describes what is known about the strategies obese people use to cope with weight stigma, which coping approaches appear to hold the most promise, and what the most pressing research needs in this area are.

Strategies that one chooses to cope with stigma can take many forms. Unlike characteristics such as race, gender, and age, which cannot be changed, obese people will sometimes lose weight. Many attempt to do so, hoping their social situations will improve. Obese persons may choose to deal with bias in social interactions by avoiding or confronting the perpetrators of stigma and choosing whether to accept, internalize, or challenge the content of the stigmatizing message or discriminatory behavior. Whether an individual adopts a stable coping style that is used across multiple situations or uses different approaches that are sensitive to specific situations, most strategies can have adaptive or maladaptive consequences depending on context. In addition, both individual and situational factors will influence the choice of coping strategy and its potential effectiveness. Variables such as gender, age, self-esteem, personality characteristics, perceived control of stigma, self-perceived problem-solving skills, and extent of social group identification can all affect coping (Puhl & Brownell, 2003).

METHODS OF COPING

Weight-Loss Attempts

To the extent to which a person believes that body weight is within personal control, attempting to reduce may be perceived as a means of avoiding weight stigma. Individuals who tend to blame themselves for being stigmatized may be more likely to employ this strategy rather than using other coping approaches to deal with bias (Miller & Major, 2000). For example, Joanisse and Synnott (1999) suggest that many obese people internalize social stereotypes about obesity, believing that weight is the cause of their problems, and engage in repeated weight-loss attempts as a way to eradicate negative social circumstances.

Although little work has examined weight loss as a coping strategy, some research suggests that obese people may perceive reduced stigma to be a desirable outcome of gastric bypass surgery. In one self-report study of patients who had obesity surgery, 87% reported that their weight had prevented them from being hired for jobs, 90% reported experiencing stigma at their workplaces, and 84% avoided public places (Rand & MacGregor, 1990). After the surgery, all patients reported reduced discrimination (stating that they had rarely or never perceived prejudice since the operation), and 90% reported increased cheerfulness and confidence (Rand & MacGregor, 1990).

A related study suggests that motivations for obtaining weight-loss surgery are rooted in both social and medical concerns. Peace and colleagues (1989) found that 59% of patients undergoing gastric restriction surgery requested the surgery for social reasons, such as embarrassment, and only 10% for medical reasons (Peace, Dyne, Russell, & Stewart, 1989). Following the operation, patients reported positive changes in their interpersonal relationships and occupational functioning.

Despite the limitations of these small, self-report studies, it is important to consider the possibility that obese persons may perceive surgery to be one way of escaping stigma. What research doesss exist suggests that people do, in fact, experience less stigma and discrimination if they lose large amounts of weight. This helps proves the obvious—that the weight is the cause of the stigma. The weakness in this literature is that what little data exist come primarily from research with surgery patients, in whom the weight change is most extreme, although there is preliminary evidence that experiences of weight stigma may prompt weight-loss among participants in behavioral weight loss programs (Latner, Stunkard, Wilson, & Jackson, 2006). It is not known whether lesser weight losses produced by nonsurgical means have a similar impact.

Confirmation/Self-Acceptance

Obese persons may react to stigma by accepting negative attributions ascribed to them by others. This approach underscores the influence of others' perceptions on one's beliefs and the possibility that stigmatized people behave or think in ways that are consistent with stereotypes. Quinn and Crocker (1998) suggest that obese individuals may confirm negative stereotypes to feel more like members of society who express these normative attitudes. It may also be a way to enhance motivation to lose weight. Given the widespread negative stereotypes, it is possible that obese people may readily come to accept societal perceptions, even if they are false. Members of other stigmatized groups (such as racial minorities or disabled individuals) are rarely directly blamed for their stigmatized status, but because obesity is so often believed to be under personal control (Crandall, 1994; Crandall & Cohen, 1994), obese individuals may be less inclined to challenge or reject stigma toward them because they believe their condition may be temporary and that losing weight is always a possibility.

Two experimental studies have illustrated the presence of confirmation as a reaction to weight stigma among obese women. In one study, male participants were instructed to engage in casual telephone conversations with female participants who were not visible to them. Males were provided with a photograph of either an obese or a normal-weight woman whom they were led to believe was their telephone partner. Results showed that during the phone conversations, obese female participants presented themselves as being similar to the stereotyped assumptions made by their phone partners and confirmed males' negative weight-related perceptions of them. The authors propose that this strategy may have been used by obese women to facilitate positive social interactions (Snyder & Haugen, 1995).

In another study, obese and nonobese women were led to believe that a male participant was rating their attractiveness as a potential dating partner. In reality, the male participant was a confederate, and women were randomly assigned to receive either positive or negative feedback from him. Heavier women responded to negative feedback by attributing this criticism to their own weight, which they perceived to be a central factor predicting social outcomes. Rather than blaming the confederate for his negative response, these women reacted by accepting his negative stereotypes (Crocker, Cornwell, & Major, 1993). More work is needed to determine whether internalizing blame versus blaming others for their attitudes have distinct outcomes for obese individuals and to what degree each of these strategies affects emotional well-being and future stigma encounters.

Degher and Hughes (1999) propose that obese persons may comply with certain social stereotypes in order to reduce negative responses and maximize acceptance by others. In their field study exploring coping methods used by obese adults in a weight-control organization, the majority of participants reported complying with the stereotype of the "jolly fat person" (Hughes & Degher, 1993).

Few studies have addressed confirmation as a coping strategy to deal with weight stigma. What work exists suggests that this strategy has potentially maladaptive consequences, including negative affect, depression, hostility, and vulnerability to low self-esteem (Crocker et al., 1993; Fuller & Groce, 1991; Quinn & Crocker, 1998).

Self-Protection

Self-protective coping strategies aim to provide a shield from stigma and to help maintain self-esteem (Crocker & Major, 1989). Preserving self-esteem may be especially important among obese individuals who have remained overweight despite previous weight-loss attempts. Self-protection can involve several individual strategies. One coping method is to attribute negative feedback to the prejudiced attitudes of others and therefore to "discredit the discreditor" (Siegel, Lune, & Meyer, 1998). Members of the National Association to Advance Fat Acceptance (NAAFA), for example, publicly attribute negative stereotypes about obese people to biased societal attitudes and instead embrace positive attributes of being obese. In some respects, a group such as NAAFA could be considered a self-help group, with the objectives of increasing self-affirmation, body esteem, and social activism. Another strategy is to minimize or devalue domains in which one's stigmatized group is perceived as inadequate and instead valuing other areas. As an example, this might involve downplaying the importance of bodily appearance and focusing instead on valued achievements unrelated to body weight, such as academic success or participation in charitable work.

Another self-protective strategy is to compare one's current status with that of others in the stigmatized group. Whereas comparing oneself with more advantaged out-groups (e.g., thinner individuals) may threaten self-esteem, making comparisons with those who are similarly stigmatized may involve less threatening comparisons (Crocker & Major, 1989). However, research on social comparisons and coping is mixed. Some work finds that comparing oneself with another person who is "worse off" will increase self-esteem among individuals who seek self-enhancement but that, when motivated by self-improvement, people tend to compare themselves with those who are performing better (Crocker, Thompson, McGraw, & Ingerman, 1987; Taylor, Buunk, & Aspinwall, 1990). Thus it is possible that self-esteem could be threatened or protected in certain situations among obese people regardless of whether they are making an upward comparison (with someone who weighs less) or downward comparison (with someone who is heavier).

Studies have not yet examined self-protective strategies of coping among obese individuals. However, research on other stigmatized groups suggests that such strategies are related to increased self-esteem only when stigmatized individuals perceive themselves to be legitimate members of a larger group that is collectively stigmatized, not without a stigmatized group membership (Crandall, Tsang, Harvey, & Britt, 2000). Thus one might predict that self-protective strategies will be most helpful if an obese person perceives that his or her stigma is part of a larger group identity.

Given that obese individuals may not want to share membership with the larger group identity of "obese people," especially if they are trying to lose weight, self-protection strategies may be less effective under these circumstances. An example of this could include typical weight-loss treatment-group settings, in which group members wish to escape the group identity and in which social comparisons may not be self-affirming. This idea has not been tested, but it would be informative for research to examine what factors increase or decrease self-affirmation, self-protection, or personal empowerment in professional and self-help treatment groups.

Another factor that may affect self-protective strategies is the perceived controllability and causality of obesity. Crocker (1999) suggests that in situations in which uncontrollable causes of obesity are highlighted, stigma is more likely to be ascribed to external biased attitudes of others rather than to personal deficiencies, thus protecting self-esteem. More research is needed to examine to what extent and under what circumstances self-protective processes are used and how social comparisons and perceptions of causality of obesity influence these responses.

Compensation

Coping with stigma can also involve strategies that attempt to compensate for negative consequences of being overweight by demonstrating competence and skill in socially valued activities (Degher & Hughes, 1999; Taub, Blinde, & Greer, 1999).

Miller and Myers (1998) describe two types of compensation strategies. Primary compensation tries to prevent biased encounters by increasing efforts and skills used in social interactions to achieve desired goals. As an example, Myers and Rosen (1999) found that obese adults reported compensating for stigma by being assertive, friendly, and outgoing in social situations to improve others' attitudes toward them. Secondary compensation is used as a strategy following a stigmatizing situation by changing one's perceived causal role in the encounter (Miller & Myers, 1998), such as blaming others for their biased attitudes rather than internalizing blame.

Although obese individuals may be aware that stigma affects their interactions, they may not be accurate in estimations of how much effort is needed to compensate sufficiently across stigmatizing situations (Miller, Rothblum, Felicio, & Brand, 1995). It may be relatively easy to compensate if weight prejudice is perceived to be low or, alternatively, to overcompensate in ways such that excessive expression of efforts (such as overly asserting oneself) could lead to negative perceptions (Miller et al., 1995; Miller & Myers, 1998). Degher and Hughes (1999) propose that compensation is most likely to be used by obese people who have been heavy since childhood. They suggest that confronting stigma for long periods of time may increase internal pressures to succeed in other areas in order to be accepted (Hughes & Degher, 1993).

There is some evidence that compensation is employed by obese persons as a coping strategy. In one study, obese and nonobese women were observed in telephone conversations with others whom they were told either could or could not see them (Miller et al., 1995). When obese women believed that they were visible, they rated themselves as more likeable and socially skilled than nonobese women (Miller et al., 1995). However, obese women gave themselves lower ratings on social skills when telephone partners could see them but only if the women believed that they were not visible to their partners. Self-ratings were not different among obese and nonobese women if they believed they could not be seen. These self-ratings suggest that obese women tried to portray themselves more positively when they believed that their visible weight might elicit negative reactions from their partners (Miller et al., 1995). More work is needed in this area to examine whether compensation strategies do in fact achieve more favorable perceptions of obese individuals.

Confrontation

An assertive coping strategy is to confront the "perpetrator" of stigma. This process involves directly challenging another person's behavior, often in an attempt to stop future stigmatizing actions (Levy, 1993). In a small self-report study of 23 obese adults, participants reported using verbal assertion and physical aggression as responses to perpetrators of stigma (Joanisse & Synnott, 1999). Responses included making formal complaints to store managers when employees were rude to them, reacting with verbal "comebacks" or insults when stigmatized by others, and using verbal threats to end relationships with others if negative comments about their weight did not stop. Physical aggression was reported less frequently, but two participants admitted responding aggressively to stigmatizing comments. Participants reported that verbally asserting their rights and challenging the perpetrator was an effective strategy in coping with biased individuals.

There is insufficient research on confrontation to determine whether this coping strategy ends further weight discrimination and can improve emotional well-being through feelings of personal empowerment. It is possible that even if confrontation strategies are unsuccessful, they may still lead to feelings of increased confidence (Levy, 1993). However, there are also potential negative consequences of confronting individuals that could have adverse emotional outcomes if obese persons do not feel prepared to assert themselves or if the behavior provokes even more aggression and stigma.

Social Activism

Some obese individuals may channel assertive responses by participating in public social groups and movements to attack weight prejudice. A well-known advocacy group, NAAFA is an example of a group that publicly challenges stigma and discrimination and promotes size acceptance. Efforts from groups such as NAAFA, especially when covered in the media, can shine light on the problem and have the potential to affect legislation, regulation, and litigation, so belonging to this kind of group might provide obese individuals with acceptance and social support.

No research has studied social activism as a specific coping strategy to deal with weight stigma, but Deaux and Ethier (1998) suggest that this may be chosen as a coping strategy when individuals believe that their stigmatized status is unalterable. Although societal messages about weight (fostered by the diet industry) perpetuate the notion that the body is malleable and that weight is controllable, many obese people remain overweight despite multiple weight-loss attempts. For these individuals, it is possible that social activism may be a more desirable strategy. Another hypothesis is that choosing this strategy may be influenced by the degree to which obese persons identify themselves with a larger social group and how they perceive their membership in the group (Deaux & Ethier, 1998). Perhaps obese individuals are more likely to participate in group-oriented coping responses over time as their experiences with stigma increase. These questions need to be tested.

Avoidance/Disengagement

In contrast to coping assertively through activism, stigmatizing encounters may lead some obese individuals to avoid and withdraw from social interactions. Individuals with poor abilities or confidence in coping strategies may be more likely to engage in avoidance reactions (Swim, Cohen, & Hyers, 1998). Avoidance can involve psychological disengagement from situations in which stigma is likely to occur. Some work suggests that disengagement from social interactions over long periods of time may result in chronic withdrawal in multiple areas of living, which may in turn decrease personal drive, interpersonal skills, and ability to succeed (Major & Schmader, 1998).

One self-report study of obese adults reported that using avoidance responses to cope with stigma was correlated with higher levels of distress (Myers & Rosen, 1999). Emotional distress increases as a result of isolation and lack of social support, which are likely outcomes of avoidance. Hughes and Degher (1993) similarly found that obese persons, in response to stigma, commonly reported avoiding social situations such as going shopping or to the beach where they felt observed. Research is needed to explore the extent to which disengagement is used by obese individuals and whether it is a useful coping strategy to reduce stigma without increasing emotional suffering.

METHODOLOGICAL ISSUES
AND RESEARCH RECOMMENDATIONS

This review provides a brief summary of coping strategies that obese individuals may implement when responding to weight stigma. Existing work has largely been descriptive, and many studies have relied on small samples, used single measures of key variables, and examined few methods of coping. There has also been considerable variation in the levels of overweight among obese persons included in these studies.

The overall lack of research on coping with obesity stigma makes it difficult to draw conclusions about the use and effectiveness of various coping strategies. It is not known whether some methods of coping are specific to weight stigma or can also be used to cope with other life stressors or whether certain strategies are used more often than others. One important avenue of research will be to compare types of coping strategies used by obese people witj those adopted by other socially stigmatized groups. The utility of specific coping strategies in other areas (such as race or gender bias) may provide leads as to what methods of coping might be most beneficial for weight stigma.

It will also be important to determine whether certain coping strategies for dealing with weight stigma result in weight loss, as well as emotional well-being, and whether the types and frequency of coping strategies used by obese individuals change with different weight categories. Table 17.1 outlines research questions on these issues that we believe are important to help move this field of study forward.

SUGGESTIONS FOR HEALTH CARE PROFESSIONALS

The research described in this chapter suggests some possible ways that clinicians and other professionals might help obese individuals who are trying to cope with stigma. It may be important to help obese individuals to obtain social support and acceptance through larger group membership, to conceptualize their stigmatized identity in ways that enhance social functioning and confidence to succeed, to foster their self-esteem and protection from harmful effects of stigma without disengaging from important areas of living, and to effectively and appropriately assert their rights when confronting perpetrators of stigma.

TABLE 17.1. Needed Areas of Research to Increase Understanding on Coping Strategies for Weight Stigma

Area of study	Specific research topic
Measurement of coping	• Definition of measurement criteria for "effective" coping strategies for weight stigma • Identification of adaptive versus maladaptive outcomes of stigma coping strategies • Development of appropriate measurement of coping strategies and their impact • Identification of multiple methods for assessing coping strategies • Distinctions between situation-specific and more global coping strategies
Stigma topics	• Relationship between frequency of stigma experiences and choice of coping strategies • Usefulness of various coping strategies in reducing future weight stigma • Stigmatizing experiences that require the most frequent use of coping strategies • Preferences for use of certain coping strategies in various stigmatizing situations • Impact of coping efforts to deal with stigma on reactions and perceptions from others
Individual characteristics	• Impact of gender on frequency and types of coping strategies used by obese persons • Relationship between age of onset of obesity and use and success of coping strategies • Association between level of obesity and frequency and types of coping tools used • Impact of self-esteem on coping strategies used by obese individuals • Relationship between personality characteristics and choice of coping strategies • Association between perceptions of responsibility for weight and coping responses • Impact of social group membership on coping strategies used by obese individuals
Clinical/ treatment issues	• Impact of coping efforts to deal with stigma on weigh-loss outcomes and eating behaviors • Impact of stigma experiences and coping efforts on decisions to obtain bariatric surgery • Relationship between the use and frequency of coping strategies and emotional well-being • Usefulness of addressing stigma as a component of therapy/treatment for weight loss • Relationship between dieting/weight-loss history and use of particular coping strategies • Impact of current dieting status on responses to stigmatizing situations • Association between binge eating and coping methods used by obese persons • Relationship between medical status (e.g., comorbid conditions) and coping tools used • Impact of current psychological functioning on use/effectiveness of coping strategies

Many of the coping strategies highlighted in this chapter could be integrated as components of self-help interventions. Providing individuals with information about different coping strategies available to them, as well as self-assessment tools to help identify which strategies may best match their personalities and stigmatizing experiences, would be an excellent first step in these efforts. For example, individuals wishing to increase self-esteem might be directed to information on self-protection coping strategies, whereas those who want to address ongoing stigma from family members might seek guidance from verbal confrontation strategies. It would also be useful to provide individuals with self-assessment tools to monitor whether their chosen coping strategies are leading to beneficial and measurable changes (e.g., increased self-esteem, decreased frequency of stigma experienced). As part of these efforts, it would be important to consider variables that may influence coping skills of clients, such as age, competency, psychosocial resources, and interaction styles (Beuf, 1990; Puhl & Brownell, 2003).

Although we cannot yet predict the relative impact of different coping approaches for dealing with weight stigma, it seems worthwhile to at least increase awareness among obese clients that different tools for coping are available to them. Sobal (1991) has outlined a framework for clinicians to address weight stigma with clients, which may also have applicability in guiding self-help interventions. The model has four components, including *recognition* (developing insight and understanding of stigma), *readiness* (anticipating and preparing for stigmatizing events through cognitive and role-play rehearsals), *reaction* (short-term and long-term coping resources), and *repair* (repair and recovery from problems resulting from stigma events). The potential applicability of this model to guide clinicians in a range of health care settings is promising, as is its potential utility for educating clients in a self-help format. However, systematic testing of this model is needed to establish its effectiveness in helping obese clients successfully cope with stigma.

Only one published treatment study (to our knowledge) has specifically targeted ways of coping with weight stigma in psychotherapy for obese clients (Robinson & Bacon, 1996). This study involved a short-term psychological treatment program for obese women, which aimed to improve their self-esteem and physical activity and to decrease depression and fat-phobic attitudes. The stigma component of this program included discussing the origins of stereotypes toward obese people, decreasing self-blame by counteracting bias toward obesity, challenging negative attitudes, and increasing assertiveness when confronted with prejudice. Participants improved on all measures at the end of treatment, including lower levels of depression and fat phobia, fewer restrictions in daily activities, and higher self-esteem. This study suggests that including components in therapy or treatment programs that address ways of coping with weight stigma may have important benefits for overweight participants. Controlled treatment studies of this kind are needed.

CONCLUSIONS

A variety of responses are available to help individuals cope with the stigma of obesity. There has been inadequate attention to this area and weaknesses in methods of existing work, but a number of promising directions for future work can be identified. We have summarized research questions to guide these efforts and to help fill key gaps in knowledge. Because coping with weight stigma is a new and understudied topic, focused efforts must examine both empirical and conceptual avenues of research and explore multiple methods of coping among obese persons and other stigmatized groups so that an accurate understanding of this problem can be achieved and effective coping tools can be disseminated.

Although obesity remains prevalent, widespread, and difficult to treat, strategies for dealing with weight stigma might one day find their place alongside weight and medical management strategies in the overall effort to protect health and well-being. It is important, therefore, to foster research on coping with bias, but even more so to change social conditions that create bias to befin with.

REFERENCES

Adams, G. R., Hicken, M., & Saliehi, M. (1988). Socialization of the physical attractiveness stereotype: Parental expectations and verbal behaviors. *International Journal of Psychology, 23,* 137–149.

Beuf, A. H. (1990). *Beauty is the beast: Appearance-impaired children in America.* Philadelphia: University of Pennsylvania Press.

Bordieri, J. E., Drehmer, D. E., & Taylor, D. W. (1997). Work-life for employees with disabilities: Recommendations for promotion. *Rehabilitation Counseling Bulletin, 40,* 181–191.

Canning, H., & Mayer, J. (1966). Obesity: Its possible effect on college acceptance. *New England Journal of Medicine, 275,* 1172–1174.

Carpenter, K. M., Hasin, D. S., Allison, D. B., & Faith, M. S. (2000). Relationships between obesity and DSM-IV major depressive disorder, suicide ideation, and suicide attempts: Results from a general population study. *American Journal of Public Health, 90,* 251–257.

Cramer, P., & Steinwert, T. (1998). Thin is good, fat is bad: How early does it begin? *Journal of Applied Developmental Psychology, 19,* 429–451.

Crandall, C. S. (1994). Prejudice against fat people: Ideology and self-interest. *Journal of Personality and Social Psychology, 66,* 882–894.

Crandall, C. S. (1995). Do parents discriminate against their heavyweight daughters? *Personality and Social Psychology Bulletin, 21,* 724–735.

Crandall, C. S., & Cohen, C. (1994). The personality of the stigmatizer: Cultural world view, conventionalism, and self-esteem. *Journal of Research in Personality, 28*, 461–480.

Crandall, C. S., Tsang, J., Harvey, R. D., & Britt, T. W. (2000). Group identity-based protective strategies: The stigma of race, gender, and garlic. *European Journal of Social Psychology, 30*, 355–381.

Crocker, J. (1999). Social stigma and self-esteem: Situational construction of self-worth. *Journal of Experimental Social Psychology, 35*, 89–107.

Crocker, J., Cornwell, B., & Major, B. (1993). The stigma of overweight: Affective consequences and attributional ambiguity. *Journal of Personality and Social Psychology, 64*, 60–70.

Crocker, J., & Major, B. (1989). Social stigma and self-esteem: The self-protective properties of stigma. *Psychological Review, 96*, 608–630.

Crocker, J., Thompson, L. L., McGraw, K. M., & Ingerman, C. (1987). Downward comparison, prejudice, and evaluation of others: Effects of self-esteem and threat. *Journal of Personality and Social Psychology, 52*, 907–916.

Davis-Coelho, K., Waltz, J., & Davis-Coelho, B. (2000). Awareness and prevention of bias against fat clients in psychotherapy. *Professional Psychology: Research and Practice, 31*, 682–684.

Deaux, K., & Ethier, K. A. (1998). Negotiating social identity. In J. K. Swim & C. Stangor (Eds.), *Prejudice: The target's perspective* (pp. 301–323). San Diego: Academic Press.

Degher, D., & Hughes, G. (1999). The adoption and management of a "fat" identity. In J. Sobal & D. Maurer (Eds.), *Interpreting weight: The social management of fatness and thinness* (pp. 11–27). New York: Aldine de Gruyter.

Eaton, D. K., Lowry, R., Brener, E., Galuska, D. A., & Crosby, A. E. (2005). Associations of body mass index and perceived weight with suicide ideation and suicide attempts among U.S. high school students. *Archives of Pediatrics and Adolescent Medicine, 159*, 513–519.

Fontaine, K. R., Faith, M. S., Allison, D. B., & Cheskin, L. J. (1998). Body weight and health care among women in the general population. *Archives of Family Medicine, 7*, 381–384.

Fuller, M. L., & Groce, S. B. (1991). Obese women's responses to appearance norms. *Free Inquiry in Creative Sociology, 19*, 167–174.

Galuska, D. A., Will, J. C., Serdula, M. K., & Ford, E. S. (1999). Are health care professional advising obese patients to lose weight? *Journal of the American Medical Association, 282*, 1576–1578.

Greenberg, B. S., Eastin, M., Hofshire, L., Lachlan, K., & Brownell, K. D. (2003). Portrayals of overweight and obese individuals on commercial television. *American Journal of Public Health, 93*, 1342–1348.

Guyll, M., Matthews, K. A., & Bromberger, J. T. (2001). Discrimination and unfair treatment: Relationship to cardiovascular reactivity among African American and European American women. *Health Psychology, 20*, 315–325.

Hughes, G., & Degher, D. (1993). Coping with a deviant identity. *Deviant Behavior, 14*, 297–315.

Joanisse, L., & Synnott, A. (1999). Fighting back: Reactions and resistance to the stigma of obesity. In J. Sobal & D. Maurer (Eds.), *Interpreting weight: The social management of fatness and thinness* (pp. 49–70). New York.

Kristeller, J. L., & Hoerr, R. A. (1997). Physician attitudes toward managing obesity: Differences among six specialty groups. *Preventive Medicine, 26*, 542–549.

Latner, J. D., Stunkard, A. J., Wilson, G. T., Jackson, M. L., & Stunkard, A. J. (in press). The perceived effectiveness of continiung care and group support in the long-term self-help treatment of obesity. *Obesity Research, 14*, 404–471.

Levy, A. J. (1993). Stigma management: A new clinical service. *Families in Society, 74*, 226–231.

Maddox, G. L., & Liederman, V. (1969). Overweight as a social disability with medical implications. *Journal of Medical Education, 44,* 214–220.

Major, B., & Schmader, T. (1998). Coping with stigma through psychological disengagement. In J. K. Swim & C. Stangor (Eds.), *Prejudice: The target's perspective* (pp. 219–241). San Diego: Academic Press.

Maroney, D., & Golub, S. (1992). Nurses' attitudes toward obese persons and certain ethnic groups. *Perceptual and Motor Skills, 75,* 387–391.

Miller, C. T., & Major, B. (2000). Coping with stigma and prejudice. In T. F. Heatherton, R. E. Kleck, M. R. Hebl, & J. G. Hull (Eds.), *The social psychology of stigma* (pp. 243–272). New York: Guilford Press

Miller, C. T., & Myers, A. M. (1998). Compensating for prejudice: How heavyweight people (and others) control outcomes despite prejudice. In J. K. Swim & C. Stangor (Eds.), *Prejudice: The target's perspective* (pp. 191–218). San Diego: Academic Press

Miller, C. T., Rothblum, E. D., Felicio, D., & Brand, P. (1995). Compensating for stigma: Obese and nonobese women's reactions to being visible. *Personality and Social Psychology Bulletin, 21,* 1093–1106.

Myers, A., & Rosen, J. C. (1999). Obesity stigmatization and coping: Relation to mental health symptoms, body image, and self-esteem. *International Journal of Obesity, 23,* 221–230.

Neumark-Sztainer, D., Story, M., & Faibisch, L. (1998). Perceived stigmatization among overweight African-American and Caucasian adolescent girls. *Journal of Adolescent Health, 23,* 264–270.

Olson, C. L., Schumaker, H. D., & Yawn, B. P. (1994). Overweight women delay medical care. *Archives of Family Medicine, 3,* 888–892.

Pagan, J. A., & Davila, A. (1997). Obesity, occupational attainment, and earnings. *Social Science Quarterly, 78,* 756–770.

Paul, R. J., & Townsend, J. B. (1995). Shape up or ship out? Employment discrimination against the overweight. *Employee Responsibilities and Rights Journal, 8,* 133–145.

Peace, K., Dyne, J., Russell, G., & Stewart, R. (1989). Psychological effects of gastric restriction surgery for morbid obesity. *New Zealand Medical Journal, 102,* 76–78.

Price, J. H., Desmond, S. M., Krol, R. A., Snyder, F. F., & O'Connell, J. K. (1987). Family practice physicians' beliefs, attitudes, and practices regarding obesity. *American Journal of Preventive Medicine, 3,* 339–45.

Puhl, R., & Brownell, K. D. (2001). Obesity, bias, and discrimination. *Obesity Research, 8,* 788–805.

Puhl, R., & Brownell, K. D. (2003). Ways of coping with obesity stigma: Review and conceptual analysis. *Eating Behaviors, 4,* 53–78.

Puhl, R. M., Henderson, K. E., & Brownell, K. D. (2005). Social consequences of obesity. In P. Kopelman, I. Caterson, & W. Dietz (Eds.), *Clinical obesity and related metabolic disease in adults and children.* Malden, MA: Blackwell.

Quinn, D. M., & Crocker, J. (1998). Vulnerability to the affective consequences of the stigma of overweight. In J. K. Swim & C. Stangor (Eds.), *Prejudice: The target's perspective* (pp. 125–143). San Diego: Academic Press.

Rand, C. S., & MacGregor, A. M. (1990). Morbidly obese patients' perceptions of social discrimination before and after surgery for obesity. *Southern Medical Journal, 83,* 1390–1395.

Register, C. A., & Williams, D. R. (1990). Wage effects of obesity among young workers. *Social Science Quarterly, 71,* 130–141.

Robinson, B. E., & Bacon, J. G. (1996). The "if only I were thin . . . " treatment program: Decreasing the stigmatizing effects of fatness. *Professional Psychology: Research and Practice, 27,* 175–183.

Roehling, M. V. (1999). Weight-based discrimination in employment: Psychological and legal aspects. *Personnel Psychology, 52,* 969–1017.

Rothblum, E. D., Brand, P. A., Miller, C. T., & Oetjen, H. A. (1990). The relationship between obesity, employment discrimination, and employment-related victimization. *Journal of Vocational Behavior, 37*, 251–266.

Siegal, K., Lune, H., & Meyer, I. H. (1998). Stigma management among gay/bisexual men with HIV/AIDS. *Qualitative Sociology, 21*, 3–24.

Sobal, J. (1991). Obesity and nutritional sociology: A model of coping with the stigma of obesity. *Clinical Sociology Review, 90*, 125–141.

Snyder, M., & Haugen, J. A. (1995). Why does behavioral confirmation occur? A functional perspective on the role of the target. *Personality and Social Psychology Bulletin, 21*, 963–974.

Swim, J. K., Cohen, L. L., & Hyers, L. L. (1998). Experience everyday prejudice and discrimination. In J. K. Swim & C. Stangor (Eds.), *Prejudice: The target's perspective* (pp. 37–59). San Diego: Academic Press.

Taub, D. E., Blinde, E. M., & Greer, K. R. (1999). Stigma management through participation in sport and physical activity: Experiences of male college students with physical disabilities. *Human Relations, 52*, 1469–1483.

Taylor, S. E., Buunk, B. P., & Aspinwall, L. G. (1990). Social comparison, stress, and coping. *Personality and Social Psychology Bulletin, 16*, 74–89.

Teachman, B., Gapinski, K., & Brownell, K. D. (2001, February). *Stigma of obesity: Implicit attitudes and stereotypes.* Poster presented at the meeting of the Society for Personality and Social Psychology, San Antonio, TX.

Teachman, B. A., & Brownell, K. D. (2001). Implicit anti-fat bias among health professionals: Is anyone immune? *International Journal of Obesity, 25*, 1525–1531.

Weiler, K., & Helmes, L. B. (1993). Responsibilities of nursing education: The lessons of Russel v. Salve Regina. *Journal of Professional Nursing, 9*, 131–138.

Wiese, H. J., Wilson, J. F., Jones, R. A., & Neises, M. (1992). Obesity stigma reduction in medical students. *International Journal of Obesity and Related Metabolic Disorders, 16*, 859–868.

Index

Abs Diet, evaluation of, 48–49
Action stage of change, physical activity and, 61, 62t, 65t
Addiction, *Overcoming Binge Eating* (Fairburn, 1995) and, 107
Adiposity rebound, 275
Aim for a Healthy Weight website, 143–144
American Academy of Pediatrics, childhood obesity prevention and, 283t
American College of Sports Medicine (ACSM) recommendations regarding physical activity, 57
Amino acids, protein and, 337
Anorexia nervosa
  body image and, 118, 133
  Internet-based interventions and, 152
Antidepressants
  binge-eating disorder and, 75
  bulimia nervosa and, 111–112, 113, 114
  night eating syndrome and, 321–322
Anxiety disorders, night eating syndrome and, 311
Appearance assumptions, *The Body Image Workbook* (Cash, 1997), 122
Appetite. *see also* Appetite-focused cognitive-behavioral therapy for binge eating
  binge eating and, 325–326, 327–328
  self-monitoring of, 332–335, 333f
Appetite-focused cognitive-behavioral therapy for binge eating, 325–327. *see also* Cognitive-behavioral therapy
  components of, 329–330
  overview, 330–340, 331f, 333f, 339t, 342
  self-help and, 340–342

Assertiveness, *Getting Better Bit(e) by Bit(e)* (Schmidt and Treasure, 1993) and, 96
At-risk children
  assessing parents and caregivers of, 272–274, 273f, 274f
  defining, 266–272, 268f, 269f
Atkins for Life diet, evaluation of, 44–46
Attachment, guided group support and, 218
Automatic thoughts
  binge eating and, 329–330
  Getting Better Bit(e) by Bit(e) (Schmidt and Treasure, 1993) and, 96
  night eating syndrome and, 319–320
Avoidance coping strategy, 355–356

B

Behavior change strategies, childhood obesity prevention and, 280–282
Behavior modification strategies
  maintaining weight loss and, 31
  Trevose Behavior Modification Program (TBMP), 232–233
Behavioral factors in SCT, physical activity and, 58, 59f
Behavioral interventions
  binge eating and, 329–330
  childhood obesity prevention and, 275–280, 278t, 279t, 280–282
  dietary intervention, 253–255
  goal-setting and, 251–253
  long-term effects of, 207–213, 209t–211t
  for minority populations, 258–260
  motivation and, 257–258

Behavioral interventions (*continued*)
    overview, 206, 243–244, 248–249, 260
    physical activity and, 255–257
    problem solving and, 250–251
    self-monitoring and, 244–248, 253–
        254, 256–257
    social support and, 249–250
    theoretical foundation of, 244
Behavioral Risk Factor Surveillance
        System (BRFSS), 56–57
Behavioral weight loss
    binge-eating disorder and, 75
    overview, 223–224
Behaviors during maintenance. *see also*
        Maintaining weight loss
    calorie consumption and, 23, 24t, 25t
    in dieters in the general population, 10
    in National Weight Control Registry
        (NWCR), 7
Behaviors during weight loss. *see also*
        Weight loss
    calorie consumption and, 22–23, 24t,
        25t
    in general population, 8–9
    in National Weight Control Registry
        (NWCR), 6–7
Behaviors, *The Body Image Workbook*
        (Cash, 1997) and, 123
Beverage consumption
    Atkins for Life diet and, 45–46
    childhood obesity prevention and, 279
    creating a healthy food environment
        and, 296
    dietary guidelines regarding, 27–28, 30
Bibliotherapy
    binge-eating disorder and, 77
    body-image disturbances and, 120–123
    The Body Image Workbook (Cash,
        1997) and, 120–123
    bulimia nervosa and, 94–100, 100–
        106, 106–112
    *Bulimia Nervosa and Binge-Eating: A
        Guide to Recovery* (Cooper, 1993,
        1995) and, 100–106
    effectiveness of, 12–15
    Getting Better Bit(e) by Bit(e) (Schmidt
        and Treasure, 1993) and, 94–100
    Overcoming Binge Eating (Fairburn,
        1995) and, 106–112
Biggest Loser Club, as an Internet-based
        intervention, 156t
Binge eating. *see also* Binge-eating
        disorder
    appetite-focused model of, 330–332,
        331f

bulimia nervosa and, 92–93
computer-assisted intervention for,
    166–174
Getting Better Bit(e) by Bit(e) (Schmidt
    and Treasure, 1993) and, 95
Internet-based interventions and, 151
Overcoming Binge Eating (Fairburn,
    1995) and, 109
role of appetite in, 327–328
Binge-eating disorder. *see also* Appetite-
        focused cognitive-behavioral
        therapy for binge eating; Binge
        eating
    appetite-focused model of, 330–332,
        331f
    comparing self-help treatment to
        pharmacotherapy, 83–85, 84f
    computer-assisted intervention for,
        166–174
    enhancing self-help treatment for, 82–
        83
    need for guided self-help treatments
        for, 75–76
    night eating syndrome and, 316
    nonspecialist delivery of guided self-
        help for, 80–82
    overview, 73–74, 85–86, 325–327
    role of appetite in, 327–328
    treatment literature for, 74–75
    treatment studies for, 76–80, 80f
    weight loss and, 85–86
Blood glucose levels
    benefits to losing weight and, 243
    carbohydrates and, 26, 338–340,
        339t
    glycemic index and, 29
    OPTIFAST and, 35
Blood pressure
    OPTIFAST and, 35
    physical activity and, 56
Body dysmorphic disorder, 118–119
Body for Life for Women, evaluation of,
        47–48
Body image. *see also* Body-image
        disturbances
    bulimia nervosa and, 113
    cognitive-behavioral therapy for, 120–
        123, 129–131
    development and processes of, 119–
        120
    Getting Better Bit(e) by Bit(e) (Schmidt
        and Treasure, 1993) and, 95–96
    Internet-based interventions for, 141–
        144, 144–152
    overview, 118–119, 134–135

self-help for, 127–129, 131–134, 131–134

treatment of childhood weight problems and, 292, 294–295

Body-image desensitization, body image and, 121–122

"Body Image Diary", 121

Body-image disturbances. *see also* Body image

cognitive-behavioral therapy for, 120–123, 124–126, 129–131

overview, 118–119, 134–135

self-help for, 127–129

treatment outcome research, 124–126

Body-image investment, 118, 128

Body-Image Therapy: A Program for Self-Directed Change (Cash, 1991), 124–125, 129

The Body Image Workbook (Cash, 1997), 120–123, 126

Body mass index

defining at-risk children for obesity and, 267–268, 268*f*, 269*f*

treatment of childhood weight problems and, 292–293

Bottle feeding, childhood obesity prevention and, 275–277

Breast feeding, childhood obesity prevention and, 275–277

Breathing exercises, night eating syndrome and, 316–317

Bulimia nervosa. *see also* Appetite-focused cognitive-behavioral therapy for binge eating

appetite-focused model of, 330–332, 331*f*

body image and, 118, 133

Bulimia Nervosa and Binge-Eating: A Guide to Recovery (Cooper, 1993, 1995) and, 94, 100–106

computer-assisted intervention for, 166–174

Getting Better Bit(e) by Bit(e) (Schmidt and Treasure, 1993) and, 94–100

Overcoming Binge Eating (Fairburn, 1995) and, 94, 106–112

overview, 92–94, 325–327

role of appetite in, 327–328

self-help for, 112–115

Bulimia Nervosa and Binge-Eating: A Guide to Recovery (Cooper, 1993, 1995)

empirical studies of, 104–106

overview, 94, 100–106

Bulimic Investigatory Test (BITE), 94

Bulletin boards, online, obesity treatment and, 153, 156, 160

C

Calorie consumption

10–characteristic method of evaluating a diet and, 22–23, 22*t*, 24*t*, 25*t*

childhood obesity prevention and, 276–277

creating a healthy food environment and, 298, 298*t*

dietary intervention and, 253–254

in dieters in the general population, 8–9

in dieters in the National Weight Control Registry (NWCR), 7

fluids and, 27–28

low-calorie diets, 27–28, 193–194, 195

medically supervised programs, 188–189

night eating syndrome and, 311, 315–316

in popular diets, 36*f*

very-low calorie diets, 188–189, 191, 193–194, 195

Cancer, as a comorbidity of obesity, 30

Carbohydrates

appetite-focused model and, 338–340, 339*t*

Atkins for Life diet and, 44

Curves and, 46–47

dietary guidelines regarding, 26, 28–29

Cardiac changes, low-calorie diets and, 25*t*

Cardiovascular disease, as a comorbidity of obesity, 30

Center for Disease Control (CDC) recommendations, regarding physical activity, 57

Change, processes of

assessing parents and caregivers of at-risk children and, 272–274, 273*f*, 274*f*

physical activity and, 60–63, 62*t*, 63*f*

Characteristics of self-guided dieters, in National Weight Control Registry (NWCR), 5–6

Childhood experiences, *Getting Better Bit(e) by Bit(e)* (Schmidt and Treasure, 1993) and, 96

Childhood obesity prevention. *see also*
    Prevention of obesity
  assessing parents and caregivers of at-
    risk children, 272–274, 273*f*, 274*f*
  behavior change strategies, 280–282
  critical periods for, 275
  defining at-risk children for, 266–272,
    268*f*, 269*f*
  overview, 265–266, 282–284, 282*f*,
    283*f*
  target behaviors for, 275–280, 278*t*,
    279*t*
Childhood treatment of weight problems
  challenges for parents, 290–291
  creating a healthy food environment
    and, 296–301, 298*t*
  creating a supportive environment and,
    294–295
  goal-setting and, 291–294
  overview, 289–290, 304
  physical activity and, 301–304
  weight bias and, 295–296
Children at-risk for obesity. *see also*
    Childhood obesity prevention;
    Childhood treatment of weight
    problems
  assessing parents and caregivers of,
    272–274, 273*f*, 274*f*
  defining, 266–272, 268*f*, 269*f*
Cholesterol levels, OPTIFAST and, 35
Clothing preference, treatment of
    childhood weight problems and,
    294–295
Cognitive-behavioral therapy. *see also*
    Appetite-focused cognitive
    behavioral therapy for binge eating
  binge-eating disorder and, 74–87, 325
  body image and, 120–123, 124–126,
    127–129, 129–131, 131–134, 134–
    135
  bulimia nervosa and, 93–94, 99, 114
  computer-assisted, 167
  Internet-based interventions and, 146
  for night eating syndrome, 312–322,
    313*f*, 314*t*, 315*f*, 316*f*
Cognitive errors, *The Body Image
    Workbook* (Cash, 1997) and, 122–
    123
Cognitive restructuring
  body image and, 133
  The Body Image Workbook (Cash,
    1997) and, 122–123
  bulimia nervosa and, 113
  maintaining weight loss and, 31
Cohesion, group, 214–215, 217

Colon cancer, physical activity and, 56
Commercial weight loss programs
  costs of, 184*t*
  effectiveness of, 11–12
  Internet-based interventions and, 156*t*,
    158, 195–197
  medically supervised programs, 182*t*,
    184*t*, 188–195
  nonmedical commercial programs,
    181–188, 182*t*, 184*t*
  organized self-help programs, 197–
    199
  overview, 179–181, 181*t*, 199–200
Commonsense test, 10–characteristic
    method of evaluating a diet and,
    33
Compensation coping strategy, 353–354
Compensatory metabolic responses,
    maintaining weight loss and, 225
Compliance with self-help programs,
    Getting Better Bit(e) by Bit(e)
    (Schmidt and Treasure, 1993) and,
    97–98
Composition of macronutrients and
    micronutrients in a diet
  10–characteristic method of evaluating
    a diet and, 22*t*, 25–30
  Abs Diet and, 48
  Atkins for Life diet and, 45–46
  French Women Don't Get Fat diet and,
    49
  during maintenance phase, 28–30
  OPTIFAST and, 35
  SlimFast diet and, 38
  South Beach Diet and, 39
  Ultimate Weight Solution diet and, 42
  during weight-loss phase, 25–28
Computer-assisted self-help. *see also*
    Internet-based interventions
  for bulimia nervosa and binge eating,
    166–174
  obesity treatment and, 153
  overview, 139, 166–167, 172–174
Confirmation coping strategy, weight
    bias and, 350–351
Confrontation coping strategy, 354
Contemplation stage of change, physical
    activity and, 61, 62*t*, 65*t*
Continuing care. *see also* Maintaining
    weight loss; Posttreatment weight
    gain; Relapse prevention
  costs of, 235
  overview, 226–230, 235–236
  Trevose Behavior Modification
    Program (TBMP), 230–235

Coping skills
 night eating syndrome and, 316–317
 research recommendations, 356
 weight bias and, 349–356, 357t, 358–359
Coronary heart disease, physical activity and, 56
Cost of a diet
 10–characteristic method of evaluating a diet and, 22t, 32–33
 Abs Diet and, 48
 French Women Don't Get Fat diet and, 49
 OPTIFAST and, 36, 38
 SlimFast diet and, 38
Cross-cultural considerations
 behavioral interventions and, 258–260
 defining at-risk children for obesity and, 270–272
 Internet-based interventions and, 147
 maintaining weight loss and, 227–229
Curves diet, evaluation of, 46–47
Customization of a weight-loss plan, 10–characteristic method of evaluating a diet and, 22t, 33

D

Dehydration
 carbohydrates and, 26
 low-calorie diets and, 25t
 South Beach Diet and, 41
 Ultimate Weight Solution diet and, 42
Depression
 benefits to losing weight and, 243
 body image and, 119
 night eating syndrome and, 311
 treatment of childhood weight problems and, 292
 weight bias and, 348
Diabetes Prevention Program
 clinical trial done by, 11–12
 minority populations and, 258–259
 overview, 249
 problem solving and, 250–251
 relapse and, 223–224
Diabetes, type 2
 benefits to losing weight and, 243
 as a comorbidity of obesity, 30
 OPTIFAST and, 35
 physical activity and, 56
Diagnostic and Statistical Manual of Mental Disorders (DSM-IV)
 binge-eating disorder and, 73–74
 bulimia nervosa, 92

Diagnostic criteria, binge-eating disorder and, 74
Diet pills, in dieters in the general population, 9
Diet supplements, in dieters in the general population, 9
Dietary behavior, self-monitoring of, 245–247
Dietary guidelines
 10–characteristic method of evaluating a diet and, 22t, 33
 comparing popular diets using, 40f
 composition of macronutrients and micronutrients in a diet and, 25–26
 Internet-based interventions and, 144
 OPTIFAST and, 35
Dietary Guidelines for Americans (U.S. Department of Health and Human Services and U.S. Department of Agriculture, 2005)
 carbohydrates and, 28
 composition of macronutrients and micronutrients in a diet and, 25–26
 on fiber, 27
 maintaining weight loss and, 31
Dietary intervention, 253–255
Dieting
 binge eating and, 325–326
 bulimia nervosa and, 95
 Bulimia Nervosa and Binge-Eating: A Guide to Recovery (Cooper, 1993, 1995) and, 103–104
 Overcoming Binge Eating (Fairburn, 1995) and, 107, 109–110
Digestion, carbohydrates and, 338
Discrimination, weight bias and, 348–349
Disengagement coping strategy, 355–356
Diuretics use, Getting Better Bit(e) by Bit(e) (Schmidt and Treasure, 1993) and, 95
Duration of self-guided diets, 10
Dyslipidemia
 as a comorbidity of obesity, 30
 physical activity and, 56

E

E-mail support
 obesity treatment and, 153, 160
 physical activity and, 67–68
Eating disorders
 body image and, 118, 131
 body-shape disturbances and, 145
 Internet-based interventions and, 147–148

Eating Disorders Inventory, 328
eDiets.com
    costs of, 184t, 196
    overview, 158, 182t, 195–196
Electrolyte imbalances, low-calorie diets
    and, 25t
Emotional support, physical activity and, 60
Empowerment, maintaining weight loss
    and, 229
Environmental factors
    contributors to posttreatment weight
        gain and, 207
    healthy food environment as a part of,
        296–301, 298t
    Internet-based interventions and, 157
    physical activity and, 58, 59f, 60
    posttreatment weight gain and, 224–226
    treatment of childhood weight
        problems and, 290, 294–295
Essential fatty acids, dietary guidelines
    regarding, 26
Ethnicity, defining at-risk children for
    obesity and, 270–272
Evaluating a diet
    10–characteristic method of, 21–33,
        22t, 24t, 25t
    overview, 50
    of popular diets, 34–50, 36f, 37t, 40t
Evolutionary perspective, toxic
    environment, 224
Exercise. see Physical activity
Expert-system approach, physical activity
    and, 64–66
Exposure and response prevention, The
    Body Image Workbook (Cash,
    1997), 123
Exposure to food, childhood obesity
    prevention and, 280–281
Expressive writing, body image and,
    133–134

F

Family. see also Childhood treatment of
    weight problems
    Getting Better Bit(e) by Bit(e) (Schmidt
        and Treasure, 1993) and, 97
    physical activity and, 303
Family-based treatment, 157. see also
    Childhood treatment of weight
    problems
Fast-food consumption
    childhood obesity prevention and,
        279–280
    creating a healthy food environment
        and, 300

Fasting
    caloric levels of, 24t, 25t
    in dieters in the general population, 9
Fat, dietary guidelines regarding, 26, 29
Fear tactics, physical activity and, 58
Feedback, online, 149–150
Feeding practices, childhood obesity
    prevention and, 275–277, 278t
Fertility, as a comorbidity of obesity,
    30
Fiber
    carbohydrates and, 28
    dietary guidelines regarding, 27, 29
Fluids
    Atkins for Life diet and, 45–46
    childhood obesity prevention and, 279
    creating a healthy food environment
        and, 296
    dietary guidelines regarding, 27–28, 30
Food avoidance, Overcoming Binge
    Eating (Fairburn, 1995), 109–110
Food choices, appetite-focused, 335–336
Food environment, treatment of
    childhood weight problems and,
    296–301, 298t
Food restriction
    appetite-focused, 335–336
    childhood obesity prevention and,
        276–277, 278t
    creating a healthy food environment
        and, 297–298
Food volume, appetite-focused, 336–337
French Women Don't Get Fat diet,
    evaluation of, 49–50

G

Gallbladder disease, as a comorbidity of
    obesity, 30
Gastric capacity, binge eating and, 328
Genetic factors, treatment of childhood
    weight problems and, 291
Getting Better Bit(e) by Bit(e) (Schmidt
    and Treasure, 1993)
    empirical studies of, 98–100
    overview, 94–100
Glucogenic amino acids, carbohydrates
    and, 26
Gluconeogenesis, carbohydrates and, 26
Glucose intolerance, as a comorbidity of
    obesity, 30
Glycemic index. see also Blood glucose
    levels
    carbohydrates and, 339, 339t
    overview, 29

Glycemic load, 339–340, 339t. see also
    Blood glucose levels
Glycogen, fluids and, 27–28
Goal-setting
    behavioral interventions and, 251–253
    The Body Image Workbook (Cash,
        1997) and, 121
    guided group support and, 217
    treatment of childhood weight
        problems and, 291–294
Group cohesion, 214–215, 217
Group goals, 217
Group self-help. see also Guided group
        support
    overview, 177
    social support and, 249–250
    Trevose Behavior Modification
        Program (TBMP), 231–232
Group treatment programs, obesity
    treatment and, 152–153
Guidance, guided group support and, 218
Guided group support. see also Group
        self-help
    costs of, 212
    future directions in, 216–218
    lifestyle interventions for the
        management of obesity and, 206
    long-term effects of, 207–213, 209t–
        211t
    overview, 205, 218–219
    structure and function of, 213–216

H

Health behaviors, maintaining weight
    loss and, 225
Health benefits to losing weight
    maintaining weight loss and, 225
    overview, 243
    treatment of childhood weight
        problems and, 293
Health care, weight bias and, 347–348,
        356–359, 357t
Health Management Resources (HMR)
    costs of, 184t, 190
    overview, 182t, 189–191, 194–195
Health problems
    10–characteristic method of evaluating
        a diet and, 22t, 30
    maintaining weight loss and, 225
    Maker's Diet and, 43
    OPTIFAST and, 35–36
    Overcoming Binge Eating (Fairburn,
        1995) and, 107
    weight bias and, 348

Herbs, Maker's Diet and, 44
Historical influences to body image, 119
Hunger cues. see also Appetite-focused
        cognitive behavioral therapy for
        binge eating
    binge eating and, 325–326
    self-monitoring of, 332–335, 333f
Hypercholesterolemia, OPTIFAST and,
        35
Hyperinsulinemia, as a comorbidity of
        obesity, 30
Hypertension
    as a comorbidity of obesity, 30
    OPTIFAST and, 35
Hypoglycemia, physical activity and, 56

I

In vivo exposure and response
        prevention, The Body Image
        Workbook (Cash, 1997), 123
Inpatient treatment, bulimia nervosa and,
        114
Institute of Medicine (IOM), physical
        activity and, 57
Instrumental support, physical activity
        and, 60
Insulin resistance, physical activity and,
        56
Internal locus of control, maintaining
        weight loss and, 230
International Obesity Task Force (IOTF),
        treatment of childhood weight
        problems and, 290
Internet-based interventions. see also
        Computer-assisted self-help
    body image and, 133
    body-shape disturbances and, 144–
        152
    obesity treatment, 152–160, 154t–
        155t, 156t
    overview, 141–144, 160–162, 195–
        197
    physical activity and, 66–68
    Student Bodies program, 145–148
Interoceptive awareness, binge eating
        and, 328
Interpersonal experiences, body image
        and, 119
Interpersonal relationships, Getting
        Better Bit(e) by Bit(e) (Schmidt and
        Treasure, 1993) and, 97
Interventions, behavioral. see Behavioral
        interventions
Investment, body image and, 118, 128

J

Jenny Craig diet
   costs of, 184t, 186
   effectiveness of, 187–188
   as an Internet-based intervention, 156t,
      158
   overview, 182t, 185–186

K

Ketosis
   carbohydrates and, 26
   low-calorie diets and, 25t

L

LA Weight Loss
   costs of, 184t, 187
   effectiveness of, 187–188
   overview, 182t, 186–187
Laxatation
   carbohydrates and, 26
   fluids and, 27–28
Laxative use, Getting Better Bit(e) by
      Bit(e) (Schmidt and Treasure,
      1993) and, 95
Lean-body-mass decrease, low-calorie
      diets and, 25t
LEARN program
   compared to eDiets.com, 158, 196
   overview, 31
   treatment studies utilizing, 79
LEARN Program for Weight
      Management 2000 and
      Maintenance Survival Guide
      (Brownell, 2000)
   compared to eDiets.com, 158, 196
   overview, 31
   treatment studies utilizing, 79
Lifestyle interventions
   long-term effects of, 207–213, 209t–
      211t
   overview, 206, 223–224
Lifestyle physical activity (LPA), 301. see
      also Physical activity
Linear-growth decrease in children, low-
      calorie diets and, 25t
Long-term treatment, obesity treatment
      and, 152
Low-calorie diets. see also Calorie
      consumption
   fluids and, 27–28
   medically supervised programs,
      195
   Medifast/TSFL, 193–194

M

Maintaining weight loss. see also
      Continuing care; Posttreatment
      weight gain; Relapse prevention
   10–characteristic method of evaluating
      a diet and, 22t
   Atkins for Life diet and, 45
   behaviors related to, 7
   benefits to losing weight and, 244
   calorie consumption and, 23, 24t, 25t
   coexisting health problems and, 30
   composition of macronutrients and
      micronutrients in a diet and, 28–30
   contributors to posttreatment weight
      gain, 206–207
   in dieters in the general population, 10
   Health Management Resources (HMR)
      and, 189
   Internet-based interventions and, 158–
      160
   lifestyle interventions for the
      management of obesity and, 206
   long-term effects of guided group
      support and, 207–213, 209t–211t
   OPTIFAST and, 38
   overview, 31, 226–230
   South Beach Diet and, 39, 41
   toxic environment and, 225–226
   Trevose Behavior Modification
      Program (TBMP), 233–235
   Ultimate Weight Solution diet and, 42
Maintenance phase, behavioral
      interventions and, 248–249. see
      also Maintaining weight loss
Maintenance stage of change, physical
      activity and, 61, 62t, 64–65, 65t.
      see also Maintaining weight loss
Maker's Diet, evaluation of, 43–44
Meal patterns. see also Night eating
      syndrome
   behavioral interventions and, 254–
      255
   bulimia nervosa and, 113
Meal planning
   bulimia nervosa and, 113
   Bulimia Nervosa and Binge-Eating: A
      Guide to Recovery (Cooper, 1993,
      1995) and, 103
   Overcoming Binge Eating (Fairburn,
      1995) and, 109
Meal replacements
   behavioral interventions and, 254
   in dieters in the general population, 9
   effectiveness of, 15–16

Health Management Resources (HMR)
    and, 189
Medifast/TSFL and, 193–194
OPTIFAST, 34–36, 191
SlimFast, 38
Media images
    treatment of childhood weight
        problems and, 294–295
    weight bias and, 348
Medications
    binge-eating disorder and, 75
    bulimia nervosa and, 111–112, 113,
        114
    night eating syndrome and, 321–322
Medifast/TSFL
    costs of, 184t, 194
    overview, 182t, 193–195
Micronutrients, dietary guidelines
    regarding, 27
Minerals, Maker's Diet and, 44
Mood disorders, 311. see also
    Depression
Mortality risks, physical activity and, 56
Motivation
    behavioral interventions and, 257–258
    physical activity and, 257
    Trevose Behavior Modification
        Program (TBMP), 233–235
Motivational interviewing
    behavioral interventions and, 258
    Internet-based interventions and, 146
Multi-impulsive patients, 99–100
Multiple attempts at losing weight,
        characteristics of self-guided dieters
        in NWCR and, 6
Muscle dysmorphia, body image and,
        118–119

N

National Association to Advance Fat
        Acceptance (NAAFA), 352, 355
National Health Interview Survey, 9
National Heart, Lung, and Blood
        Institute's Aim for a Healthy
        Weight website, 143–144
National Task Force on the Prevention
        and Treatment of Obesity, night
        eating syndrome and, 316
National Weight Control Registry
        (NWCR)
    overview, 4
    self-guided dieters in, 4–8
Night Eating Assessment, 314–315,
        315f

Night eating syndrome
    definition of, 310–311
    overview, 319–320, 323
    pharmacotherapy and, 321–322
    prevalence of, 311
    self-help for, 317–322
    treatment of, 312–322, 313f, 314t,
        315f, 316f
Nutrient deficiencies
    low-calorie diets and, 25t
    treatment of childhood weight
        problems and, 293

O

Obesity
    binge-eating disorder and, 74, 75, 85–
        86
    body image and, 131
    contributors to posttreatment weight
        gain, 206–207
    Getting Better Bit(e) by Bit(e) (Schmidt
        and Treasure, 1993) and, 96
    guided group support and, 205
    Internet-based interventions and, 141–
        144, 152–160, 154t–155t, 156t
    lifestyle interventions for the
        management of, 206
Online interventions. see Internet-based
        interventions
Online support groups, 153, 156, 160.
    see also Internet-based
        interventions
OPTIFAST
    costs of, 184t, 192
    evaluation of, 34–36, 36f, 37f,
        38
    overview, 182t, 191–193, 194–
        195
Osteoarthritis, as a comorbidity of
        obesity, 30
Outcome expectancy, physical activity
        and, 59–60
Overcoming Binge Eating (Fairburn,
        1995)
    empirical studies of, 110–112
    overview, 77, 94, 106–112
    treatment studies utilizing, 79, 81,
        83
Overcoming Bulimia program
    overview, 167–169, 173
    patient's acceptance of, 170–171
Overeaters Anonymous (OA)
    costs of, 184t, 198
    overview, 182t, 198, 199

P

Personal factors in SCT, physical activity and, 58, 59f
Personality attributes, body image and, 119
Pharmacotherapy
binge-eating disorder and, 75–76, 83–85, 84f, 86
night eating syndrome and, 321–322
Physical abuse, *Getting Better Bit(e) by Bit(e)* (Schmidt and Treasure, 1993) and, 96
Physical activity
Abs Diet and, 49
behavioral interventions and, 255–257
Body for Life for Women and, 47–48
Curves and, 46–47
in dieters in the general population, 9
in dieters in the National Weight Control Registry (NWCR), 7
French Women Don't Get Fat diet and, 49
health benefits of, 56
maintaining weight loss and, 31
Maker's Diet and, 44
night eating syndrome and, 320–321
OPTIFAST and, 36
prevalence of, 56–57
promoting via self-help approaches, 57–63, 59f, 62t, 63f
relationship of to obesity, 55–56
self-monitoring of, 245–247
South Beach Diet and, 41
theory-based approaches to, 57–63, 59f, 62t, 63–68, 63–68, 63f, 65t, 68–69
treatment of childhood weight problems and, 301–304
Ultimate Weight Solution diet and, 42
Physical characteristics, body image and, 119
Physiological factors, maintaining weight loss and, 225
Polycystic ovarian disease, as a comorbidity of obesity, 30
Popular diets, evaluations of, 34–50, 36f, 37t, 40t
Portion sizes
appetite-focused, 336
creating a healthy food environment and, 298–299
Positive reinforcements
childhood obesity prevention and, 281–282

Trevose Behavior Modification Program (TBMP), 233–235
Posttreatment weight gain. *see also* Continuing care; Maintaining weight loss; Relapse prevention
contributors to, 206–207, 224–226
overview, 223–224, 226–230
Precontemplation stage of change, physical activity and, 61, 62t, 64, 65t
Prejudice, weight bias and, 348–349
Preparation stage of change, physical activity and, 61, 62t, 65t
Prevalence rates of those dieting
defining at-risk children for obesity and, 271–272
overview, 3–4
of self-guided dieting in the NWCR, 5
Prevention of obesity. *see also* Childhood obesity prevention
critical periods for, 275
Internet-based interventions and, 151–152, 157
target behaviors for, 275–280, 278t, 279t
Proanorexia websites, 152
Problem solving
behavioral interventions and, 250–251
bulimia nervosa and, 94–95
Bulimia Nervosa and Binge-Eating: A Guide to Recovery (Cooper, 1993, 1995) and, 103
Overcoming Binge Eating (Fairburn, 1995) and, 109
Progressive muscle relaxation, 312
Protein
appetite-focused model and, 337–338
dietary guidelines regarding, 26–27, 29
fluids and, 27–28
Proximal factors to body image, 119
Psychoeducation, body image and, 132–133
Psychotherapy
body image and, 129–131
bulimia nervosa and, 114
Pyramid guidelines. *see* Dietary guidelines

Q

Quality of life
benefits to losing weight and, 243
body image and, 119
weight bias and, 348–349

R

Rate of weight loss, 10–characteristic method of evaluating a diet and, 23

Readiness to change, assessing parents and caregivers of at-risk children and, 272–274, 273f, 274f

Recording of food amounts, in dieters in the general population, 9

Regaining lost weight. see also Continuing care; Maintaining weight loss; Relapse prevention
  contributors to, 206–207, 224–226
  overview, 223–224, 226–230

Reinforcements
  childhood obesity prevention and, 281–282
  Trevose Behavior Modification Program (TBMP), 233–235

Rejection, treatment of childhood weight problems and, 295–296

Relapse. see also Continuing care; Maintaining weight loss; Relapse prevention
  contributors to, 206–207, 224–226
  overview, 223–224, 226–230

Relapse prevention. see also Continuing care; Maintaining weight loss; Posttreatment weight gain
  Atkins for Life diet and, 45–46
  The Body Image Workbook (Cash, 1997) and, 123
  bulimia nervosa and, 113
  Getting Better Bit(e) by Bit(e) (Schmidt and Treasure, 1993) and, 96
  Internet-based interventions and, 158–160
  maintaining weight loss and, 31
  Maker's Diet and, 43
  night eating syndrome and, 317
  overview, 226–230
  physical activity and, 65
  South Beach Diet and, 41

Relaxation
  body image and, 121–122
  night eating syndrome and, 316–317

Remotivation, maintaining weight loss and, 31

Restrictive feeding practices
  appetite-focused, 335–336
  childhood obesity prevention and, 276–277, 278t
  creating a healthy food environment and, 297–298

Reward, self
  creating a healthy food environment and, 296–297
  motivation and, 257–258

Role modeling, childhood obesity prevention and, 281

S

SALUT project, 169–170

Satiety. see also Appetite-focused cognitive behavioral therapy for binge eating
  binge eating and, 325–326
  mechanisms that signal, 336–337
  self-monitoring of, 332–335, 333f

School-based intervention
  body image and, 148–152
  Internet-based interventions and, 157

School environment, creating a healthy food environment and, 300

Selective serotonin reuptake inhibitors, night eating syndrome and, 321–322. see also Antidepressants

Self-acceptance, weight bias and, 350–351

Self-Assertion for Women (Butler, 1992), Overcoming Binge Eating (Fairburn, 1995), 111

Self-awareness, night eating syndrome and, 316–317, 319–320

Self-defeating thoughts, Getting Better Bit(e) by Bit(e) (Schmidt and Treasure, 1993) and, 96

Self-destruction, Getting Better Bit(e) by Bit(e) (Schmidt and Treasure, 1993) and, 97

Self-efficacy
  guided group support and, 216
  maintaining weight loss and, 229
  physical activity and, 58–59
  toxic environment and, 224

Self-esteem
  body image and, 119
  maintaining weight loss and, 229
  self-protection coping strategy and, 352–353
  treatment of childhood weight problems and, 292
  weight bias and, 356–359, 357t

Self-evaluation, body image and, 118

Self-guided approaches to weight loss
  characteristics of, 5–6
  effectiveness of, 10–16
  in general population, 8–10

Self-guided approaches to weight loss
  (*continued*)
  in National Weight Control Registry
    (NWCR), 4–8
  overview, 3–4, 16–19
Self-monitoring
  of appetite, 332–335, 333*f*
  in behavioral interventions, 244–248
  body image and, 121, 132–133
  The Body Image Workbook (Cash,
    1997) and, 121
  *Bulimia Nervosa and Binge-Eating: A
    Guide to Recovery* (Cooper, 1993,
    1995) and, 102
  of dietary and exercise behavior, 245–
    247
  dietary intervention and, 253–254
  guided group support and, 218
  night eating syndrome and, 312–314,
    313*f*, 315–316
  Overcoming Binge Eating (Fairburn,
    1995) and, 108
  overview, 244–248
  physical activity and, 256–257
  of weight, 247–248
Self-protection, coping strategies and,
    352–353
Self-regulation
  breast feeding and, 275–277
  self-efficacy and, 59
Self-reliance, maintaining weight loss
    and, 229
Self-schema, body image and, 119–120
Self-worth, guided group support and,
    218
Set Your Body Free Body Image
    Program, 146
Sexual abuse, *Getting Better Bit(e) by
    Bit(e)* (Schmidt and Treasure,
    1993) and, 96, 97
Sexual functioning, body image and, 119
Shameful feelings about weight, Internet-
    based interventions and, 149
Shape concerns, Internet-based
    interventions for, 144–152
Shapeup.org, 158
Skipping meals, 9
Sleep apnea, as a comorbidity of obesity,
    30
Sleep hygiene, night eating syndrome
    and, 317, 320–321
SlimFast, evaluation of, 38
Social activism, 355
Social anxiety, body image and, 119
Social attraction to a group, 214, 215

Social-cognitive theory
  evidence for, 63–68, 65*t*
  physical activity and, 58–63, 59*f*, 62*t*,
    63–68, 65*t*, 69
Social integration of a group, 214, 215,
    218
Social provisions model, 218
Social support
  avoidance coping strategy and, 355–
    356
  behavioral interventions and, 249–250
  guided group support and, 215–216
  Internet-based interventions and, 160
  maintaining weight loss and, 229
  night eating syndrome and, 321
  obesity treatment and, 152–153
  physical activity and, 60, 64–65, 257
  Trevose Behavior Modification
    Program (TBMP), 231–232
Socialization, body image and, 119
Socioeconomic status, defining at-risk
    children for obesity and, 270–272
South Beach Diet
  evaluation of, 38–39, 41
  as an Internet-based intervention,
    156*t*
Sports, organized, treatment of childhood
    weight problems and, 303
Stereotypes
  coping strategies and, 349–356, 358–
    359
  self-protection coping strategy and,
    352–353
Stigma. *see also* Weight bias
  coping strategies and, 349–356
  health care and, 356–359, 357*t*
  online feedback and, 149–150
  overview, 347, 359
  research recommendations, 356
  treatment of childhood weight
    problems and, 293
Stomach capacity, binge eating and,
    328
Student Bodies program, 145–148
Substance use disorders, night eating
    syndrome and, 311
Success of self-guided diets, 10
Suicidality, 348
Supplements, vitamins and minerals. *see
    also* Vitamins
  in dieters in the general population, 9
  Maker's Diet and, 44
Support groups online, 153, 156, 160.
    see also Internet-based
    interventions

T

Take Off Pounds Sensibly (TOPS)
    costs of, 184t, 197
    overview, 182t, 197–198, 199
Task cohesion, 214, 215, 217
Teasing in childhood. *see also* Weight
        bias
    body image and, 142
    extent and impact of, 348
    treatment of childhood weight
        problems and, 295–296
Telephone contact
    effectiveness of, 14–15
    Health Management Resources (HMR)
        and, 189
    physical activity and, 66
Television viewing
    childhood obesity prevention and,
        277–278, 278t, 279t
    night eating syndrome and, 321
    self-monitoring of by children, 274f
10–characteristic method of evaluating a
        diet
    overview, 21–33, 22t, 24t, 25t, 50
    using to evaluate popular diets, 34–50,
        36f, 37t, 40t
Theoretical framework for self-help
        approaches
    evidence for, 63–68, 65t
    physical activity and, 57–63, 59f, 62t,
        63–68, 63f, 65t, 68–69
Therapeutic diary, bulimia nervosa and,
        94–95
Therapists' attitudes towards self-help
        treatment, 171–172, 174
Thoughts, automatic
    binge eating and, 329–330
    Getting Better Bit(e) by Bit(e) (Schmidt
        and Treasure, 1993) and, 96
    night eating syndrome and, 319–
        320
Toxic environment, 224–226
Transtheoretical model
    evidence for, 63–68, 65t
    physical activity and, 60–63, 62t, 63–
        68, 63f, 65t, 69
Treatment. *see* Behavioral interventions
Treatment of childhood weight problems.
        see Childhood treatment of weight
        problems
Treatment of night eating syndrome,
        312–322, 313f, 314t, 315f, 316f
Trevose Behavior Modification Program
        (TBMP), 228, 230–235

U

U. S. Department of Agriculture Center
        for Nutrition Policy and Promotion
        (USDA-CNPP) website, 144
Ultimate Weight Solution diet, evaluation
        of, 41–43
USDA dietary guidelines. *see* Dietary
        guidelines

V

Very-low-calorie diets. *see also* Calorie
        consumption
    Health Management Resources
        (HMR), 189
    medically supervised programs, 188–
        189, 195
    Medifast/TSFL, 193–194
    OPTIFAST and, 191
Vitamins. *see also* Supplements, vitamins
        and minerals
    dietary guidelines regarding, 27
    Maker's Diet and, 44
    South Beach Diet and, 41
*Voluntary Guidelines for Providers of
        Weight Loss Products or Services*
        (Federal Trade Commission, 1999),
        32
Vomiting, self-induced
    appetite-focused model of, 330–332,
        331f
    bulimia nervosa and, 92–93
    Getting Better Bit(e) by Bit(e) (Schmidt
        and Treasure, 1993) and, 95

W

Water
    Atkins for Life diet and, 45–46
    childhood obesity prevention and, 279
    creating a healthy food environment
        and, 296
    dietary guidelines regarding, 27–28,
        30
Web-based interventions. *see* Internet-
        based interventions
Websites. *see also* Internet-based
        interventions
    Aim for a Healthy Weight website,
        143–144
    Internet-based interventions, 156t
    U. S. Department of Agriculture
        Center for Nutrition Policy and
        Promotion (USDA-CNPP) website,
        144

Weighing self
  in dieters in the general population, 9
  self-monitoring of, 247–248
Weight bias. *see also* Stigma
  coping strategies and, 349–356
  extent and impact of, 347–349
  health care and, 356–359, 357t
  overview, 359
  research recommendations, 356
  treatment of childhood weight
    problems and, 293, 295–296
Weight, bulimia nervosa and, 95
Weight gain, Internet-based interventions
  and, 141–144, 151
Weight loss
  Atkins for Life diet and, 44–45
  binge-eating disorder and, 85–86
  body image and, 128–129
  calorie consumption and, 22–23, 24t,
    25t
  coexisting health problems and, 30
  composition of macronutrients and
    micronutrients in a diet and, 25–28
  contributors to posttreatment weight
    gain and, 207
  in general population, 8–9
  in National Weight Control Registry
    (NWCR), 6–7

OPTIFAST and, 36
South Beach Diet and, 38–39
Ultimate Weight Solution diet and, 41–42
weight bias and, 349–350
Weight Loss Practices Survey, 9
Weight loss programs. *see* Commercial
  weight loss programs
Weight, monitoring of, 247–248
Weight problems in children. *see*
  Childhood obesity prevention;
  Childhood treatment of weight
  problems
Weight-related teasing in childhood,
  body image and, 142
Weight Watchers. *see also* Commercial
  weight loss programs
  costs of, 183, 184t
  effectiveness of, 11–12, 187–188
  as an Internet-based intervention, 156t,
    158
  overview, 182t, 183, 185, 199
*What Do You See When You Look in
  the Mirror?* (Cash, 1995), 125–126
Whole-grain foods, 28